T0215336

Seminars in the Psychotherapies

Second edition

College Seminars Series

For details of available and forthcoming books in the College Seminars Series please visit:
www.cambridge.org/series/college-seminars-series/

Seminars in the Psychotherapies

Second edition

Edited by
Rachel Gibbons
Jo O'Reilly

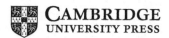

CAMBRIDGE
UNIVERSITY PRESS

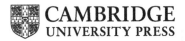

CAMBRIDGE
UNIVERSITY PRESS

Shaftesbury Road, Cambridge CB2 8EA, United Kingdom

One Liberty Plaza, 20th Floor, New York, NY 10006, USA

477 Williamstown Road, Port Melbourne, VIC 3207, Australia

314–321, 3rd Floor, Plot 3, Splendor Forum, Jasola District Centre, New Delhi – 110025, India

103 Penang Road, #05–06/07, Visioncrest Commercial, Singapore 238467

Cambridge University Press is part of Cambridge University Press & Assessment, a department of the University of Cambridge.

We share the University's mission to contribute to society through the pursuit of education, learning and research at the highest international levels of excellence.

www.cambridge.org
Information on this title: www.cambridge.org/9781108711838

DOI: 10.1017/9781108686976

First published 2007, Gaskell, The Royal College of Psychiatrists
This second edition published by Cambridge University Press & Assessment 2021

A catalogue record for this publication is available from the British Library

ISBN   978-1-108-71183-8   Paperback

....

Every effort has been made in preparing this book to provide accurate and up-to-date information which is in accord with accepted standards and practice at the time of publication. Although case histories are drawn from actual cases, every effort has been made to disguise the identities of the individuals involved. Nevertheless, the authors, editors and publishers can make no warranties that the information contained herein is totally free from error, not least because clinical standards are constantly changing through research and regulation. The authors, editors and publishers therefore disclaim all liability for direct or consequential damages resulting from the use of material contained in this book. Readers are strongly advised to pay careful attention to information provided by the manufacturer of any drugs or equipment that they plan to use.

Rachel Gibbons is a Consultant Psychiatrist, Medical Psychotherapist, Psychoanalyst and Group Analyst based in London, UK. She has worked in the NHS for the past 20 years in various psychiatric and psychotherapeutic settings. Up until February 2020, she also worked as the National Director of Therapies for the Priory Group. She is a member of the Executive Committee of the Medical Psychotherapy Faculty of the Royal College of Psychiatrists. She is the Chair of the new RCPsych working group on the Effect of Suicide and Homicide on Psychiatrists, and the Patient Safety Group. She has been working on suicide over the last 12 years and is a member of the National Suicide Prevention Advisory Group.

Jo O'Reilly is a Consultant Psychiatrist and Medical Psychotherapist working in Camden and Islington NHS Foundation Trust, London, UK, and a member of the British Psychoanalytic Society. During her 16 years in her current NHS role, she has developed a keen interest in the application of psychoanalytic ideas to psychiatric care and how this can enrich clinical understanding and support staff. She is a member of the Executive Committee of the Medical Psychotherapy Faculty of the Royal College of Psychiatrists and vice chair of the Specialist Advisory Committee contributing to curriculum development and training nationally. She has extensive experience in supervision, consultation and reflective practice within mental health care, developing activities locally and nationally which contribute towards a more psychotherapeutic approach to psychiatry.

Contents

Section 2. Work in Practice

Section 3. Contemporary Developments

Contributors

Gwen Adshead
Consultant Forensic Psychotherapist. West London and CNWL. Member of the Institute of Group Analysis

Anthony W. Bateman
Visiting Professor UCL, Honorary Professor in Psychotherapy University of Copenhagen, Consultant to Anna Freud Centre

William Burbridge-James
Consultant Psychiatrist in Medical Psychotherapy.
Essex Partnership University NHS Foundation Trust. Psychoanalyst. Chair of the Specialist Advisory Committee Medical Psychotherapy Faculty Royal College of Psychiatrists.

Adam Dierckx
Consultant Medical Psychotherapist, Greater Manchester Mental Health NHS Foundation Trust

Maria Eyres
Consultant Psychiatrist in Medical Psychotherapy. Psychoanalytic Psychotherapist (BPC), DocHealth Academic Secretary Royal College of Psychiatrists Medical Psychotherapy Faculty Royal College of Psychiatrists.

Jason Hepple
Honorary Psychotherapist Medical Directorate Summerset Foundation Trust.

Simon Heyland
Consultant Psychiatrist in Medical Psychotherapy
Birmingham & Solihull Mental Health Foundation Trust

Tennyson Lee
Consultant Psychiatrist in Medical Psychotherapy
Honorary Senior Lecturer, Wolfson Institute, Queen Mary University of London
Deancross: Tower Hamlets Personality Disorder Service, Mile End Hospital, London

Frank Margison
Gaskell Psychotherapy Service, Greater Manchester Mental Health NHS Foundation Trust

Miomir Milovanovic
Consultant Psychiatrist in Medical Psychotherapy, Psychoanalyst

C Susan Mizen
Consultant Psychiatrist in Psychotherapy, Adult Directorate Devon Partnership NHS Trust

Maria Papanastassiou
Consultant Psychiatrist North East London FT NHS Foundation Trust. Group Analyst.

Steve Pearce
Honorary Senior Clinical Lecturer, Oxford University
Consultant Medical Psychotherapist, Oxford Health NHS Trust

Tim Read
Emeritus Consultant Psychiatrist Royal London Hospital. Director Institute of Psychedelic Therapy. Group Analyst.

P. J. Saju
Consultant Medical Psychotherapist, Drury Lane Health and Wellbeing Centre, South West Yorkshire Partnership NHS Foundation Trust, Wakefield

Phil Stokoe
Organisational Consultant Philip Stokoe Associates. Psychoanalyst.

Sue Stuart-Smith
Consultant Psychiatrist in Medical Psychotherapy.

Joanne Stubley
Consultant Medical Psychotherapist and Lead Clinician Trauma Service Tavistock Clinic, Psychoanalyst.

Margot Waddell
Visiting Lecturer Tavistock and Portman NHS Foundation Trust. Psychoanalyst. Child Analyst.

Jessica Yakeley
Consultant Psychiatrist in Forensic Psychotherapy. Director, Portman Clinic. Director of Medical Education. The Tavistock and Portman. NHS Foundation Trust. Psychoanalyst.

Foreword

It is more than 25 years since I first bought the first editions of the seminar series while preparing for the Membership of the Royal College of Psychiatrists (MRCPsych) exams as a trainee psychiatrist. I have subsequently developed an interest in education and how we learn. Now, as Dean of the Royal College of Psychiatrists I find myself responsible for many aspects of psychiatric education in the UK. Since studying for my own membership exams, much has changed in our field. What has not changed, however, is the primacy of George Engel's biopsychosocial model which puts the patient and their utterly unique set of circumstances centre stage in our thinking [1, 2].

Throughout my career, I have always appreciated the breadth and depth of specialist knowledge that the world of mental health offers its students, from the impact of social policy, through the cellular biology of neuroscience to psychological theories of mind. The intellectual rewards of exploring this Aladdin's cave of knowns and unknowns are extraordinarily rich, particularly in a rapidly changing and advancing world.

Understanding who people are and how they have become is at the heart of what we do as psychiatrists. This book sets out key concepts of psychological development and how we relate to others and the world around us.

Working with other human beings is never straightforward, and all who work in health and social care will be too familiar with the mental and emotional stress in working with people who themselves are hurting, perplexed and distressed. Having paradigms in which to examine and explain our own reactions, at the sharp end of this work, is essential in containing our own anxiety and maintaining a sense of well-being. This book is full of thoughtful descriptions of how concepts such as countertransference and projective identification relate to everyday practice and the importance of finding reflective space for supervision and peer support.

In common with the rest of medicine, psychiatric training is supported by educational and clinical supervision which is designed to facilitate educational progression and maintain patient safety. However, also enshrined in our General Medical Council approved curricula is the unique concept of psychiatric supervision. I am extremely proud of the recognition within our specialty of the importance of high-quality supervision which plays a critical role for trainees in developing strategies for resilience, well-being, maintaining appropriate professional boundaries and understanding the dynamic issues of therapeutic relationships. It also supports the development of leadership competencies and is necessarily informed by psychodynamic, cognitive and coaching models [3].

This supervision is different from psychotherapy supervision, which is critical for those undertaking any form of psychotherapy with people. However, psychiatric supervision owes its existence to the rich tradition of psychoanalysis which helps inform modern therapeutic practice. It is key in delivering modern recovery-focussed, person-centred care.

These concepts deserve to have a wide audience, far beyond the bounds of psychiatry, and will be of interest and importance to all doctors and those in the health and care sector who wish to excel in understanding the heart of therapeutic relationships. After all, the quality of the therapeutic relationship between patient and doctor or client and therapist remains predictive, not only of a good outcome in talking therapies [4], but also in care in general [5].

Despite our intentions to bring our best selves to work, the relational nature of what we do inevitably exposes our own emotional vulnerabilities and anxieties as caregivers. This book is a very helpful starting place to understand defence mechanisms and the systems we create around patients to try to contain these.

Many will identify with my own vivid memories of the initial rollercoaster of emotions starting out in medical practice; trying to make sense of complex interactions between myself, patients, staff and the organisations I worked for. I remember clearly the sense of relief when I became aware a little later of the existence of an academic paper 'Hate in the Countertransference' [6]. It was much later still that I read it and became aware of who it was by, but for a while, the mere knowledge of the title of Winnicott's 1949 paper gave me permission to also bring my human self to work. Subsequent psychotherapy training and supervision has arguably been the single most important training experience which enabled me to make sense of an often confusing and disturbing work environment as a psychiatrist in training, and now as a consultant general adult psychiatrist.

This book eloquently covers formulation, that is, understanding patients' difficulties in psychodynamic terms. It will be useful to those starting out on psychotherapy training or simply wanting to understand their patients better. It describes the process of psycho-dynamic therapy in understandable terms and covers important, but often avoided, topics of patient discontinuation, therapeutic boundaries and helpful advice on referring patients for therapy. It describes underpinning theories and a practical description of all therapies likely to be encountered in modern practice within NHS or public health settings. As such it will be of interest to those exploring different therapeutic modalities, as part of training.

Underpinned by evidence throughout, the book describes essential psychotherapeutic aspects of psychiatric disorders encountered in everyday practice in general psychiatry including depression, psychosis, trauma, personality disorders, medically unexplained symptoms and self-harm. It also covers children's mental health and psychiatry within forensic settings.

After initial training, it frequently becomes clear that working with patients is often the more straightforward part of what we do as clinicians. Understanding organisational dynamics within complex systems can be perplexing, and at times overwhelming, to the practitioner starting out. Having psychodynamic paradigms as clear reference points can help practitioners reflect and make sense of their interactions and emotional responses, within systems. Developing a well-honed ability to reflect is essential to maintaining compassion which is critical not only for the people we work with as patients, but also for colleagues and importantly for ourselves [7]. As Joan Erikson, the lesser-known partner of the famous psychoanalyst Erik Erikson, put it 'The more you know yourself, the more patience you have for what you see in others' [8].

The final chapter of the book takes an Eriksonian approach in describing opportunities for psychotherapeutic development throughout the various career stages of a psychiatrist from medical student to retirement. It describes many of the areas of challenge and opportunities for personal growth throughout a typical working life. This is an underacknowledged and seldom discussed area which will be helpful for those at the beginning of their careers as well as those established in practice and those approaching retirement and beyond. 'Lots of old people don't get wise, but you don't get wise unless you age', Joan Erikson sagely said [8].

As a clinician, my focus is on supporting patients achieve their potential as they work towards their own goals for what recovery means to them. As an educationalist, my focus is on learning and supporting students, trainees and colleagues achieve their true professional potential. Understanding the barriers that get in the way of learning is fundamental to both processes. There is often necessary pain and mistakes involved in learning, but the rewards of subsequent growth as a result are immense [9].

As I reflect on my own journey as a psychiatrist I feel immensely privileged to have been trusted to glimpse and explore the inner worlds of others. I am grateful to have had wise mentors and colleagues who have provided educational support to develop the advanced communication skills demanded of psychiatrists in order to do their best to understand the thinking and emotional life of their patients.

For some reading this book, it will be full of new and exciting concepts and information. For others, like me, it may provide a refreshing reminder of why, despite its challenges, the field of psychiatry and mental health is unsurpassed in providing endless intrigue and academic curiosity.

This edition of *Seminars in the Psychotherapies* goes a long way to providing psychiatrists and health and care professionals at all stages of their career with key and relevant knowledge which applied wisely will help many attempting to solve problems inherent in being human.

Dr Kate F. Lovett
Dean, Royal College of Psychiatrists
February 2021

References

1. Engel GL. The need for a new medical model: a challenge for biomedicine. *Psychodyn Psychiatry* 2012; 40(3): 377–96.

2. Royal College of Psychiatrists. *Person-Centred Care: Implications for Training in Psychiatry.* College Report CR215. London: RCPsych, 2018.

3. Royal College of Psychiatrists. *A Competency Based Curriculum for Specialist Core Training in Psychiatry.* London: RCPsych, 2013. Updated April 2020.

4. Lambert MJ, Barley DE. Research summary on the therapeutic relationship and psychotherapy outcome. *Psychotherapy* 2001; 38(4): 357–61.

5. Kaplan SH, Greenfield S, Ware JE Jr. Assessing the effects of physician-patient interactions on the outcomes of chronic disease. *Med Care* 1989; 27(3): S110–27.

6. Winnicott DW. Hate in the countertransference. *Int J Psychoanal* 1949; 30: 69–74.

7. Ballatt J, Campling P. *Intelligent Kindness: Reforming the Culture of Healthcare.* London: RCPsych Publications, 2011.

8. Goleman D. Erikson, in his own old age, expands his view of life. *New York Times,* June 14, 1988.

9. Dweck CS. *Essays in Social Psychology. Self-Theories: Their Role in Motivation, Personality and Development.* New York: Psychology Press, 2000.

Preface

Knowledge of the self is the mother of all knowledge. So it is incumbent on me to know myself, to know it completely, to know its minutiae, its characteristics, its subtleties, and its very atoms.
Khalil Gibran

Working in mental health puts us in touch with the complexity, depth, creativity and turmoil of the human mind. We are at the emotional coal face, privileged to be encountering the fundamental unknowability and strangeness of the internal world. How much we make of this opportunity depends on how open or closed we are to the experience. Our patients communicate their disturbance powerfully and the working environment can be challenging and exhausting without meaningful understanding. To explore one's own mind, and to be receptive and knowledgeable about the unconscious processes that underlie all mental activity, allows us to learn from this experience. Working in this area then becomes more creative, enjoyable, productive, and of lower personal risk. It feeds rather than depletes.

To remain 'mentally well' is an enormous challenge and many of us will join our patients in having periods of sustained mental distress in our lifetime. The reasons for any psychological or psychiatric breakdown are multifactorial and each person has their own vulnerabilities based on their particular circumstances and formative experiences. We are not only individuals, we function within groups, intimate relationships, family networks, and larger social and global arenas, a matrix of emotional connections which profoundly affects our mental health. This complicates and diversifies a reductionist biological perspective and makes for a much deeper, richer, understanding of our human struggle.

We both identify ourselves as biopsychosocial or psychodynamic psychiatrists. We have worked within frontline mental health services for many years. In addition to our psychiatric training, we are also psychoanalysts, and have undertaken further psychotherapy trainings. When we were starting out as trainee psychiatrists there was a division, or split, between the three conceptual pillars addressing the aetiology of mental distress: the biological, the social and the psychological. Biological ideas about the origins and treatment of mental illness were given precedence over psychological or relational factors. This was a strong reaction to the earlier preference for psychoanalytic understanding; and a resistance to bringing together different perspectives. Within this medical, action-based, approach to mental distress, psychiatrists saw themselves as medical doctors. They viewed their task as gathering information and identifying symptoms in the service of making a diagnosis and prescribing a range of primarily pharmacological interventions.

During our careers we have seen significant shifts in the understanding and treatment of mental illness. There has been a gradual rapprochement between the biological, social and psychological, and a recovery of the understanding that mental health is a holistic discipline. The central role of unconscious processes in mental life, and the importance of life experiences, relationships and the quality of early nurture in shaping the mind are now widely accepted. Currently within mental health there is new diversity, open-mindedness and curiosity about the person behind the psychiatric presentation. Examples of this more holistic approach include the adoption in many services of Open Dialogue as a psychologically based approach to treating psychosis, and the neuroscientific advances evidencing the fundamental role of early relationships in brain development. This contemporary approach to mental disorder, as illustrated in this book, prioritises the central importance of relationships in emotional life, psychological functioning and psychiatric breakdown. Emphasis is also placed on viewing symptoms as communications suffused with meaning requiring understanding and beyond the therapeutic reach of pharmacological interventions alone.

We have aimed to make this book accessible and relevant to all mental health staff interested in the psychological and relational aspects of their work. We have included the current mainstream psychological models, their theoretical underpinnings and a guide to the psychotherapeutic treatments derived from these approaches. The scope and complexity of these models provides a rich understanding of how the mind develops and functions; a necessary basis for understanding the form the breakdown takes when the balance of the mind is disturbed. We have included chapters showing how key psychological theories can enrich our understanding of a range of mental disorders, and the various forms psychiatric breakdown may take, from self-harm to psychosis, mood disorders to personality difficulties. Further chapters focus upon the emotional impact of working with mental distress and how this intensity of these encounters can inform a psychotherapeutic approach to psychiatry. For readability and consistency babies are referred to as he and the primary carer as the mother – while fully recognising that we all start lives as babies and both men and women play crucial roles in the early nurture of our children.

We are grateful to all the leading contemporary clinicians who have contributed chapters to this book. Many are medical psychotherapists (trained in medicine, psychiatry and psychological therapy), who are currently working within mental health services. Their trainings in psychological treatments and extensive clinical experience gives theoretical depth and breadth to their writing and they have brought their sections to life with a range of vividly described clinical scenarios.

This book was completed during the 2020 coronavirus pandemic and was influenced by the profound psychological and social change in our attitudes, behaviours and habits that followed. There has been a paradigm change and the pandemic has shed light on areas of dysfunction, prejudice, discrimination and inequality in society. The necessity of collective endeavour has been powerfully underlined, and the risks of isolation and disconnection have become increasingly apparent. We have seen how anxiety and fear can exacerbate splits and create conflicts. The worldwide spread of this new disease has shed light on the need to come together, to overcome unhelpful divisions and to challenge false dichotomies.

We hope this book contributes to the practice of psychiatry and the understanding of the mind. Trainees will find much of what they need to know for their developing clinical skills, their exams and for undertaking therapeutic work within these pages. More experienced clinicians and psychotherapists will also find new and creative approaches to the clinical dilemmas routinely faced working within the fascinating territory of the human mind.

Part I

Therapy Theory and Practice

Chapter

1

Psychodynamic Theory: The Development of a Model of the Mind

Jo O'Reilly

This chapter aims to describe the key contributions that psychoanalytic theory has made to our understanding of the mind.

The practice of psychiatry and the development of psychological treatments rest upon how we understand the mind and emotional life. As clinicians working with patients with difficulties in how they feel, relate and think we need an understanding of psychic life in healthy and more disturbed states, just as practitioners of physical medicine need to understand bodily processes in sickness and in health.

Since the late nineteenth century psychoanalytic theory has provided a platform from which a series of models of the mind have evolved. An underlying and fundamental tent of this approach is that most of mental functioning occurs at an unconscious level; a finding now widely supported within psychology and neuroscience [1]. The unique contributions of a psychoanalytic approach seek to elucidate and to understand the form and nature of these unconscious processes, both in healthy and more disturbed states of mind. Furthermore, clinical techniques derived from psychoanalysis such as free association and dream interpretation are specifically aimed at identifying unconscious mental processes and psychoanalysis has a great deal to offer a systematic study of the unconscious. Although the terms psychodynamic or psychoanalytic tend to be used in association with psychotherapeutic treatment, a psychoanalytic approach refers to a school of thought able to provide insights into the workings of the mind far beyond the treatment approaches derived from it.

The limits of rational thought and considered volitional action in explaining emotional life are blindingly evident from the complexities, extremities and non-common-sensical nature of much of human behaviour. Being driven by powerful emotional forces which we may struggle to fully know or to understand is intrinsic to human life. Our need to love, to connect and to relate contrasts with acts fuelled by hatred, cruelty and alienation. We can function in both highly creative and deeply destructive ways and a coherent model of mental life requires the capacity and vision to address this paradox. Psychoanalytic thinking draws upon the intensity and passion of early life, when the infant's survival is dependent upon his ability to secure a nurturing attachment, and to regulate and to manage his primitive terrors, as the starting point from which to consider the management of psychic energy throughout life. In taking a developmental perspective psychoanalysis seeks to identify the influencing factors determining how we feel, relate and behave from infancy and throughout life. This enormously ambitious project provides a means to consider how the internal world is formed at an individual and unique level, and also how we behave in groups and within society.

The development of psychoanalytic theory has a fascinating history involving the evolution of ideas seen as provocative, enlightening, disturbing and controversial within the contexts of the times within which they have emerged. This chapter will introduce some of the key ideas and thinkers contributing to this body of work. Additional reading will be recommended at the end of the chapter for those who wish to further their explorations of this rich and complex subject.

Despite differences in emphasis and at times conflicts about key ideas, all schools of psychodynamic thought are concerned with both unconscious and conscious aspects of mental life and the interplay and tensions between them. A defining belief of a psychoanalytic perspective is that the unconscious forms a vast substructure underpinning the conscious mind and exerting pressures and influences upon it; all behaviour and subjective experience is therefore seen as having unconscious determinants.

Sigmund Freud: The Neurologist and Pioneer of the Unconscious

Dreams are the Royal Road to the Unconscious
Sigmund Freud, 1900 [2]

Sigmund Freud (b. 1856, Freiburg, d. 1939, London) trained in medicine and neurology; his early research interests lay in the area of brain damage linked with aphasia. He realised the limits of the mechanistic localisation-based theories in understanding the cases he saw and his first published book *On Aphasia* represented an early attempt to incorporate a dynamic and psychological model of the mind into the world of neurobiology [3]. His rejection of an anatomical brain model as adequately explaining his patients' symptoms was further fuelled by the cases he observed under the care of the renowned neurologist Charcot in the Salpêtrière asylum in Paris in 1885. He became deeply interested in the study of hysteria, recognised that paralyses, physical maladies, dreams and parapraxes of the patients he encountered could only be explained by models of disturbance of psychological function and that mental function could not be located within an anatomical structure. Furthermore, he recognised these symptoms as expressions of experiences consciously forgotten which could be remembered under hypnosis, a striking realisation captured by his words '*hysterics suffer mainly from reminiscences*' [4].

Freud's private practice as a neurologist enabled him to study patients and their symptoms in detail. The case of Anna O, a young woman who presented with a host of physical symptoms including a cough, paralyses, disturbances of speech and sight and fainting fits after her father's death, led him to conclude that traumatic experiences can be repressed and continue to reside in an area of the mind which is entirely unconscious, yet these experiences make their voices heard by re-emerging as symptoms. If the trauma can be remembered and spoken about – a process he called **catharsis**, there is no further need of the physical symptoms that resolve accordingly. This formed the basis of what he referred to as **the talking cure**. Drawing on his background in physical sciences Freud developed the idea of a mental apparatus that, in common with other bodily systems, aims to maintain a steady homeostatic state against internal psychic energy that is seeking discharge. He saw the mind as being dominated by instinctual drives to ensure basic needs were expressed and met which he considered as largely residing in the unconscious – a vast substructure underpinning the volitional conscious mind and with a distinctive nature and functioning [5].

As a scientist Freud continually modified his ideas on the basis of clinical observation and experience, leading to a series of theoretical models and emergence of developing clinical techniques. His early work included the use of hypnosis, which he later abandoned in favour of **free association,** or encouragement of the patient to speak openly and freely about whatever comes to their minds. Free association has been called the **fundamental rule** of psychoanalysis and assumes that everything that emerges in thoughts and communications has meaning. Further clinical techniques followed such as dream interpretation, the neutral stance of the therapist and a way of listening, all of which sought to access and to tune into the workings of the unconscious as they reveal themselves in everyday life [6].

Hence the scene was set for the exploration of this vast territory; the unconscious aspects of the mind to which Freud devoted much of his subsequent career. Although in parts controversial, challenging and, in common with all great advances in understanding, modified by later discoveries, it is remarkable how much Freud's ideas have contributed to our understanding of mental processes. Like Darwin and Einstein, Freud changed the paradigms through which we understand ourselves – the modern world is familiar and comfortable with the concept of unconscious processes and how they may affect our emotional and social functioning. More contemporary discoveries within neuroscience support his finding that the vast majority of mental life occurs at an unconscious level.

In keeping with his medical training, Freud's ambitions lay in developing a general theory of the mind from which pathology could be understood. But he was interested in more than just illness; he also sought to understand the breadths and depths of human functioning at its most creative and destructive, from the individual to societal level, from sadism to war, from infancy to schizophrenia; the scope of his work was vast and his writing prolific.

Freud's evolving models of the mind followed his shift in thinking from the anatomical to the psychological. His earliest **topographical model** divided the mind into three parts – the **conscious**, the **unconscious**, serving as a reservoir of instinctual urges and repressed memories, and the **preconscious**, representing areas of the mind requiring attention and prompting to make themselves consciously known. However, the topographical model ran into difficulties and in 1923 Freud introduced a major revision with the **structural theory** of the mind in which the conscious, unconscious and preconscious are all understood as dynamic, fluid qualities of mental processes as opposed to discrete areas of the mind. The structural theory divides the mind into the **id**, the **ego** and the **superego** in which mental processes are grouped together in terms of their functional significance [7].

Within Freud's structural theory of the mind the id is entirely unconscious and holds the basic instinctual urges such as aggression and sexuality. (More recent findings from the developing world of neuropsychoanalysis dispute this as the affective states from them seem to be conscious [8].) Psychological processes of the id are primitive and entirely different to rational thought. Referred to as **primary process thinking** the mental life of the id knows no shame, guilt or inhibition and operates entirely under the reign of the **pleasure principle**. In the magical land of primary process thinking logic is disregarded, opposites can co-exist without conflict, external reality is ignored and instant gratification of all urges and appetites with avoidance of all pain and discomfort is the aim, resorting to hallucinatory wish fulfilment or magical thinking to avoid frustration. Primary process activity is evident in the play of young children, revealed in glimpses in mental and verbal slips and more fully in dreams and psychosis. The id was referred to by Freud as the **seething cauldron** of unacceptable impulses such as the desire to kill or insatiable cravings for sexual satisfactions.

Unimpeded by input from perceptual organs about external reality, the id functions under the sway of its own wishes and appetites.

Instinctual urges and the vast resource of psychic energy seeking discharge from the id require active management and are censored by the **superego** which functions as a conscience, repressing what it considers to be morally unacceptable and supporting the ego in making realistic judgements and decisions. Freud conceptualised the superego as socially conditioned and developing from the internalisation of parental attitudes and approval. The **ego** has the task of mediating between external reality, the superego and the needs and demands of internal needs and urges. The ego strives to function in keeping with the **reality principle**, ensuring both executive thoughts and motor actions are able to negotiate and manage the expectations, opportunities and limitations of the external world while also relating to the appetites and needs of the id.

The ego develops as the central aspect of the psyche; it comprises both conscious and unconscious aspects and is the seat of thought. Ego structures are informed by the perceptual organs about external reality; it controls motility and is tasked with managing the passions of the id, which it does with varying degrees of success. Balancing the primitive appetites and survivalist instincts of the id alongside the pressures of the superego, which can be unduly harsh or tolerant, is a precarious task for both the individual and for social groups and behaviours. Freud wrote about the tension between these processes on the world stage and how in Europe the First World War showed that the deep human instinct to kill overwhelmed the use of negotiation and diplomacy [9].

Hence our psychological functioning is constantly challenged and informed by pressures from the unconscious, which contains the most primitive and survival-oriented drives and urges, and from the prohibitions and limits of the superego which strives to regulate them. According to Freud the mind's ability to function depends on the balance between these different forces, most of which are beyond conscious awareness. An overly powerful superego, for example, can lead to punitive ways of seeing oneself, excessive self-criticism and self-inhibition, while an excess of id, or an ego too fragile to manage the forces of id, means the ability to function in keeping with the demands of external reality is threatened.

Freud saw psychological symptoms as expressions of unconscious conflict between unconscious urges and conscious behaviour. He referred to this as **psychic determinism** – that our feelings, thoughts, behaviours and symptoms are inherently filled with meaning how is beyond conscious awareness. As he wrote in 1895 '*dreams are never concerned with trivia*' [2] – we may like to see ourselves as rational and in control, or at the mercy of random and arbitrary experiences, but in psychodynamic theory our internal and experiences and the situations we find ourselves in are full of meaning. The best jokes for example may have some primary process in them and often have an aggressive component, the laughter discharging the underlying aggressive wish. **Freudian slips** in speech and the forgetting of undesirable realities may all be signs that a wish from the unconscious has gained entry into the conscious mind in disguised form, so the lapse is far from meaningless and may reveal powerful unconscious urges.

In Freud's early work with patients with conversion disorders he found that the repressed knowledge of childhood sexual trauma seemed to be the foundation of his patients' symptoms, which became known as the **seduction theory** [10]. This emphasised the causative impact of abuse in adult cases of hysteria and obsessional neurosis and placed trauma and nurture at the heart of his early theories. However, for reasons not fully elucidated, but seemly linked to the frequency with which sexual material emerged during his work with his patients, Freud turned his attention to developing ideas about childhood sexual curiosity and urges, abandoning the seduction theory. This remains one of the most controversial areas of his work with far-reaching consequences for psychoanalysis. Criticisms followed that the child's actual experience and the prevalence of childhood sexual abuse was denied and neglected in his subsequent theories [11]. However, Freud's ideas about childhood sexuality led to his discovery of key concepts such as the transference, repetition compulsion, and personality development. Freud saw infantile sexuality as different to mature adult sexuality and described **stages of psychosexual development**, meaning that different areas of the body become the focus of instinctual sexual energy or **libido**, depending on the prevailing developmental preoccupations [12].Hence in the first year **or oral stage** satisfaction via feeding means the main source of pleasure is the mouth, the **anal stage** (1–3 years) refers to the acquisition of bowel control through toilet training and the **genital stage** (3–5 years) refers to anxiety about the genitals and recognition of difference. Each stage has its associated nature and functions and if not satisfactorily navigated the individual may become fixated at certain stages with implications for character development (it has become common parlance for example to describe people as being 'anal' in keeping with this idea).

Freud used material from his own dreams to further his understanding of the unconscious and discovered strong feelings of love for his mother and jealousy towards his father in this analysis. He believed these to be universal themes and linked this discovery to the **Oedipus Myth** in which Oedipus unwittingly kills his father and marries his mother. Freud saw this myth as capturing a universal developmental challenge and central to psychological development – the unconscious rivalry and murderous wish towards the same sex parent, with a desire for exclusive ownership of the other. The term **Electra complex** was used to describe a similar constellation of unconscious desire in girls. Freud thought that oedipal issues come most overtly to the fore between three and five years of age, such as may be expressed in acceptable form by the 'daddy's girl' type behaviours of a daughter or 'mummy's little man' of a son. He considered that the development of healthy superego function depended in part on a satisfactory resolution of anxieties linked with oedipal urges, allowing adult sexuality to be enjoyed within societally accepted parameters and at the same time free from excessive inhibition.

Although issues arising from oedipal urges and anxieties continue to play a central role in psychoanalytic theory, there have been marked departures and developments from this earlier model – most strikingly by Melanie Klein. Recognition and negotiation of triangulation in relationships and the experience of exclusion is seen as a key developmental challenge, alongside the universal longing for the exclusive love of another and intense hatred when this is denied.

Defence Mechanisms

Humankind cannot bear too much contact with reality
T S Eliot

The struggle for the ego to manage instinctually based urges, and the demands and challenges provided by privations, losses, frustrations and traumatic experiences in external reality means the mind needs to be able to manage potentially overwhelming urges, emotions and anxiety. To preserve its capacity to function the mind has developed a wide range of **defence mechanisms** – in essence these are the mind's tactics employed against the pressures of unacceptable desire or unbearable experiences and are mobilised in response to anxiety. Defences are unconscious, universal, constantly in action, and adaptive. They allow the ego to think by titrating contact with both painful reality and primitive impulses from the id.

In more extreme forms however defensive functioning can develop into more problematic behaviours, distortions of reality or psychological symptoms. The latter may develop when an unacceptable urge from the id, or an experience repressed beyond conscious knowledge, cannot be adequately defended against, and a compromise has to be reached between the unconscious forces and the failing defence – usually this means that the unacceptable impulse or experience may present in a sufficiently disguised form to be consciously acceptable. This can become the basis of a neurotic disorder, phobia, psychosomatic complaint or conversion symptom. Defensive organisations can also become excessively rigid and dominate mental functioning to the extent they become entrenched in the personality, such as in obsessional, anankastic or borderline personality organisation.

Defence mechanisms are historically categorised in relation to the stage of development when they are most commonly prevalent, although all forms can continue to be operative throughout life; they overlap and are interdependent on one another – we all operate under the influence of a community of defensive activities that relate to and inform each other. The immature defences for example are most frequently deployed in infancy and early childhood and are also powerfully operative in psychotic and borderline states. The more mature defences are generally seen as more adaptive and also importantly as the source of much or man's creative endeavours in channelling the energy from id impulses towards alternative means of expression. Table 1.1 illustrates some common defence mechanisms, based on Freud's early conceptualisations, but added to and modified by subsequent psychoanalysts.

Freud and Transference/Countertransference

The processes of transference and countertransference refer to how the minds of people interact and impact on one another through unconscious means. These are ubiquitous processes that inform our perceptions and responses to others and allow us to intuit about another's state of mind. In infancy when at our most dependent and vulnerable, the mind is exquisitely sensitive to the reactions and responses of others; this is key to survival. The quality of these early essential and nurturing relationships powerfully affects our unconscious expectations of, and responses towards others. These early templates continue to be added to and modified throughout life and are present to varying extents in all our interactions and relationships. Someone with secure and nurturing early relationships for example may respond to an angry interaction with calmness and confidence, whereas if early life has been characterised by neglect and fear then the perception of threat may be more easily triggered and the response may be to feel threatened or paranoid. Freud recognised and named the transference in his early work, initially seeing it as a form of resistance against therapeutic change, later seeing it as a potential path to unconscious material. Use of the transference and countertransference remain cornerstones of psychoanalytic technique, although as ubiquitous processes the power and effects are not confined to the consulting room and powerfully inform how we perceive and respond to others at an unconscious level.

Table 1.1 Psychological defence mechanisms

	Meaning
Primitive/Immature defences	
Repression	The unconscious forgetting of what is unbearable to know about
Denial	Refusal to accept a threatening reality
Projection/Projective identification	Expulsion of any thoughts, qualities or feelings which the individual rejects about himself
Splitting	The binary separation of good and bad experiences
Idealisation/Denigration	Seeing something or someone as all good, perfect and the Attribution of entirely bad qualities to another
Regression	Reverting back to an earlier stage of development to avoid responsibilities, demands and conflicts associated with current stage of life
Acting out	Taking action to avoid painful affect
Reaction formation	Assuming an attitude diametrically opposed to a repressed wish
Somatisation	The location of emotional tension or pain into the body and focus of concern becoming on physical symptoms
Schizoid	Avoiding relating to others and substituting gratifying fantasy
Dissociation	Temporary loss of awareness of reality, state of extreme detachedness, loss of memory and loss of identity e.g. in extreme trauma
More mature defences	
Displacement	Avoiding conflict by expression towards a substitute person or object
Identification	The qualities of another person become part of one's own identity
Identification with the aggressor	Becoming the threat oneself to master fear of being the victim
Introjection	Internalising the qualities of another to avoid awareness of loss
Intellectualisation	Use of theoretical abstract concepts in order to manage and distance oneself from painful feelings
Isolation of affect	Separating an idea from its accompanying affect to make it more acceptable
Rationalisation	Justification made to explain away a thought, feeling or experience unbearable to know about
Sexualisation	Turning an encounter or experience into an exciting and sexualised experience as a defence against intimacy and anxiety

Table 1.1 (cont.)

	Meaning
Undoing	Negation of shameful urges revealed through a behaviour using excessive activities to undo them
Mature defences	
Altruism	Prioritising other's needs beyond one's own
Ascetism	Excessive self-discipline as a defence against greed or anxiety
Anticipation	Worrying ahead for perceived painful events
Sublimation	'Purification' of urges with a sexual or aggressive component into a socially acceptable form
Suppression	Consciously diverting the mind away from anxiety or pain
Humour	The making bearable of painful events through comedy and irony

Freud has been hailed as one of the great thinkers of all time and has been a hugely influential figure on our cultural, societal and clinical landscapes. He was however a man of his times and many of his ideas have been considerably modified by subsequent theorists. He did not tolerate dissent and some of his early collaborators fell out of favour. He has attracted criticism including from leading feminists [13] for his rather limited theory of the sexual development of women, and he had little to say about the role of mothers or of the importance of early nurture; he admitted he did not understand women very well. He did however make a huge contribution towards understanding the struggles and conflicts inherent in emotional life, highlighted the significance of unconscious mental processes and linked the biological with the complexity of psychological life. Having witnessed the horrors of the First World War, and fleeing the Nazis for London during the second, he did not pull back from a full and frank appraisal of all the urges, creative and destructive, and the cruelty inherent in human behaviour and was entirely committed to seeking ways to understand all aspects of the mind. In emphasising the importance of ego function in controlling the impulses of the id he provided psychological ways to understand the danger when thought breaks down and is replaced by action fuelled by primitive urges seeking gratification. As part of his legacy he left a metapsychology of a scale unmatched by any other model.

Anna Freud

Freud's younger daughter, Anna (b.1895, Vienna, d.1982, London) became a leading figure in the psychoanalytic world, and a pioneer in child psychoanalysis. From her extensive experience she developed further ideas about ego development and the defences, emphasising the interplay between the internal and the external worlds, and first described the defences of **identification with the aggressor and altruism** [14]. The Anna Freud Centre in London remains as testament to her ideas and clinical contribution.

Carl Jung

Until you make the unconscious conscious, it will direct your life and you will call it fate.

Carl Gustav Jung (b.1875, d.1961, Zurich Switzerland) was a psychiatrist who worked with Bleuler in schizophrenia research before developing a close collaboration with Freud. Despite the excitement and closeness of their early relationship, developing differences in theoretical approaches led to the irretrievable breakdown in their professional and personal friendship, a schism with repercussions lasting into contemporary times in terms of limiting potential cross-fertilisation of ideas. Jung felt that in addition to the psychic structures that Freud had identified there was a spiritual dimension to internal experience that had central importance and which could not be reduced to Freudian drives. Jung emphasised the importance of **symbolism** in our individual and **collective psyche** finding common themes in myths from around the world. He postulated a **collective unconscious** populated by **archetypes** – universal themes of meaning that lies beneath and transcend our personal ego structures.

Jung's thinking was profoundly influenced by **synchronicity** – the concurrence of an event and an inner experience, which are connected by a sense of meaning for the individual experiencing them. He introduced the concept and his personal experience of these meaningful coincidences in everyday life led him to the conclusion that there was a **causal order** that linked the inner world of the mental with the outer world of the physical through their meaning.

At the apex of Jung's hierarchy of archetypes is the **Self**. The Self is a mysterious concept that can be understood in prosaic terms as the best possible version of ourselves and which involves a unification of the conscious and the unconscious aspects of the psyche. Jung coined the term **individuation** to describe the death rebirth process and psychological transformation that marks the transition from ego to Self in advanced stages of ego development. The **anima** (and its masculine version the **animus**) occupied a central role in Jung's model as the archetypal feminine that has to be owned and integrated by ego structures for individuation to progress [15].

Jung was considered one of the great thinkers of the twentieth century although his ideas have been less influential in modern psychiatry and psychotherapy. He described his own *confrontation with the unconscious* in his autobiography and how the material that emerged in this personal crisis shaped his subsequent work, referred to subsequently as a creative illness [16]. Jung thought of psychotherapy as a developmental journey of psycho-spiritual maturation and Jungian depth psychology provided for many a modern method of accessing the spiritual power of the deep psyche at a time when traditional religion was losing its relevance.

Melanie Klein

The study of the adult neurosis led Freud to discover the child in the adult, the study of children led Mrs Klein to the infant in the child [17].

Melanie Klein (b. 1882, Vienna, d. 1960, London) further developed ideas about unconscious processes from her groundbreaking psychoanalytic work with infants and young children. While Freud extrapolated backwards from his work with adults in developing ideas about early development, Klein used her understanding of infantile and primitive psychological processes and raw states of affect to generate ideas about adult psychic life. She placed early emotional experience as central to the development of adult psychic life. Klein's direct observations of infants with their mothers, and perhaps her own experiences as a mother herself, led to the recognition that the mother's state of mind provides the primary emotional environment for the child – and of the child as being *relationship seeking* from birth. This heralded an intense interest in early experiences of care in psychoanalysis and a huge advance in our understanding of emotional development and the role of early relationships.

Klein had an extreme gift for recognising how children use play to create scenarios in keeping with their conscious and unconscious preoccupations. She developed the **play technique**; using a selection of toys and drawing materials children would be encouraged to play freely in their therapy sessions – seen as the equivalent of free association for adults. The child's play was recognised as being full of meaning, the toys and activities representing key figures and emotional issues in symbolic form, and as worthy of the same level of serious consideration by the analyst as the verbal expressions and dreams of adult patients. She recognised how anxieties, emotional urges, Oedipal issues and conflict were expressed and to an extent worked out in this way. This gave access to the unconscious world of the child and both confirmed some of Freud's findings while adding some unexpected new discoveries about the unconscious.

Klein differed from Freud in seeing the infant as seeking to communicate and to relate to others from their earliest days, not simply to satisfy instinctual needs. From this viewpoint she saw feelings, both emotional and physical, as being experienced in terms of *a relationship with another* in early life. She used the term **object** to refer to the people to whom the infant primarily relates. According to Klein in infancy this relating is towards *parts* of the other – their lap, breast, arms etc., and these have not yet been put together in the infant's mind to form a whole person. She wrote of the breast as representing the nurturing capacity of the other [18].

After birth the infant is no longer cocooned within the regulatory homeostatic mechanisms of the mother's bodily processes and is faced with an external reality in which he is separate and has to find ways to secure his own survival. He faces hunger, cold, frustration and aloneness for the first time and is entirely dependent on care in order to live; he is not able to move, feed or protect himself. Klein recognised the intensity, desperation and passion with which the infant seeks to relate and also how he interprets all his experiences in relational terms – every feeling is experienced in relation to another. Fortunately for the infant the mother's state of mind is usually exquisitely tuned into the intensity of his need and the nature of her response is key to emotional development.

Klein saw **unconscious phantasy** as the basis of mental life and as evidenced in infancy and in children's play. Unconscious phantasy differs from fantasy, which is a conscious process of mental retreat into daydreaming in response to frustration. Unconscious phantasy refers to the unconscious mental representation of somatic experience in early life and gives it meaning in relational terms. For example, after a satisfying feed the pleasurable experience of a full tummy may be accompanied by a phantasy of a wonderfully sustaining object held within the infant. Klein also recognised innate destructive urges and feelings of rage and fear, which are unmodified and primitive at the start of life. This includes **envy**, which Klein recognised as the destructive and to an extent constitutional urge to destroy the goodness of the other [19]. In addition she suggested the infant has an innate unconscious knowledge about sexuality, and the parental relationship. She saw the Oedipal situation as key to the development of the mind and the child as being aware of triangular situations that he is excluded from in the earliest months of life. She saw issues of aggression, sexuality, omnipotence and attempts to find creative solutions in her observations of children's play and drawings.

Klein developed the idea of there being two positions of central importance in early life – the **paranoid-schizoid and depressive positions** [20]. In the first days and weeks of life the infant has to find ways to deal with powerful emotions, and good and bad experiences in the external world, overwhelming anxiety including fear of non- survival, and innate destructive urges. He does this initially through processes of **splitting** and **projection. Splitting** refers to a binary division of experiences into good and bad; these are absolute states with no ambiguity or uncertainty. Klein stressed the importance of this for healthy development and as the infant's first attempt to structure his experiences. By **projecting** unwanted and troublesome urges and affects into the external world the infant is able to inhabit a benign state of mind in which he can safely settle and feed. However, by projecting aggressive urges outside of the self the external world can become a threatening and dangerous place leading to fear of attack and persecutory anxiety, ideas helpful in understanding paranoid states of mind.

These ideas help to explain the everyday intensity of infantile emotional life, easily observed in the persecuted screams of a hungry baby, signalling a terror that his very life could be endangered, and the absolute bliss and total state of trust after a satisfying feed which may closely follow this – both are absolute and extreme states entirely disconnected from each other in early life. Within these states the baby is relating to both the utterly wonderful and absolutely terrifying aspects of his own internal phantasies rather than the reality of an understood external world. His internal experience has become the entire reality. Through unconscious phantasy the infant experiences his bodily sensations and affects as being caused by benign or malignant objects – a hunger pain for example as an attack from a hostile persecutor who is attacking his tummy. This is also referred to as **part object relating** – the mother is related to in parts, and there is no connection in early life between the bad/attacking mother who abandons him to persecutors and the loving and nurturing one. The key anxiety in the paranoid-schizoid position is persecutory – having projected fear of annihilation into the world around there is a terror of attack from outside. The term **projective identification** adds depth to the concept of projection and includes the process by which the object is changed by the projection – so the person who is the target of the projection of hostility and aggression may in turn become angry themselves.

As the infant develops, he starts to recognise the mother who frustrates his wishes and has her limitations is the same as the loving mother upon whom he is entirely dependent – the parts start to come together to form a whole. This heralds the **depressive position** that Klein saw as evident from three to six months of age [21]. The mother starts to become a whole object in the infant's mind – with the painful realisation this is also the mother whom the infant has so hated and felt such aggression towards. This allows the development of feelings such as concern, guilt for the infant's own aggression towards the mother he so loves and needs, responsibility and a desire to make things better through **reparation.** These are necessary and normal emotions to tolerate and bear – the depressive position is not the same as depression but the associated anxiety in depressive position functioning is depressive in nature and in keeping with both loving and needing the object. Holding both love and hatred together can be difficult to bear and to integrate and working this through requires repeated **mourning** as previous positions are given up and reparation is made for the hatred which has been felt. Defences may be launched against the painful work of depressive position functioning. **The manic defence** involves denial of the object's importance with denigration, omnipotence and avoidance of guilt **and obsessional defences** involve control and repetitive activities towards undoing aggressive acts. Children's play is rich in material supporting these ideas, using toys as **symbols** to express and resolve themes of love and hatred, aggression and reparation.

Hence Klein described and differentiated between two basic groups of anxieties and defences; the paranoid-schizoid position characterised by splitting leading to idealisation and denigration and the co-existence of extremes of good and bad within the individual, projection and projective identification in which parts of the self are experienced as located in others, and poor integration of the ego in which there is no memory of a good object when absent. In this state of mind there can be confusion between self and other and the ability to symbolise is impaired leading to concrete thinking; there is no 'as – if' when paranoid-schizoid functioning predominates.

Hallmarks of depressive position functioning include experiencing the self and others in an integrated way, as having both resources and limitations, being able therefore to hold ambivalent and conflicting experiences in mind. This involves an ability to tolerate mourning and guilt and ownership of one's own aggression, needs and dependency.

A key feature emphasised by Klein and subsequent theorists [22] is that a continuous movement occurs between the two positions and throughout life; we can all fluctuate from more depressive positions of mind in which we function in more integrated ways and with secure senses of ourselves and others to more fragmented states in which we can feel more persecuted and it is harder to hold a perspective and the capacity to think. Klein also opened the idea that psychotic anxiety and processes are present from early life. She contributed significantly to the understanding of the psychological processes underlying paranoia and psychosis seeing these as having their psychological antecedents in early, primitive and normal psychological processes (see Chapter 14).

Klein's theory of projective identification, in which the mother is used to contain some part of the baby's emotional state, informed early ideas about the importance of **containment** in psychic development. If the mother is able to adequately contain her baby, to receive him and to feel with him, to process and to understand the projected emotions the infant experiences, he **introjects** an experience of being calmly understood. Over time the infant gradually develops his capacity to do this for himself – to become increasingly independent and *self-contained*. In contrast if the mother appears damaged, overwhelmed, non-responsive or retaliatory, his guilt and despair increase.

Criticisms of Klein include that she focussed too exclusively on the internal experiences of the baby and not enough on external reality, although she did emphasise how the actual state of the mother is key. Her ideas formed the basis of **object relations theory**, giving psychic form to the architecture of unconscious processes, in which the internal world is populated by representations and phantasies about internal and external feelings and experiences, and brought the importance of early life and the quality of early nurture to the forefront of psychoanalytic thinking [23].

Donald Winnicott

There is no such thing as a baby [24]

This startling statement illustrates Donald Winnicott's emphasis on the primal importance of the infant–mother relationship, without which the infant cannot continue to exist. He emphasised the importance of the mother's state of mind, her receptivity and responses towards her baby as providing his entire environment in early life and introducing the term **primary maternal preoccupation** to describe the infant's need for a non-intrusive awareness of, and exclusive focus upon his communications [25]. This has been likened to the state of mind of an analyst when listening to their patient.

Donald Winnicott (b. 1896, Devon, d. 1971, London) was a paediatrician and a psychoanalyst who saw thousands of children with their mothers in the paediatric hospital and clinics he ran at Paddington Green Children's Hospital. He further developed Klein's object relations theory and saw the emotional and relational aspects of the baby's environment as key to healthy development. He introduced the term **good enough mother** as able to provide sufficient emotional holding or a **facilitative environment** for the infant to explore, organise and satisfy their basic needs – both physical, emotional and relational [26]. Under good enough conditions the baby is able to develop what Winnicott described as **a true self** with a secure sense of their own identity. However, if the baby's sense of themselves becomes impinged upon by the mother's own emotional needs then a **false self** may develop which colludes with perceived pressure to be a certain kind of object for another – with parts of the true self kept hidden [27]. An example may be an excessively good child with a disturbed mother, who keeps their own angry and aggressive urges concealed although these may be expressed in other ways – or through psychopathology. Winnicott emphasised the importance of **play** for both adults and the developing child – and the importance of potential space for **transitional phenomena** to occur towards the infant being able to creatively explore the environment which includes the use of **transitional objects,** often used to describe a toy or blanket which may be used towards the process of separation from the primary object. He wrote of the importance of an early merged state of **illusion** in which the infant may creatively feel he can create the breast or required other, and the importance of **disillusionment** in relinquishing this in order to negotiate weaning and a sense of a separate self. Winnicott also developed ideas about delinquent and antisocial behaviours, described as a sign of hope that actual deprivation in the external environment had occurred and was being protested about [28].

Wilfred Bion

The purest form of listening is to listen without memory or desire [29]

Wilfred Bion (b.1897, India, d.1979, UK) was a decorated tank commander in the First World War and trained as a physician and then a psychiatrist in the 1940s. The two world wars were massive stimulants to the development of his ideas and during the Second World War he worked as a psychiatrist at the military hospital in Northfields where he further developed his ideas. Bion observed from experience in active combat how group cohesion was maintained if men could unite against a common enemy and went on to incorporate group activities and therapy at Northfield Hospital and the Tavistock Institute of Human

Relations in London. He developed further ideas about group processes and group therapy and his ideas about 'Basic Assumptions' in groups have been described as the 'metapsychology' of groups (see Chapter 11).

After training in psychoanalysis Bion's achievements continued to be highly original and illuminating. In the 1940s he was one of several hugely talented psychoanalysts to be analysed by Melanie Klein and he became deeply interested in the analysis of psychotic patients. In 1970 he moved to Los Angeles and his work there became powerfully influential in Latin America but became increasingly outside the mainstream of psychoanalyst thought in Europe.

Bion's major contributions included ideas about the key importance of the maternal environment for development, detailing further some of the processes identified by Winnicott. He described **maternal reverie** and **maternal receptivity to projective identification** from the baby as being of crucial importance in allowing the baby to develop their own reflective capacity [30]. His highly original ideas about the psychological processes involved in thinking transformed psychoanalytic theory. He saw thoughts as *already existing* in the infant but requiring the **alpha function** of another to come into realisation. This is achieved through projective identification of the unprocessed sensory data or **beta elements** into the mother who through her own mature processing and state of **maternal reverie** is able to contain and return them in modified form as **alpha elements** – which the baby is able to experience as understood thoughts. He called this process **container-contained**. He applied these ideas to the ability to learn, to psychotic processes [31] and to the psychoanalytic process between patient and analyst, emphasising the importance of how to listen and to be receptive in the consulting room.

Attachment Theory

Attachment is a unifying principle that reaches from the biological depths of our being to its furthest spiritual reaches
Jeremy Holmes [32]

Further gains in understanding internal emotional experience, the influences upon psychological development in childhood and of how powerfully unconscious psychological processes drive and repeat behaviours were achieved through the work of John Bowlby (1907–90, London) and James and Joyce Robertson in the 1950s. This involved the observation of children and their parents separated in hospital and residential care. Their descriptions and films of distressed children separated from their parents, at a time when parents were routinely advised to leave their children during hospital admissions, have radically changed how we now think about this and how paediatric services are organised, with parents now encouraged to stay with their unwell children [33].

Bowlby emphasised the survival needs of the infant as being entirely dependent upon their attachment to a caregiver; we need to attach securely and to be able to bind this attachment securely in the earliest hours and days of infancy. The success with which this is achieved determines not only survival but the template for all further relating as these early patterns, laid down when the mind is most vulnerable and its sensitivities most heightened, are repeated throughout life in subsequent relationships and psychological resilience. Bowlby drew upon biological and ethological models as opposed to the prevailing psychoanalytic ideas of the time. The realities and limitations of the actual caregiving relationships are brought to the fore and strongly emphasised in attachment theory. The emphasis is on

Table 1.2 The main patterns of attachment

Attachment pattern	Behaviour after separation
Secure	Infant seeks proximity and welcomes mother back
Insecure avoidant	Infant ignores the mother's absence and return
Insecure ambivalent	Distressed, clingy, then rejecting behaviour
Insecure disorganised	Incoherent response – source of safety is also a source of threat with fear of the mother

real-life experiences and the development of robust rating scales to investigate attachment patterns has allowed for systemic assessment and categorisation of attachment patterns, linked with the responsiveness and nurturing ability of the primary caregiver [34].

Key to attachment theory is that security in childhood is relationship specific, security is related to the parent's sensitivity and response towards the child's state of mind, and that classification of a child's attachment patterns at the age of one has predictive power for later psychosocial development. Infant security can be assessed at one year in a standardised test situation, **the Strange Situation**, in which two brief separations and reunions between the child and the mother are observed [35]. On the basis of the child's behaviour their attachment pattern can be categorised as shown in Table 1.2.

There is evidence that secure attachment can be protective when faced with adversity in later life and in social relating, and that disorganised attachment can be predictive with regard to later life stress management, and conduct problems [36]. Separation from attachment figures leads to panic, and loss to despair that may be of key significance in understanding depression in adult life [37]. Adult attachment patterns can also be rated and evaluated using the Adult Attachment Interview and it has been shown that there is a high correlation between the parental representation of attachment and the child's behaviour at one year. Assessment patterns of the expectant mother as rated during pregnancy are able to predict with 70–80 per cent certainty what the attachment pattern of the infant will be at one year, seeming proof of the importance of the maternal environment both pre- and post-natally on psychological development [38].

In addition to changing the culture and practices in child care, institutions, family courts and hospitals, attachment theory has provided a measureable means to address the importance of mother–infant relating in early life, how this is repeated through generations and how this relates to psychological resilience and relationship patterns in later life. It has stimulated a huge amount of research including the work of Peter Fonagy and Mary Target into the ability to **mentalize** [39] and has demonstrated how powerfully unconscious psychological processes, linked to early experiences of nurture and the mother's own internal world, drive and repeat behaviours.

Conclusion

This chapter has described some of the contributions of psychoanalytic theory towards our understanding of the human mind. There are widely diverging ideas, arguments and controversies which continue to surround these ideas, as well as highly creative discoveries and research activities proliferating from them. Advances in research in social, cognitive and affective neuroscience confirm the importance of early nurture, unconscious processes and relationships in brain development [40]. Psychoanalysis has revolutionalised our understanding of the mind and provided penetrating insights into unconscious mental processes, psychological development, psychic determinism and the limits of rationality in human activity and how we relate. Furthermore, clinical techniques designed to reveal unconscious processes have been specifically developed and modified. While the model continues to be revised and to evolve, psychoanalysis provides the most far-reaching, coherent and comprehensive framework we have in seeking to understand and to investigate the complexity of human emotional life and behaviour. No other theory has come close in aiming to illuminate and to explore the psychological processes underpinning the vast terrain of the mind, to explain man's destructiveness and creativity, the importance of thought and relationships, and in linking biological need with psychic contents. Psychoanalysis has also formed the bedrock for a diaspora of psychological treatments based upon psychoanalytic under-standing, some of which will be described as this collection of essays unfolds.

References

1. Miller GA. The magical number seven plus or minus two: some limits on our capacity for processing information. *Psychol Rev* 1956; 63(2): 81–97.

2. Freud S. The interpretation of dreams. In J Strachey, ed., *The Standard Edition of the Complete Psychological Works of Sigmund Freud, Volume IV (1900): The Interpretation of Dreams (First Part)*. London: Hogarth Press, 1953. (Original work published 1900)

3. Freud S. *On Aphasia: A Critical Study*. London: Imago, 1953.

4. Freud S, Breuer J. Studies on hysteria. In J Strachey, ed., *The Standard Edition of the Complete Psychological Works of Sigmund Freud, Volume II (1893–1895): Studies on Hysteria by Josef Breuer and Sigmund Freud*. London: Hogarth Press, 1955. (Original work published 1895)

5. Freud S. The unconscious. In J Strachey, ed., *The Standard Edition of the Complete Psychological Works of Sigmund Freud, Volume XIV (1914–1916): On the History of the Psycho-Analytic Movement, Papers on Metapsychology and Other Works*. London: Hogarth Press. 1957; pp. 159–216. (Original work published 1915)

6. Freud S. Papers on Technique. In J Strachey, ed., *The Standard Edition of the Complete Psychological Works of Sigmund Freud, Volume XII (1911–1913): Case History of Schreber, Papers on Technique and Other Works*. London: Hogarth Press, 1958. (Original work published 1912)

7. Freud S. The ego and the id. In J Strachey, ed., *The Standard Edition of the Complete Psychological Works of Sigmund Freud, Volume XIX (1923–1925): The Ego and the Id and Other Works*. London: Hogarth Press. 1961; pp. 1–66. (Original work published 1923)

8. Solms M. The conscious id. *Neurospsychoanalysis* 2013; 15: 5–85.

9. Freud S. Thoughts for the time on war and death. The disillusionment of the war. In J Strachey, ed., *The Standard Edition of the Complete Psychological Works of Sigmund Freud, Volume XIV (1914–1916): On the History of the Psycho-Analytic Movement, Papers on Metapsychology and Other Works*. London: Hogarth Press. 1957; pp. 275–288. (Original work published 1915)

10. Freud S. The aetiology of hysteria. In J Strachey, ed., *The Standard Edition of the Complete Psychological Works of Sigmund Freud, Volume III (1893–1899): Early Psycho-Analytic Publications*. London:

Hogarth Press. 1953; pp. 187–222. (Original work published 1896)

11. Masson JM. *The Assault on Truth: Freud's Suppression of the Seduction Theory.* New York: Farrar, Straus, and Giroux, 1984.

12. Freud S. Three essays on the theory of sexuality. In J Strachey, ed., *The Standard Edition of the Complete Psychological Works of Sigmund Freud, Volume VII (1901–1905): A Case of Hysteria, Three Essays on Sexuality and Other Works.* London: Hogarth Press. 1953; pp. 125–248. (Original work published 1905)

13. de Beauvoir S. *The Second Sex.* 1949.

14. Freud A. *The Ego and the Mechanisms of Defence.* London: Routledge Press, 1966.

15. Jung CG. *The Archetypes and the Collective Unconscious,* 2nd ed. London: Taylor & Francis, 1991.

16. Jung C. *Memories, Dreams, Reflections: An Autobiography.* New York: Random House, 1965.

17. Segal H. *Klein.* London: Karnac Books. 1989; p. 55.

18. Klein M. *The Psycho-Analysis of Children.* London: Hogarth Press, 1932.

19. Klein M. Envy and gratitude. In *The Writings of Melanie Klein.* Vol. 3. *Envy and Gratitude and Other Works.* London: Hogarth Press. 1957; pp. 176–235.

20. Klein M. Notes on some schizoid mechanisms. In M Klein, P Heimann, S Isaacs, J Riviere, eds., *Developments in Psychoanalysis.* London: Hogarth Press. 1952; pp. 292–320.

21. Klein M. Mourning and its relation to manic depressive states. In *The Writings of Melanie Klein.* Vol. 1. *Love, Guilt and Reparation.* London: Hogarth Press. 1935; pp. 344–89.

22. Steiner J. The equilibrium between the paranoid-schizoid and depressive positions. In *Clinical Lectures on Klein and Bion.* The New Library of Psychoanalysis 14. Brunner-Routledge reprinted 2003.

23. Klein M. Our adult world and its roots in infancy. *The Writings of Melanie Klein.* Vol.

3. *Envy and Gratitude and Other Works.* London: Hogarth Press. 1959; pp. 247–63.

24. Winnicott DW. Discussion at a Scientific Meeting of the British Psychoanalytic Society. Circa 1940

25. Winnicott DW. Primary maternal preoccupation. In *Collected Papers: Through Paediatrics to Psycho-Analysis.* Tavistock Publications 1958/Karnac Books 1987; pp. 300–6.

26. Winnicott DW. Transitional objects and transitional phenomena. In *Playing and Reality.* London: Routledge Classics. 1991; pp. 1–34.

27. Winnicott DW. The concept of the false self. In *Home Is Where We Start From.* London: Penguin Books 1986; pp. 65–70.

28. Winnicott DW. Aspects of juvenile delinquency. *The Child the Family and the Outside World.* London: Penguin Books. 1964. Reprinted 1991; p. 227.

29. Bion WR. Notes on memory and desire. In *Melanie Klein Today.* Vol. 2. 1967. The New Library of Psychoanalysis. Reprinted 2001.

30. Bion WR. A theory of thinking. In *Second Thoughts.* London: Heinemann. 1967; pp. 110–19. Reprinted in 1990 Marefield.

31. Bion WR. Attacks on linking. In *Second Thoughts* London: Heinemann. 1967; p. 93 Reprinted in 1990 Marefield.

32. Holmes J. *John Bowlby and Attachment Theory.* London: Routledge, 1993.

33. Robertson J and J. *Separation and The Very Young.* London: Free Association Books, 1989.

34. Bowlby J. *A Secure Base: Clinical Implications of Attachment Theory.* London: Routledge, 1988.

35. Ainsworth M, Blehar M, Waters E, Wall S. *Patterns of Attachment: A Psychological Study of The Strange Situation Test.* Hillsdale NJ: Lawrence Erlbaum Associates Inc, 1978.

36. Sroufe LA. Psychopathology as an outcome of development. *Dev Psychopathol* 1997; 9 (2): 251–68.

37. Solms M. Depression: A Neuropsychoanalytic Perspective. *Int Forum Psychoanal* 2012; 21: 207–13.

38. Fonagy P, Steele H, Steele M. Maternal representations of attachment during pregnancy predict the organization of infant–mother attachment at one year of age. *Child Dev* 1991; 62: 891–905.

39. Fonagy P, Target M. Playing with reality: I. Theory of mind and the normal development of psychic reality. *Int J Psychoanal* 1996; 77: 217–33.

40. Solms LM. The Neurobiological underpinnings of psychoanalytic theory and therapy. *Front Behav Neurosci* 2018; 12: 294.

A Psychodynamic Approach to Psychiatry

Jo O'Reilly

A psychodynamic approach to psychiatry provides an overarching coherent conceptual framework from which all other treatments can be prescribed.
Gabbard [1]

The practice of psychiatry is an extraordinarily complex task. Mental disorder produces bizarre and illogical symptoms, our patients may behave self-destructively and engage in harmful relationships, activities which seem puzzling to the rational mind. Despite the distressing and disabling effects of mental illness the most carefully considered treatment plans may be met with resistance and refusal to engage. Working with disturbed states of mind allows privileged access to the deeper workings of the human psyche which may be fascinating and difficult to comprehend. The emotional impact of the work is often deeply involving and intense.

Meeting this multilayered task draws deeply on our skills and resources and requires a conceptual framework with the depth and range to accommodate this complexity. This chapter describes how a psychodynamic approach to psychiatry can helpfully contribute to this framework and enhance clinical understanding as the basis of treatment. Psychodynamic psychiatry rests upon psychoanalytic theory and key concepts underpinning this approach will be outlined. These ideas will be illustrated by case examples to show how the application of a psychodynamic approach deepens and enriches everyday psychiatric care.

Key Concepts in a Psychodynamic Approach to Psychiatry

So what does the term psychodynamic psychiatry mean? In general terms a psychodynamic perspective enables the importance of relationships, psychological development, life experiences and constitutional factors to be integrated and considered together in understanding the development and presentation of mental disorder. The key underlying principles can be summarised as follows:

1. A focus upon the unique personal biography of the individual presenting to mental health services
2. Symptoms are viewed as having meaning, however curious they may seem
3. Psychological mechanisms in disturbed states of mind are seen as continuous with, and more extreme versions of, normal functioning
4. Psychiatric breakdown is recognised as occurring along pre-existing fault lines in the psyche in keeping with developmental vulnerability
5. The ability to mourn is recognised as key to psychological development and difficulties with the mourning process predispose to the development of symptoms and breakdown, which is often triggered by loss events

6. Unconscious mental processes are powerfully expressed in mental disorder and attending to the transference, countertransference, projection and splitting significantly enhances clinical understanding
7. Countertransference enactments can define the way in which patients are managed
8. Emotional and psychological aspects of containment are key to psychiatric care
9. Resistance to change perpetuates mental illness as symptoms may be performing an important function
10. Psychodynamic and biological factors interact and influence the expression and form of psychiatric symptoms

A Biopsychosocial Approach to Psychiatry

It is much more important to know what sort of patient has the disease than what sort of disease the patient has

William Osler [2] (1848–1919)

Although writing as a physician, William Osler recognised the importance of attending to the person with the illness rather than the physician limiting his interest to the pathology of the disease process.

This resonates with what we hold dear in psychiatry, the branch of medicine most overtly directed at the person as a whole and their life experience. A fundamental idea in contemporary psychiatry is that an integrated biopsychosocial approach is the most helpful way to understand mental disturbance.

In addressing the psychological aspects of psychiatric presentation, a psychodynamic model provides a model of the mind which takes a primary interest in the personal biography of the patient presenting to services. In addition, the recognition of unconscious processes and exploration of how they operate can shed light upon the meaning conveyed in psychiatric symptoms. Our patients become more understandable if their preoccupations and beliefs are seen as more extreme or bizarre means to both express and manage disturbing internal responses to the painful realities of life common to us all, such as loss, deprivation, limitation and trauma.

> Ms P's father had left the family when she was 13 years old and moved to another country. Upon hearing at the age of 19 that he had remarried and had another daughter Ms P presented to psychiatric services expressing delusional beliefs that she was marrying Prince Harry and that Paul McCartney would be the vicar.

In this case the content of Ms P's delusions seems highly meaningful when her personal biography is taken into account. A wedding and the presence of a man with another family are central to the material. In addition, an understanding of primary process thinking helps to understand her symptoms as being driven by the wish fulfilment seeking and reality denying forces of the unconscious. The painful experience of being left and replaced by her father is transformed into the delusion that she is to become a highly envied wife and daughter herself, a princess in the eyes of the world, able to secure the undivided attention of a father figure who has left his family to attend to her at her wedding.

Her symptoms could therefore be seen as an attempt to both express and to compensate for the losses and hurt she has experienced and to find a solution which circumnavigates a painful reality. The external reality has been replaced in her mind by a preferable situation of her own creation. Such an approach considers the underlying issues behind her break-down, enriches the case formulation and fosters treatment which conveys understanding and curiosity about the contents of her mind, her key relationships and her life experience. It also allows staff to recognise her vulnerability to feelings of rejection and replacement and to sensitively consider these issues in her relationships with staff in her ongoing care.

Psychodynamic Psychiatry and Biology

In the last 2 decades, it has become obvious that child abuse, urbanization, migration, and adverse life events contribute to the etiology of schizophrenia. . . .. Just as the lungs process air, so the brain processes external stimuli; consequently its healthy function can be harmed by noxious factors in the social environment.

Professor Robin Murray [3]

A range of factors contributes to the development and expression of mental disorder. The relative influence of biological, psychological and social factors will vary on a case by case basis and between different conditions. There may be powerful genetic influences or drug-induced factors in the development of schizophrenia for example, but the psychotic process is still occurring in the context of the person's history, relationships, attachment pattern and emotional internal world with all its unique sensitivities. These factors combine to influence the vulnerability factors, the nature of the symptoms, the relationships formed with the treating team and the course the condition takes.

Research findings in a range of fields, from neuroscience to attachment theory, have shown the brain to be a responsive, plastic and dynamic structure that adapts, develops and functions in the context of relationships. Constitutional factors combine with experiences of nurture and emotional attunement and are shaped further by trauma and other external experiences contributing in a dynamic manner to the development of the brain and personality [4–7].

Research has also shown how conscious thought is a limited resource and that much of mental life occurs outside conscious awareness [8]. The limited capacity of conscious memory means that much of our experience is stored in the unconscious on the basis of past similar experience and meaning, and we respond to situations in the present based upon recognition of patterns familiar to us. The psychoanalytic concept of the transference addresses a similar phenomenon with relationships describing how we respond to the present on the basis of internalised past patterns of relating [9].

Mental life can be thus viewed as a complex dynamic system in which biological substrates of the brain, conscious and unconscious aspects of the mind and external experiences are in constant conversation with each other. A unique individual internal world therefore develops which is in constant dialogue with the genome, the neurocircuitry of the brain and external reality. In mental disorder and psychiatric breakdown, the causal factors, the meaning of the situation for the individual concerned and the form the symptoms take depend upon the interaction and balance between these aspects of the system on a unique and highly personal basis.

A psychodynamic approach to psychiatry takes a holistic approach in addressing the biological factors, psychological processes and relational issues in mental disorder. This provides a comprehensive framework, emphasising emotions, relationships and meaning, from which all aspects of treatment, including the use of medication and need for medical investigation, can be considered.

The Unconscious

The ego is not master in its own house

Sigmund Freud [10]

The understanding of mental disorder is deepened by exploring the unconscious layers of the mind, and the mechanisms, structures and processes by which early history, repressed memory and emotional biography are stored and expressed; the underlying tissues and physiology of the psyche as it were.

Key points about the unconscious:

1. Most mental activity occurs at an unconscious level. As clinicians this means even our most considered and rational thought processes are guided and informed also by pressures from the unconscious substructures of the mind. How we perceive situations in the external world, how we make decisions, how we feel and act largely beats to the rhythm of an unconscious score which we have limited conscious access to

2. All behaviour, symptoms and actions have meaning at an unconscious level, no matter how paradoxical and nonsensical they may seem

3. Unconscious processes operate differently to rational conscious thought and are more in keeping with primary process activity, characterised by replacement of external by psychical reality, wish fulfilment, tolerance of contradiction, timelessness, avoidance of pain and magical thinking (see Chapter 1)

4. Our defensive organisations strive to maintain an equilibrium between pressures emanating from the unconscious and the external world

5. When defences become overwhelmed symptoms can reveal the workings of the unconscious. A similar process happens in sleep when we dream

6. Unconscious processes may be floridly revealed in states of mental disturbance

In psychiatry, the most significant issues and key developmental events shaping the personality are available in the patient's history, routinely gathered in mental health services. The key interpersonal issues are also manifest in the relationships formed and behaviours expressed towards staff. Mental health staff are therefore extremely well placed to make a comprehensive formulation about their patient's difficulties; there is a richness of information available to them from the spoken histories from patients and families, and their own observations from within the team.

Symptoms and behaviours presenting to mental health services are brimming with information about unconscious processes. These may seem bizarre and incomprehensible as the psychological processes of unconscious operate differently to rational thoughts, but, like dreams, they have meaning. The manner in which a patient may relate to and emotionally impact upon staff contains vivid and immediate material which is also key to formulation and understanding. In disturbed states of mind the restraining function of the defensive organisation is challenged and unconscious emotional forces can ricochet around inpatient units and community team, powerfully affecting management.

Ms S was admitted with a relapse of a psychotic illness under Section 3 of the Mental Health Act. Prior to the admission her young children were taken into care. She constantly accused staff of neglect and not meeting her needs; they felt persecuted and inadequate, leading to frustration, irritation and a tendency to avoid contact with her on the ward. When able to consider their feelings towards her as containing important information about her own feelings of guilt and failure at not having been able to adequately care for her children, feelings of sympathy, interest and concern re-emerged in the team.

Ms S's case illustrates how meaningful emotional states in an inpatient setting can be projected into staff, unconsciously steering management and requiring recognition and understanding.

Psychodynamic Psychiatry, Early Development and Paranoia

Psychoanalytic theory views the psychological mechanisms of pathological states as more extreme versions of normal function. This means that the potential seeds of mental breakdown reside in all of us and the degree to which these become manifest depends on a range of factors. In states of heightened anxiety and psychological distress more primitive forms of mental function come to the fore. Thus, developmental issues and transitions not satisfactorily negotiated or resolved earlier in life can reveal themselves in the form that the psychological disturbance takes. An understanding of psychological development can help to recognise when early wounds and difficulties are exposed as part of the patient's presentation to mental health services.

Psychoanalytic theory emphasises the importance of early development in shaping adult personality. In early life the nature of the attachment relationships, the experiences of emotional attunement and containment of primitive and intense emotional states are internalised to form psychological structures in the mind. These internal templates, or 'objects' in psychoanalytic terms, inform how we later relate to the world and shape our response to challenges in external reality. The ability to manage primitive psychological urges, anxiety and appetites depends both upon constitutional factors and on the regulatory capacity of the external nurturing environment. The capacity to recognise feelings as distinct from reality (e.g. I am frightened rather than the world is dangerous) requires the capacity to symbolise to become established, along with the ability to think without the mind becoming overwhelmed and fragmented; and this is crucial in psychological development. The development of a secure sense of one's own identity requires an ability to psychologically separate from the dependency of infancy, a challenge revisited in adolescence; thus patterns of dependency, difficulties with separation and hostility towards authority figures may indicate challenges with this complex process. Oedipal issues of longing for exclusive relationships, intolerance of exclusion and disappointment, the impact of traumatic life experiences and boundary violations and loss are key to determining the resource and vulnerability within the internal world. Issues related to these challenges may be forcefully expressed in how patients in disordered states of mind interact with mental health teams.

Some of these processes can be well illustrated if we look at the common symptom of paranoia.

In early life paranoid anxieties are understood by the *paranoid-schizoid position* as serving a useful purpose in separating and preserving good experiences by projecting unbearable states of anxiety and frustration into the outside world [11] (see Chapter 1).

This psychological mechanism is universal and necessary in early life but in more extreme form underlies paranoid mental states. In mental disturbance or intense stress, normal projective processes can intensify into paranoid ideation in which the bad feelings projected outwards are experienced as persecutory threat. If the anxiety is sufficiently high, the suspicion of persecutory anxiety can develop into delusional conviction, where there is a visceral certainty of danger and of others intent to harm. So paranoid states presenting to psychiatric services are based on an extreme form of normal psychological processes, which can be traced developmentally. The return to more extreme and primitive forms of mental functioning ubiquitous to us all helps to explain why paranoia is such a common symptom in a range of mental health disorders. It also means that there is often an understandable kernel of truth at the heart of the paranoid belief – as Freud also wrote 'There is not only method in madness . . .but also a fragment of historical truth' [12].

> Mr B had been severely neglected as a baby by his parents and as a result had been brought up in the care system. He worked as a hospital porter in the same hospital for many years. He had struggled to maintain close relationships and was socially isolated although he was on superficially friendly terms with other hospital staff. He presented to psychiatric services in a floridly agitated and paranoid state having started a hunger strike at home. He was severely malnourished at the point of admission and spoke of a conspiracy by his managers to abuse him sexually then leave him to die. This had been triggered by a reorganisation of services in which his job was threatened and he felt his managers had treated him as a problem to be got rid of.

It seems Mr B had repeated his childhood presentation to services in a seriously neglected state, a direct repetition of his past in the present. The threat of losing his job had triggered an eruption of intense emotion and the re-emergence of traumatic material and allowed the effect of disrupted attachments in his early life to become vividly apparent; perhaps then too he had felt he was a problem to be got rid of and a vulnerability to seeing himself in this way had always resided somewhere within him. The accompanying distrust which may have also lain quietly within him had become floridly manifest as a paranoid delusional state as he was threatened with the loss of his secure base at work; as Freud wrote he was not entirely mistaken but the extreme reaction and paranoia with which he met the events in the present was informed by long-standing and understandable developmental experiences.

Childhood Adversity, Pre-existing Fault Lines and Psychiatric Breakdown

If we throw a crystal to the floor it comes apart along its lines of cleavage . . . predetermined by the crystal's structure . . .. Patients are split and broken structures of the same kind

Sigmund Freud [13]

The incidence of psychiatric breakdown, as well as physical illness increases in line with adverse childhood experience [14]. In addition to crude disturbances in early relating such as parental loss, abuse and neglect, the fine-grained repeated patterns of relating with their unique characteristics and limitations are also internalised. A model of the internal world populated by these experiences with their resources, blind spots and fragilities can be helpful in seeing the mind as having pre-existing fault lines that may determine the timing and nature of a psychiatric crisis. In stable states of mind the ego and defensive organisation is more or less able to contain these areas of psychological vulnerability and more destructive aspects of relating; but when the fault lines are stressed these unresolved issues come powerfully to the fore. Implicit to this is the idea that the breakdown or illness reveals in more florid form underlying problematic parts of the personality.

The idea of the mind having pre-existing faultiness is helpful in situations when diagnostic conflicts emerge in clinical management. If the mind has a series of potential cracks, a range of relational and psychological issues may become expressed in highlighted form during a crisis all of which may settle once agitation has settled and recovery is underway.

> Once admitted to an inpatient unit Mr B was suspicious of staff on the ward, secretive and accusatory towards others that he came across, although opinion was divided about this and other staff members experienced him as being warm and likeable. Discussion of whether he had an underlying personality disorder and should be referred to specialist services for personality disorder ensued. However, as he settled on the ward and medication helped him to become less agitated and paranoid he became more friendly and open towards others; as his psychosis receded his usual reserved but sociable personality functioning was restored.

To quote from Ovid 'Anything cracked will shatter at a touch' [15]. This can be a helpful reminder in psychiatry that breakdown occurs in keeping with long-standing vulnerabilities, which may be largely buried in the unconscious until life events touch upon these points of fragility, triggering psychiatric breakdown along a number of fault lines and presentation to services in keeping with past experience and developmental adversity. Recognition of such fault lines also offers an opportunity for treatment to address the underlying issues and to decrease future vulnerability.

Mourning and Psychiatric Illness

One day this pain will be useful to you
Ovid [16]

The ability to accept the reality of loss, to grieve and to recover and adjust to new life situations is of profound importance in mental health. Psychoanalytic theory extends the concept of loss to recognise that for every developmental step or decision taken, there is loss to face and idealisation to relinquish. A toddler able to walk independently loses a degree of closeness on the mother's lap, and in adult life every decision or change, however positive, closes the door on other possibilities. Psychoanalytic theory places the ability to mourn as being of central importance in the development of the psyche. Mourning is a necessary process in coming to terms with reality, with the recognition of the opportunities, deprivations and losses life presents us with and the acceptance of the qualities, limitations and vulnerabilities of ourselves and others.

People in need of care from psychiatric services have often experienced profound, sometimes multiple losses. Presentation to services may be triggered by a loss event and difficulties in mourning may underlie a range of mental disorders, from depressive, anxiety, manic and psychotic states [17]. Obsessional and compulsive symptoms, with the repeated need to do and to undo actions, and anxiety states in which perseveration and rumination may replace decision and action may all express underlying conflicts and difficulties with loss when the ability to mourn is fragile.

In daily psychiatric practice an understanding of the loss events associated with a deterioration in mental state can unlock entrenched patterns of presentation and deepen clinical understanding. A model of recovery in which painful emotions such as grief and sadness are hopeful and necessary signs of mourning can also assist staff to support the process and not to become anxious that low mood, tearfulness or prolonged sadness are invariably indicative of depression. Staff can then be encouraged to support the need to mourn and not to pathologise the associated emotional pain.

> Ms P was admitted to a psychiatric ward in an intractable manic state after the breakdown of her marriage. Her feelings of invincibility and omnipotence were placing her at risk in her sexual behaviour and daily functioning. She was an attractive, flirtatious and likeable woman and was often amusing. Her mania seemed somehow contagious, staff liked working with her and spoke positively of her talents, potential and future plans, despite the persistence of her manic state. Although triggered by loss, the mania also disguised her underlying devastation and inability to come to terms with the end of her marriage. Her manic symptoms expressed a strong intolerance for any contact with painful emotions and the countertransference powerfully pulled staff away from seeing her as rejected or hurt. There was a risk that the crucial psychological issue of her loss being not addressed in her management, while her mania resisted treatment efforts and seemed set to take a chronic course.

Just as there can be no progress in life without mourning the loss of what has been left behind, the ability to grieve is also important in the recovery from crisis and breakdown and in allowing adaptation to new circumstances.

The Transference and Countertransference in Psychiatry

There is no present or future – only the past, happening over and over again – now.
Eugene O'Neill [18]

The term **transference** refers to the repetition of the past in the present in relationship terms. Experiences in early life lead to persistent patterns of mental organisation and pattern recognition determines how we perceive and respond to circumstances in the present, based upon these internalised templates. The transference is an unconscious process that helps us understand how different individuals perceive similar encounters differently. It also addresses the underlying dynamics by which clinical encounters can become transformed into challenging relationships in keeping with the patient's internalised experiences of nurture, care and authority.

The **countertransference** is the unconscious emotional response elicited by others through the process of projection; it informs our 'gut feelings' or how we intuit something about another's emotional state. **Projection** is the unconscious mechanism through which feelings are externalised into others around us, for example by attributing one's own hostility to another and denying any aggression within oneself. Projection has both an **evacuative** aspect and a **communicative** aspect. The evacuation is a means of getting rid of aspects of the self deemed undesirable, and the communicative aspect is how we let others know about our own emotional states. **Projective identification** [19] refers to an identification with the projection, which alters the other in some way. This may be caused by the sheer force of the projection or it may be due to the projection hooking onto the recipient's own vulnerabilities and needs. These unconscious forces shape the clinical relationship so that it becomes an arena in which the nature of historic formative relationships become re-enacted.

Transference and countertransference phenomena are ubiquitous. They suffuse all our interactions and relationships. We perceive, expect, and respond to others based upon pre-existing pattern recognition in a similar way to how our visual system interprets the world based upon prior learning. These processes can obfuscate, distort and blind us to present realities. In psychiatric breakdown, when the restraining function of the defensive organisation is challenged and contact with external reality is loosened, transference and countertransference phenomena may be powerfully and freely expressed, so that the past may become potently replayed in the present. A consultant psychiatrist returning from leave described how it seemed 'the pilot light was lit' as soon as she walked onto the ward after a week away, to receive an unrelenting barrage of hostility and accusation from a patient whose own mother had been experienced as neglectful and as prioritising her own needs above those of her children.

As this example illustrates, patients relate to staff within mental health teams in keeping with their past experiences of nurture, neglect and care. Many patients presenting to mental health services have experienced adversity in these early relationships when at their most vulnerable and dependent and are unconsciously programmed to have difficult relationships with carers; often testing out and provoking a particular kind of response from staff which mirrors past experience. In severe states of disturbance this can become concrete; a borderline patient for example can *know* staff are neglecting them and a paranoid patient may be *convinced* that the team means them harm.

Powerful projective processes emanating from disturbed states of mind mean that staff have powerful feelings elicited in them towards their patients and are unconsciously acted upon to play their part in these repetitions. These emotional responses can provide helpful diagnostic material and potential therapeutic tools towards a better understanding of the patient's internal world. Countertransference responses based upon projection will necessarily contain feelings that are uncomfortable and painful – such as rage, hatred, frustration, disgust – and staff may be anxious that such feelings are somehow unprofessional. The opposite is true however, these are just the feelings that the patient feels they have to disown, and these projected feelings require naming and understanding as part of their presentation. Ignoring these feelings or judging them as unprofessional or unhelpful ignores crucial information and depletes clinical care.

Mr D, aged 24, had a diagnosis of paranoid schizophrenia but his relapses always occurred in response to cannabis use, the effects of which he seemed very sensitive to. His admissions followed a pattern of settling quickly on the ward, responding well to staff and complying with management plans. As soon as he was discharged he smoked cannabis again, despite his stated intentions not to. He then became unwell again and was readmitted to the ward. His increasingly frustrated consultant felt both fond of him but also deeply frustrated, felt he was put in a role to constantly nag at him and to issue instructions about what he should do. After one ward round he exasperatedly said to staff that it was as if he was Mr D's father and felt like washing his hands of him. This realisation of the role he had been unconsciously allocated in Mr D's life was very helpful – he had grown up with a single mother after his father left when he was two, and he had lacked a father figure after his grandfather had died when he was eight. It was possible then to reformulate the presentation as having developed a transference relationship with his consultant that provided him with aspects that he had lost; a father figure to help him to navigate the challenges of adolescence. He also elicited a powerful wish to give up on him as perhaps he felt his father had done. When this understanding was incorporated into the case formulation a management plan was made which reflected the importance of this transference relationship, with the allocation of a male key worker able to take on aspects of this role in an ongoing way in the community.

This case illustrates that in addition to biological factors affecting Mr D's mental state, his relapses and presentations were filled with unconscious meaning in which the relationship with his consultant, through the transference, was key. This was sensitively recognised and responded to by the consultant psychiatrist when he unwittingly voiced his countertransference, allowing clinical care to be more in keeping with communications from the transference and countertransference processes in a helpful way.

Countertransference, Enactments, Traps and Opportunities

If psychiatry is practised without due attention paid to the countertransference, clinical management will be influenced by the pull of these emotional responses and there is a risk that the present situation becomes fertile ground for replication of past experiences of unempathic or harmful relating. The suicidal patient who elicits a countertransference of disinterest, or the manic patient whom the team struggle to take seriously are examples of this. The countertransference can powerfully influence how patients are responded to by staff, impede or distort clinical decision-making and can lead to iatrogenic harm. Despite the best conscious intentions to help the patient, clinical care can unwittingly find itself beating to the rhythm of unconscious processes, which may constantly replay past patterns of inadequate care, boundary violations and conflict.

A common example may be when rigid referral criteria and frequent rejections by clinical teams, changes in key workers and rushed discharge plans may repeat damaging patterns of disrupted attachments or rejections in early life. Freud referred to this process as the **repetition compulsion** [20] by which the past is constantly repeated in the present through unconscious processes bypassing conscious recognition and becoming action. The concept of the repetition compulsion is helpful in understanding how childhood experiences of violence and other boundary violations are commonly repeated in adult relationships despite the conscious wish to avoid them at all cost; these patterns or damage are repeated both *despite* and *because of* the childhood abuse.

Countertransference enactments may also be powerfully brought to life in psychiatry when extreme and risky behaviours mean that physical restraint and administering treatment against the patient's will are necessarily part of clinical care.

Mr J had been brought up in the care system and had been abused physically and sexually by a highly organised group of men. He developed a psychotic illness in his late teens with command hallucinations telling him to harm himself and others. The decision to restrain and to sedate him with intramuscular injections filled staff with intense anxiety that they were repeating patterns of coercive abuse; equally if not medicated when acutely disturbed he would severely self-harm leaving staff feeling they had severely neglected him. The team needed support to disentangle their countertransference responses and to think through the clinical management and when restraint was necessary and indicated in order to keep him safe, as opposed to repeating patterns of abuse or neglect.

Countertransference enactments are inevitably common in health care and should be anticipated given the powerful effects of the repetition compulsion and the disturbing impact of working with mental disorder. Importantly these enactments also provide information to be understood rather than be defensively seen as evidence of unprofessionalism, although this can be a by-product if insufficient attention is paid to lapses in team functioning. As unconscious mental processes are in the driving seat it is rarely immediately apparent when a countertransference enactment may be happening. A key to recognising that one may be operating based more upon a countertransference response rather than a fully processed management plan is noticing when you are in some way acting differently to usual practice – such as making oneself unusually available to a patient, not adhering to the usual management plan or disregarding the history and attending only to immediate concerns. This requires a non-defensive openness to considering one's own practice and a culture which supports ongoing reflection and a degree of self-scrutiny within clinical teams.

Inclusion of the countertransference response as part of the mental state examination is one way to routinely develop the clinical skills of the team. The questions below can be helpful ways to prompt consideration of the countertransference as an ordinary part of clinical care.

- How do I feel about this patient?
- How do other team members feel about this patient?
- Am I doing what I would normally do, or is my clinical management different to my usual practice?
- Am I finding it difficult to think and instead feel pulled into taking a particular position or holding onto a position of certainty?
- Am I seeing a complex situation as simple?
- How are the patterns of relating in the patient's history being enacted in the relationships created in the team?
- What information may the countertransference provide about the experiences the patient cannot bear to know about themselves?

Splitting and Psychiatric Services

Splitting, or the keeping apart of good and bad aspects of experience, is a further example of how psychological processes from early states of development can come to the fore at times of crisis and psychiatric breakdown. Splitting originates from the need for the newborn baby to organise his experiences into crude categories of good and bad, allowing good experiences free from disruption. This allows a previously screaming baby to settle and to feed as feelings of frustration and rage are split from conscious awareness and distance is created between these feelings and the present situation.

Splitting is seen commonly in mental health disorders such as borderline and narcissistic personality disorder and paranoid states, where it is accompanied by concrete black and white thinking and the persecutory anxieties which Melanie Klein linked with paranoid-schizoid functioning.

Within psychiatric teams these processes can dominate how the patient perceives and responds to staff, creating havoc and division between and within teams. An understanding and degree of tolerance for the underlying psychological mechanisms as a means to allow some good experience can be crucial in containing the situation that can feel very uncomfortable for the staff involved. It is painful and anxiety provoking to be the recipient of hostile projections and to become the 'bad' team member. Clinical care is enabled in these situations if splitting processes are recognised and seen as being based upon anxiety and unconsciously led by the patient's need to locate bad feelings in certain team members in order to develop a better rapport with others. At the heart of splitting is an inherent fragility and difficulty managing the reality of others with their strengths and limitations, as whole rather than part objects (see Chapter 1). Patients can be described as manipulative as if this is based upon rational thinking rather than a psychological necessity in brittle states of mind.

> *Ms C was admitted to an adolescent inpatient unit with bulimia and escalating self-harm. On the ward she quickly developed an extremely positive relationship with the consultant psychiatrist but was harshly critical of the junior doctor, describing her as useless, uncaring, unavailable and incompetent. The ward recognised this as a distortion of the reality; in fact the junior doctor was much more freely available than the consultant and was keenly motivated to help her patient. Staff saw this as perhaps the only way that Ms C could initially relate in a positive way to the consultant, by locating all frustration and criticism in the junior doctor. The development of an idealised relationship with the consultant allowed some positive interactions and seemed to allow her to follow some of the consultant's advice. Over time a treatment aim was to bring together the consultant psychiatrist and the junior doctor into joint meetings with the patient and to find a way to address her frustration with the limited availability of the consultant and also the ways in which the junior doctor was able to offer understanding and treatment.*

The understanding and tolerance of the splitting process meant that the team did not fall into the trap of becoming divided themselves, and were able to see the importance of bringing the splits together as part of the process of recovery and development. It also enabled the junior doctor to understand this clinically rather than as a personal attack. If there is not sufficient resource or understanding to address splitting processes, then services can become split and take up positions of certainty leading to escalating conflict and accusations between teams rather than jointly sharing aspects of the difficulty.

Containment and Psychiatric Practice

Containment has its origins in the early relationship between infant and caregiver, when the baby is entirely dependent upon another to recognise, understand and meet his emotional and physical needs. Just as hands, arms and laps provide physical holding and care, the mother's mind needs to receive, to hold and to process raw states of emotion. Through the process of projection the mother feels the baby's feelings too, and is therefore in a position to understand, to sooth and to work out what to do. Containment requires another to be able to experience the emotions without becoming overwhelmed, and to be able to think under the pressure of intense states of affect – no mean feat when faced with the desperate screams of a hungry frustrated baby or toddler. Repeated experiences of emotional containment lead to the baby becoming able to recognise feelings as being feelings and not the entire reality; the beginning of being able to symbolise, to think and to therefore render understandable and manageable his emotional experiences (see Chapter 1).

These processes continue throughout life; at times of crisis we all need to express our distress to another – to find a shoulder to cry on, or to let off steam. At such times we are dependent on the other's ability to receive and to understand these feelings so we can recover back to ourselves. Containment is also a key part of what is required and offered within mental health care. Just as the care of a baby or young child requires the mother to nurture a space within her to hold the baby's projections, mental health care needs to provide a space to hold the emotional experience of the patient and to be supported to do so.

Emotional containment is not a passive or easy process. A mother may feel pushed to the limits of her resources by the intense feelings expressed by her baby; she may struggle to contain the projected affects and need support from others herself. Containment requires the ability to stay with highly anxious and distressed states of mind without taking recourse in action, cutting off emotionally or becoming emotionally dysregulated oneself. Within mental health services, particularly on inpatient units, projected emotional material can have powerfully disturbing effects and staff can also struggle not to become detached, defensively unavailable or overwhelmed.

Psychiatric breakdown and relapse commonly occur as the mind's response to an external reality which has become unbearable and the defensive organisation is no longer able to maintain its steadying function. As it becomes more disturbed and less self-contained, the vulnerable mind releases powerful projections into the outside world and people within it, in part to titrate what it can bear to know about. The accompanying emotions that are discharged can impact upon the team and organisation like emotional shrapnel. This is key to what psychiatric teams experience; forceful projections that can disrupt the team's emotional responses and their ability to think. Staff need support in order to carry out the vital emotional work of containment required under these conditions. If the projections become embedded this may affect the ability of the team to function in their usual way.

Containment in psychiatry is hence a key part of psychiatric practice. Despite the wide range of interventions offered by mental health teams to their patients the importance of relationships and the psychological aspects of containment can be under-recognised and undervalued. An example of this is the way in which continuity of care can be disrupted by insufficient consideration of the effects of staff changes that disturb patient's attachments. Key to containment is an open and receptive state of mind that is able to enquire thoughtfully and with curiosity into the nature of the difficulty, and to take appropriate action if required.

Aspects of Containment in Psychiatry

Table 2.1 Type of containment example

Physical	Medical examination and investigation, medication, Mental Health Act, observations, management of leave, physical restraint
Relational	Gathering information from a range of sources, engagement with family, offering a relationship with mental health teams and key workers, awareness of early attachment issues and how this may be manifest in relationships with those in a caring role, careful management of changes in staff and how this may be experienced
Emotional and psychological	Encouraging an open, curious and receptive state of mind including recognition of unconscious processes and countertransference issues, being able to think under pressure, use of external supervision and reflective practice to support a culture of psychologically informed case management
Organisational	Provision of suitable physical spaces for outpatient and inpatient treatment, setting up multidisciplinary teams, support for reflective practice, constructive use of regulatory processes to monitor breaches in care and to learn and to understand from them

Treatment Resistance, Envy and the Negative Therapeutic Reaction

Resistance to change is an ordinary human characteristic; resistance is a key focus of psychotherapy and pervades daily psychiatric practice. It takes a wide range of forms; in severe form it becomes embodied in the 'revolving door patient', and inpatient units may have difficulties with such patients detained under the Mental Health Act who seem to refuse all steps towards recovery. Non-compliance with medication, failure to engage with services and vigorous adherence to psychotic beliefs all have resistance to change at the heart of their activities. Resistance defends the patient's illness, opposes all efforts towards acquiring insight and maintains symptoms. Even the most distressing seeming symptoms, the most harmful repetitive compulsions or persecutory delusions, may be experienced as preferable to an external reality which feels unbearable, as some of the clinical vignettes in this chapter illustrate. Resistance avoids painful emotions such as anxiety, grief, shame, failure, rejection and isolation. Even the most paranoid patient is never alone with delusions of surveillance and conspiracy that are directed at them personally.

It can be enormously helpful if mental health staff routinely *expect* to meet resistance and are encouraged to address it as an ordinary part of treatment. We talk all too often only to the part of the patient who seems in agreement with the plan only to be thwarted by the unnamed part which is entirely opposed to change. There are a number of forms resistance takes, which psychoanalytic theory can be helpful in understanding.

Freud coined the term **negative therapeutic reaction** to describe how patients he treated could seem to get worse in response to feeling understood [21]. This is an important concept in psychiatry as it means that a seeming deterioration in a patient's mental state may be a response to the empathy and supportive treatment offered by the team, as opposed to a sign that their understanding of the case or management plan are wrong and need changing. It may not work precisely *because* of the care and accuracy of the understanding offered. It can seem a puzzling concept to understand for the rational mind and once more an understanding of unconscious processes and the workings of the internal world can be helpful. Freud linked the negative therapeutic reaction to unconscious guilt in which the continued suffering of the patient is seen as a necessary punishment that can never be relinquished by allowing any signs of recovery. Klein's ideas about **envy**, a quality she considered to have a constitutional basis, can also deepen our understanding of this phenomenon [22]. Recognition of the other's goodness and resources, and the patient's own needs and dependency upon them are met with hatred and attacked, so the team's therapeutic effort and kindness may be met by an increase in symptoms and perpetuation of the condition.

Iris was an inpatient on an eating disorders unit after developing severe anorexia nervosa after the death of her brother. The team recognised the enormous impact of this loss upon her and saw it as central to understanding her presentation and destructiveness. She engaged well in the sessions with a psychotherapist towards talking about her brother and the sessions seemed helpful towards understanding her better. On return to the wards however her eating disorder symptoms with associated vomiting and purging worsened. It was helpful to conceptualise this not as a sign that the team's understanding was wrong, but that it was precisely because of the good contact and understanding that she reacted in this way. By conceptualising this as a negative therapeutic reaction the team were able to discuss with Iris her response to feeling understood and hatred of the longing for the help of another this stirred up.

What Difference Does a Psychodynamic Approach Make to Me as a Clinician?

As outlined in this chapter, a psychodynamic approach has the potential to enhance and enrich psychiatric care in a number of ways, summarised below.

1. Faultiness conferring vulnerability to mental disorder and relapse are considered in the case formulation. The underlying issues can be recognised, understood and addressed as the basis of clinical understanding and treatment

2. An emphasis is placed upon the relational aspects of care. Attachment issues, splitting processes, projection, transference and countertransference issues are powerfully recreated within mental health care and express key information about the patient's internal world. Allowing the powerful effects of these processes to be recognised and understood enables staff to make use of all material available to them, deepens the case formulation and enhances the clinical skills of staff

3. Recognition and understanding of countertransference projections and the repetition compulsion reduces re-enactments of harmful patterns of relating in the present. This also relieves staff from uncomfortable countertransference projections

4. The emotional and psychological aspects of containment are given due emphasis in managing mental disorder

5. An understanding of primary process thinking in the unconscious allows the psychological mechanisms underlying mental disorder to be studied and understood, and meaning to be found in psychiatric symptoms

6. The team is supported to maintain an open and curious mind set

7. Treatment resistance is seen as a central challenge to psychiatric care as the symptoms may be performing an important psychological function. This also allows staff to be realistic about what is achievable to terms of treatment and to avoid omnipotence and subsequent feelings of failure

8. In seeking the meaning expressed in symptoms the challenges faced by patients become inherently more understandable. This humanises the practise of psychiatry, keeps the focus firmly upon the person with the illness, adding strength to a person centred approach to care

References

1. Gabbard G. *Psychodynamic Psychiatry in Clinical Practice*, 5th ed. Washington DC: American Psychiatric Publishing. 2014; p. 8.

2. Silverman ME, Murray TJ, Bryan CS (eds.). *The Quotable Osler*. Philadelphia: American College of Physicians, 2007.

3. Murray RM. Mistakes I have made in my research career. *Schizophr Bull* 2017; 43(2): 253–6.

4. Weaver IC, Cervoni N, Champagne FA et al. Epigenetic programming by maternal behaviour. *Nat Neurosci* 2004; 7: 847–54.

5. Bremner JD, Randall P, Vermetten E et al. MRI based measurement of hippocampal volume in PTSD related to childhood physical and sexual abuse. *Biol Psychiatry* 1997; 41: 23–32.

6. Gabbard GO. A neurobiologically informed perspective on psychotherapy. *Br J Psychiatry* 2000; 177: 117–22.

7. Buchheim A, George C, Gündel H, Viviani R. Editorial: Neuroscience of human attachment. *Front Hum Neurosci* 2017; 11: 136.

8. Solms M. The scientific standing of psychoanalysis. *BJPsych Int* 2018; 15(1): 5–8.

9. Solms ML. The neurobiological underpinnings of psychoanalytic theory and therapy. *Front Behav Neurosci* 2018; 12: 294.

10. Freud S. A difficulty in the path of psycho-analysis. In J Strachey, ed., *The Standard Edition of the Complete Psychological Works of Sigmund Freud, Volume XVII (1917–1919): An Infantile Neurosis and Other Works*. London: Hogarth Press. 1955; p. 143. (Original work published 1917)

11. Bell D. *Paranoia, Ideas in Psychoanalysis*. Cambridge: Icon Books, 2003.

12. Freud S. Constructions in analysis. In J Strachey, ed., *The Standard Edition of the Complete Psychological Works of Sigmund Freud, Volume XXIII (1937–1939): Moses and Monotheism, an Outline of Psycho-Analysis and Other Works*. London: Hogarth Press. 1964; p. 268. (Original work published 1937)

13. Freud S. New introductory lectures on psycho-analysis. In J Strachey, ed., *The Standard Edition of the Complete Psychological Works of Sigmund Freud, Volume XXII (1932–1936): New Introductory Lectures on Psycho-Analysis and Other Works*. London: Hogarth Press. 1960; p. 59. (Original work published 1932)

14. Edwards VJ, Holden GW, Felitti VJ, Anda RF. Experiencing multiple forms of childhood maltreatment and adult mental health: results from the adverse childhood experience study. *Am J Psychiatry* 2003; 160(8): 1453–60.

15. Ovid. Metamorphosis.

16. Ovid. The Amores

17. Freud S. Mourning and melancholia. In J Strachey, ed., *The Standard Edition of the Complete Psychological Works of Sigmund Freud, Volume XIV (1914–1916): On the History of the Psycho-Analytic Movement, Papers on Metapsychology and Other Works*. London: Hogarth Press. 1957; pp. 243–58. (Original work published 1917)

18. O'Neill E. *A Moon for the Misbegotten*. 1943.

19. Rosenfeld H. Contribution to the psychopathology of psychotic states; the importance of projective identification in the ego structure and the object relations of the psychotic patient. In *Melanie Klein Today*. Vol. 1. *The New Library of Psychoanalysis*. 1971.

20. Freud S. Remembering, repeating and working through (further recommendations on the technique of psycho-analysis II). In J Strachey, ed., *The Standard Edition of the Complete Psychological Works of Sigmund Freud, Volume XII (1911–1913): Case History of Schreber, Papers on Technique and Other Works*. London: Hogarth Press. 1958; p. 147. (Original work published 1914)

21. Freud S. The ego and the id. In J Strachey, ed., *The Standard Edition of the Complete Psychological Works of Sigmund Freud, Volume XIX (1923–1925): The Ego and the Id and Other Works*. London: Hogarth Press. 1961; p. 49. (Original work published 1923)

22. Klein M. *Envy and Gratitude and Other Works 1946–1963*. London: Hogarth Press, 1975.

Referral for Psychodynamic Psychotherapy: Processes and Considerations

Jo O'Reilly

I find it useful to suppose that there is something I don't know but would like to talk about
Bion [1]

For the patient, a referral to psychodynamic psychotherapy services is a highly meaningful and intensely personal experience. It offers potential to uncover the deeper issues behind whatever is troubling them and to explore areas of their emotional life beyond their conscious awareness. It is a bold step for the patient to cross this threshold, involving painful realisations and profound readjustments to their understanding of themselves and others. Alongside these challenges are the potential gains of improved mental health and function and the achievement of lasting changes in their relationships. This chapter will outline some of the issues important to consider in making and progressing such a referral.

The context within which the service is working determines the task and the available responses to a referral. This chapter will focus upon the referral processes from the perspective of a psychodynamic psychotherapy service for adults, located within an NHS Mental Health Trust.

For the referrer, the underlying reasons for making a referral may vary considerably. The psychodynamic psychotherapy service is a means to access expertise in understanding complex clinical presentations and the impact of unconscious factors in clinical care. In this context a broad approach to considering referrals is indicated, which seeks to provide a response in keeping with the underlying request. A model described as *referring to* and *referring away* will be introduced to consider both conscious and unconscious factors in the referral process. Clinical examples will illustrate the main points raised.

Risks and Potential Benefits of Progressing to Consultation

Not all referrals received into the service will progress to a consultation. It is an important part of the task from the outset to consider what a psychodynamic consultation may mean for the patient.

The offer to meet with a therapist may well be the first encounter for the patient with a psychoanalytically informed approach to their lives, relationships and sources of emotional distress. Perhaps this will be the first time that links have been consciously made between past experiences and present difficulties. For others it may involve a revisiting of issues that have been uncovered and partially processed in previous treatments. For some recent events may have revealed the emotional residue of past hurts or traumas that have lain relatively dormant until that point. The consultation is almost inevitably a powerful experience. The quality of sensitive attention paid by the therapist is likely to resonate with early experiences of nurture, longing, attunement and deprivation. It is likely that a strong transference response will be elicited which will shape their experience of the therapist. The focus upon the underlying issues behind the surface presentation means that intense feelings may emerge and deep suffering be revealed; sadness, grief, anxiety, relief, rage, shame, confusion and gratitude may all be expressed in what is often a profoundly moving experience. The patient may never have been listened to, or challenged in this way; although the full detail of what was said may be lost, the emotional experience is rarely forgotten.

At the same time, it is important to recognise that the psychodynamic consultation is an active intervention and not a neutral experience. Long-standing ways of seeing oneself in relation to others will be challenged and the patient's defensive organisation against threat and intolerable psychic pain will be mobilised. However sensitively this is handled, it is inherently a destabilising and 'invasive' process into the internal world of the patient [2]. Learning is always painful and anxiety provoking as it exposes what you do not know. Bion wrote 'if there aren't two frightened people in the room ... then there was not much point in turning up to find out what you already know' [3]. Each consultation is a unique encounter; in approaching the unconscious neither therapist nor patient knows what will emerge and to an extent this is likely to be disturbing for both parties.

Bion also wrote of the 'emotional storm' created when two characters meet, which captures [4] the intense and immediate impact of one person upon another during a therapeutic encounter. Many patients referred for psychodynamic psychotherapy struggle with emotional closeness and the anxieties this can provoke. The intimacy of the psychodynamic consultation is likely to bring this to life and may uncover the very sources of fear and distress underlying the need for their defences. It is the responsibility of the service, along with the referrer, to consider whether to offer the consultation or whether there may be other responses that may be less disturbing and more in the patient's best interests.

The Clinical Context

The context within which the work is undertaken necessarily informs the task. An NHS psychodynamic psychotherapy service located within a mental health trust is embedded in a network of mental health services. The task here is multifaceted and includes:

- The provision of a psychodynamic consultation and treatment service to patients, many of whom may have required psychiatric care and may have significant psychological vulnerability and social disadvantage. There will potentially be access to other psychological therapies, such as cognitive behavioural therapy (CBT), trauma-focussed or mentalisation-based treatments. A range of mental health teams and crisis services may provide containment and support during therapy if required
- To apply a psychodynamic perspective to emotional distress, complex presentations and countertransference responses, thus developing clinical understanding as the basis of treatment for patients under the care of GPs and mental health teams. This is likely to involve case discussions and supervision rather than direct patient contact
- To provide a training role to a range of staff, from medical students, trainee psychiatrists, to honorary staff such as group and individual psychotherapists in training. This will to an extent shape the range of treatment vacancies available
- To increase the overall capacity of the organisation to contain anxiety and emotional distress. Working with disturbed states of mind means projected states of distress disturb staff and may adversely affect clinical care through unprocessed

countertransference reactions. Such processes inevitably arise in mental health care and need to be metabolised and understood. This maybe addressed through reflective practice and clinical panels within the organisation.

Referring *To* and Referring *Away*

Psychodynamic psychotherapy services within the NHS tend to require referrals from colleagues, such as GPs, psychology services, mental health staff or other health professionals, rather than patients referring themselves. This immediately raises the question of whether the wish for treatment is driven primarily by the patient's own concerns or by the concerns of the referrer. This requires careful consideration as psychodynamic psychotherapy places considerable demands upon the patient who needs to be committed to the process of change and able to withstand the emotional turbulence this entails. There is anecdotal evidence that referrals from clinicians with little experience of psychotherapy may do better than those from referrers who themselves are very enthusiastic about its potential benefits.

In practice there is a spectrum of reasons driving referrals to psychodynamic psychotherapy services. At one end of the spectrum there may be a patient seeking to explore their underlying developmental issues in order to better understand their current difficulties and whose situation indicates this is a potentially realistic and timely endeavour. This scenario could be seen as *referring to* a service which seems likely to be able to provide the type of treatment required. Other referrals may originate from an experience of being disturbed in some way by a clinical encounter or difficulty in the relationship between the patient and the clinician. Such countertransference reactions can powerfully impact upon clinical care and the role of the psychotherapy service may be to address this difficulty rather than necessarily take the patient on for treatment. At the extreme this may be a wish to *refer away* if the clinical contact has become unbearably disturbing with limited space to process complicated projections.

Most referrals fall somewhere between these positions, hopefully arising from some shared and realistic understanding and agreement between the patient and the referrer. How best to respond may be indicated by where on this spectrum the driving forces behind the referral lie. This is illustrated in the examples below.

←————————————————————→

Referring away	*Referring to – previous*
Mr A is a litiginous patient for whom all previous attempts at treatment have led to complaints, escalating accusations currently directed at the GP for not doing enough. History includes growing up in the care system after neglect and violence in his family, and long-standing court proceedings against the children's home where he was placed, as well as previous employers. The GP who feels highly anxious, persecuted and pressured to offer more and more by the patient wonders if a better understanding of the underlying issues may be helpful – psychodynamic psychotherapy being one of the few services he had not previously been referred to.	Mr B had engaged in anger management sessions at a charity offering support for violent men after angry outbursts had led to the loss of his job and marital difficulties. He had learned to control his temper but was distressed when a link was made in these sessions between his own behaviour and the bullying behaviour he had been exposed to from his father as a child. He wished to explore this further and to try to become more patient to his partner and own children, recognising his own internalised bullying father was damaging relationships in his own family.

Helpful predictors of outcome for referrals include the pattern of previous engagement with services, along with evidence of the patient's capacity to reflect about themselves and to consider their own contributions to their difficulties. It is also important for psychotherapy services to resist omnipotent beliefs they may be able to offer some kind of special treatment that will be able to change entrenched and unproductive patterns of relating to services. For Mr A, a further referral will almost inevitably provide further fuel for the process of continuing complaint and grievance and there is little to suggest he will be able to use the consultation in a constructive way. The escalating complaints suggest an ongoing dependence on projecting inadequacy into services with nothing to indicate an ability to tolerate any self-scrutiny; the need for change for Mr A is firmly located in the external world and he continues to relate to services on the immovable assumption that they will be deficient and negligent. A helpful and realistic response may be to offer a consultation to the GP and others involved in his care to recognise and understand the nature of the pressures they are under, the role they are being allocated and the limits of what they can do.

In contrast, Mr B has shown he can engage in treatment towards making positive changes and is able to face painful realities about himself, suggesting psychodynamic psychotherapy may be a helpful process.

Factors to Consider When Proceeding with a Referral

Patients referred for psychodynamic psychotherapy tend to have long-standing difficulties. Childhood adversity and abuse are very common in their histories. Difficulties in establishing and maintaining supportive and nurturing intimate relationships in adult life are often a painful consequence of these experiences. Psychodynamic psychotherapy is primarily a relational treatment, whether offered in groups or individually, shedding light upon the unconscious determinants of these difficulties as they are revealed in treatment within the transference relationship/s. This means treatment also faces the patient with precisely the situations that they find most difficult, raising intense anxiety about trust, authority figures, personal boundaries and the risks of exposing vulnerability to another. Past trauma may resurface vividly during the treatment. The individual's attitude, defences, resources and psychological frailty in relation to these experiences determine whether they can withstand the emotional strain of treatment. It is important to resist the simplistic view that long-term developmental difficulties point towards the need for a long term and hence psychodynamic therapy, as this may not be realistic for the patient.

The process of exploration requires a capacity for open self-scrutiny to consider the ways in which one may be unconsciously contributing to the difficulties. Childhood adversity may result in a very wide range of psychological difficulties and supportive or symptom-focussed treatments such as the support of a multidisciplinary team, CBT or counselling may be more in keeping with the clinical presentation than psychodynamic psychotherapy.

> Mr C 'I couldn't engage in the group at all at the time. All I could see were the school bullies looking at me. I was straight back in that playground. After the treatment for PTSD and anxiety I know now that the fear was coming from me and wasn't about the others in the group, so I would like to give it another try.'

Childhood abuse, disrupted attachments and boundary violations can elicit powerful countertransference reactions and difficulties containing anxiety within clinicians and clinical teams. Referral patterns may both indicate a need for support for the team in processing projected disturbance and run the risk of unintentional repetition of patterns of rejection and broken relationships. It can be enormously helpful for the psychotherapy service to see beyond the referred patient at these times and to respond to the underlying distress in the team behind the referral.

> Ms D had experienced severe childhood violence and multiple separations from her parents and subsequent parental figures. Her adult life was characterised by involvement in abusive relationships, a highly chaotic lifestyle and self-harm in relation to feelings of rejection and frustration. This occurred despite the best efforts of mental health services. While it seemed clear her childhood experiences of neglect and abuse continued to be re-enacted in her relationships in adult life, it was also apparent that her low tolerance of frustration and distress meant psychodynamic psychotherapy would be too anxiety provoking for her to manage currently. It was thought that the risk of repeating another experience for her of feeling rejected and unwanted if seen for a consultation was high and this was shared with the referring team. It was agreed that the ongoing containment and support of the community mental health team, with supervision from the psychotherapy service to help to process the countertransference responses and contain anxiety in the team would be a more helpful intervention.

There can be misunderstanding and uncertainty about who to refer to psychodynamic psychotherapy services and written guidance for referrers can be helpful (see Appendix 3.1). For complex cases it is particularly helpful for the referrer and the service to have a discussion prior to making the referral. This allows dilemmas to be shared, realistic expectations to be discussed and alternative treatments to be considered. In addition, it addresses the risks of splitting between teams which may recreate early experiences of unresolved conflicts and difficulties coming to terms with painful realities. This discussion can also be helpful in offering a stepwise approach to treatment, considering what to prioritise next in their management. This potentially offers a realistic message of hope rather than a model based on acceptance or rejection, which may repeat previous experiences of unmet need or perceived failure.

NHS therapy services are almost always time-limited and special consideration needs to be given to referrals made at the ending of a previous treatment. There needs to be a gap before making a referral to psychotherapy services after another treatment has ended. This allows the benefits gained from the therapy underway to be consolidated, unresolved issues to emerge and mourning the therapeutic relationship that has just ended. The gains and limitations of the previous therapy, along with feelings about the ending need to be addressed as part of the ending process. Onward referral from another team reportedly ending on a very positive note can commonly result in displaced anger and hostility being expressed towards the next service, indicating negative aspects of the transference may not have been sufficiently acknowledged in the previous treatment.

Side Effects and Contraindications

Psychodynamic psychotherapy is not a panacea and like all treatments has side effects. It is not indicated for all cases presenting in psychological distress linked to developmental adversity. Treatment involves a necessary challenge to the usual defences which strive to achieve a degree of psychic equilibrium. These defences may lead to problematic behaviours and symptoms such as somatisation, obsessionality or emotional detachment which may worsen if emotional distress increases. The process requires of the patient some capacity to manage frustration and retain some experience of helpful therapeutic contact between sessions. The ways in which someone has behaved at times of crisis in the past, and the symptoms they may have developed when their habitual defensive structures have become overwhelmed, provide an essential guide to the possible decompensations which may occur during psychotherapy. A history of seriously self-destructive and risky behaviour, or serious psychiatric breakdown may mean it is unlikely to be in the patient's best interest to proceed with a treatment which may destabilise an already fragile internal world. In addition, any current situation or stressor which seriously limits the space for self-reflection may indicate that the current crisis needs to settle before considering a referral.

The role of psychiatric diagnosis in considering whether to refer to psychodynamic psychotherapy services is limited but not irrelevant. The consultation can be a helpful way to formulate the problem and understand the symptoms in dynamic terms. Freud advocated for looking beyond the patient's illness to their whole personality [5]. He also wrote that *'one cannot overcome an enemy who is absent or not within range'* [6] recognising both the necessity and the risk of psychoanalytically based treatments in bringing the disturbance more alive and into the treatment. This means there may be risk of temporary disruption in the patient's daily life during therapy. Patients who become suicidal, psychotic, addicted or violent in response to increased anxiety are likely to do so again when their habitual defences and perceptions are challenged. As with all treatment, the risks of intervening need to be carefully weighed up against the potential long-term benefits of the therapy, and forward planning for management of increased disturbance may provide essential containment and support for the work.

> Mr E had a diagnosis of bipolar affective disorder and had required inpatient treatment on two occasions. His mother had died when he was eight and he could see no way forward for himself unless he could process some of his early experiences and better understand his vulnerability to depression and mania. He had never felt able to address his feelings when young as he had perceived his father as too distressed to be able to help him. After careful consideration and working closely with the community mental health team (CMHT) it was agreed to offer him individual psychotherapy. He engaged very well but experienced episodes of mood elation and severe depression during his therapy, especially when his therapist was away. It was anticipated prior to the start of treatment that this pattern of breakdown would emerge within the transference relationship in therapy, and the CMHT, the crisis team and psychotherapist were able to prepare and to contain the situation, with his key worker offering increased contact when needed. Mr D and others involved in his care came to understand better his underlying need for support in order to be able to mourn his losses. After a lengthy period of both individual and then group therapy he became able to grieve. He required no further admissions and was functioning better in many areas of his life and relationships.

Table 3.1 shows some of the features of a patient's presentation which would suggest that psychodynamic psychotherapy as a treatment was currently contraindicated, likely to be harmful or unlikely to achieve anything helpful.

Pitfalls, Projections and Misperceptions

As with all interfaces between services, referrals work best when there is a good understanding between referrer, patient and the psychotherapy service about the treatment provided

Table 3.1 Referral for psychodynamic psychotherapy, contraindications and reasons for caution

Presentation	Reason for caution	Suggested response
Harmful substance misuse or dependence	Likely to worsen during therapy	Substance misuse services, with evidence of sustained ability to maintain sobriety and abstinence, e.g. minimum of 6 months depending on chronicity and severity of the dependency, abstinence before considering re-referral
Current crisis in essential housing, financial, immigration or medical needs	Lack of mental space to reflect and address longer-standing issues	Social support towards resolving these issues
Ongoing involvement in court proceedings	Scrutiny of the courts, especially if child custody issues, means there is understandable pressure to present well. Adversarial processes mitigate against open reflection	Return to psychotherapy service once court proceedings are over
Patterns of behaviour in response to frustration or anxiety which are dangerous to self or others,	These will likely increase during treatment	Psychological approaches focussed upon behavioural change
Serious risk of recurrent psychiatric breakdown requiring hospital admission	Risk this will recur during treatment	Liaison with psychiatric team to consider what is in the patient's best interest
Extensive previous engagement with psychotherapy leading to nothing changing	Further therapy likely to be of no benefit	Support the referred towards limiting the expectations of what services can provide and help the patient to realistically come to terms with their situation
Current engagement in ongoing psychological treatment	Risk of acting out a split between services and undermining ongoing treatment	Support patient to discuss their wish to leave with present therapist
Biologically based impairment to the brain which is central to the presentation	Impaired ability to process complex thoughts and emotions	Social support and other forms of psychological treatment, e.g. memory services

and when it is indicated. A lack of knowledge or understanding between any of the involved parties can lead to a frustrating experience on all sides. The potential friction can be heightened when mental health services increasingly struggle to offer consistent longer-term input to patients and the psychotherapy service can be seen as the service best able to provide this.

In selecting which referrals to take forwards, psychotherapy services can be vulnerable to being seen as precious and unhelpful. There may also be idealistic views about what can be provided, such as cases who have gained little from shorter-term treatments who are referred as if longer-term intervention is the solution, despite the lack of evidence that the patient is able to engage in treatment towards making positive change. The attitudes within the psychotherapy service too may add to potential misunderstandings; many psychotherapists have made considerable personal sacrifices and investments in their psychoanalytic training. They can feed into an unhelpful dynamic with referring services if they hold an overly idealised view of their model and locate lack of understanding or 'unsuitability' in the referrer or the patient. Psychodynamic psychotherapy is a relatively specialised intervention with costs and side effects as well as potential benefits for patients; like all treatments it is indicated for certain presentations, is helpful in some cases, and not for others.

The training role of NHS psychotherapy services, and reality of scant resources tends to shape the available treatment vacancies. Carefully selected cases may be seen under super-vision by medical students, trainee psychiatrists, other mental health staff seeking to develop their skills as well as individual and group therapists in training. This means there may be more difficulty in finding treatment for those needing to see an experienced therapist as opposed to a patient who may benefit from seeing a clinician at an earlier stage in their training.

As part of a mental health trust, psychodynamic psychotherapy services have a key role in supporting the work of colleagues in a range of other mental health teams who may be facing intense clinical pressures. There is a potentially fertile interface between the referrer who knows the patient and the psychotherapy service's ability to shed light on some of the clinical challenges by adding a psychodynamic perspective. This requires a broader remit and attitude towards referrals than that of selection of suitable cases for treatment. No one likes to be told that their referrals or patients are 'not suitable' and a willingness to engage with the pressures the referrers are working under can improve clinical care within the organisation as a whole.

Cultural Issues, Blind Spots and Limitations to the Model

Psychodynamic psychotherapy has been largely based upon Western patterns of family relationships and expectations. This includes attitudes towards sexual behaviour, and some form of adolescent rebellion as part of a separation process from the family of origin. There are however many other cultures in which this is not the expectation and there can be an inherent risk of pathologising patterns of family behaviour which may differ from the therapist's own training model and background. It may be very difficult for a therapist to understand the lived experience of those from other races or cultures different to their own. We all have our cultural blind spots and lack of sensitivity based on the limitations of our own experiences.

In theory, a psychodynamic approach can be helpful as it emphasises therapist neutrality and the importance of not imposing one's own agenda. Bion described how *'the purest form of listening is to listen without memory or desire'*, emphasising the importance of the therapist putting aside any form of personal agenda or school of thought in order to fully hear what is troubling the patient [7]. In prioritising issues such as reflective capacity and curiosity about one's internal world the ability to benefit from a psychodynamic approach is not dependent upon social class, educational level or cultural background [8] and such treatments have a potentially wide applicability across class, racial, cultural and other social groups.

These issues highlight how important it is to really listen to what is the problem in the patient's perspective and to recognise how our own ideas of normality and development are based upon the culture within which we have been raised, which may differ profoundly from what lies uppermost in our patient's mind. A key question for the referral and consultation process is the extent to which such differences can be addressed and thought about between therapist and patient; the impact for example of seeing a therapist from a cultural background perceived as privileged as opposed to their own as being material important to consider in the work.

A common challenge for NHS psychodynamic psychotherapy services is to reflect the treatment needs of their local communities. As an example patients from black, Asian and other minority ethnic backgrounds tend to be under-represented in the referrals. Reasons for this are likely to be complex but it may also be that services are not adequately sensitive and open to the needs of their population. The psychotherapy service may need to more actively consider how they may be perceived, and the kind of difficulties they are seen as being able to help with, to uncover any misperceptions or hear feedback suggesting any adverse experiences from patients or referrers. The long-standing impact of childhood adversity on the internal world of an individual transcends issues of class, culture or race but is also experienced through the lens of class, culture and race. It is important that the caseloads of psychotherapy services reflect their local demographics and to openly consider what potential barriers to therapy may be active if this is not the case.

The Gathering of Information and Patient Self-Report Questionnaire

As with all forms of referrals for treatment, a decision cannot be made without access to the relevant information. Referrals for psychotherapy need to contain full details of the patient's history, issues they are struggling with, relationships, risk, previous treatments and current functioning. If this information is lacking in the referral it is important to liaise further with the referrer rather than make a decision based upon partial information.

Many psychodynamic services send a self-report questionnaire to the patient once a decision has been made to progress the referral. This performs a number of functions; it allows the patient themselves to opt in (or out) and collects detailed information so that the consultation can focus more on the interaction and dynamic processes in the room. Implicit in the gathering of details about childhood experiences is the idea that their present difficulties have their origins in the past. This is helpful preparation for the patient prior to the consultation.

It should be explicit in the information sent with the questionnaire that the offer of a consultation is not contingent on a fully completed form being returned to the service. The questionnaire should not be seen as an obstacle to accessing treatment for those who cannot or do not wish to put their experiences and feelings in writing to an unknown other, and in these instances, patients are encouraged to let the service know.

Once the self-report questionnaire is completed, or the patient has otherwise contacted the service to confirm their own wish to be seen, the scene is set to offer the consultation interview. This will be described further in Chapter 4.

Conclusion

A psychodynamic approach, with its emphasis on the unconscious aspects of the mind, provides a model leading to a range of psychodynamic treatments as well as a means of understanding psychological disturbance and psychiatric symptoms. The referral process is an important interface that serves a number of functions.

This chapter has described some of the factors to consider for patients in making and progressing such referrals, discussing potential benefits, reasons for caution, the importance of liaison with colleagues as well as contraindications. The psychodynamic consultation is outlined as a crucial but challenging encounter with the potential for new insights and understanding for some, but overly exposing and unhelpful for others (see Chapter 4 for further details of a psychodynamic consultation).

The task of the psychodynamic psychotherapy service in the mental health trust is however multifaceted. It has an important role to play in enhancing the overall clinical understanding and ability to process unconscious processes more widely in the organisation. Some referrals may be generated by complex dynamics behind the patient's presentation which are disturbing and troubling to teams. A model described as *referring to* or *referring away* has been introduced to draw attention to how much the countertransference response of the referring clinician may be motivating the referral. There is a range of possible responses the psychotherapy service can offer to their colleagues beyond seeing the referred patient and this model can support the service in maintaining an adaptive response.

References

1. Aguayo J, Malin BD. *Wilfred Bion: Los Angeles Seminars and Supervision*. London: Karnac Books, 2013.

2. Milton J. Why assess? Psychoanalytic assessment in the NHS. *Psychoanal Psychother* 1997; 11: 47–58.

3. Featherstone W. *Being and Becoming According to Bion*. Academia. Edu.

4. Bion WR. Making the best of a bad job (1979). In F Bion, ed., *Wilfred Bion; Clinical Seminars and Other Works*. London: Karnac Books. 2000; pp. 321–32.

5. Freud S. On Psychotherapy. In J Strachey, ed., *The Standard Edition of the Complete Psychological Works of Sigmund Freud, Volume VII (1901–1905): A Case of Hysteria,* *Three Essays on Sexuality and Other Works*. London: Hogarth Press. 1953; p. 263. (Original work published 1904)

6. Freud S. Remembering repeating and working through (further recommendations on the technique of psychoanalysis). In J Strachey, ed., *The Standard Edition of the Complete Psychological Works of Sigmund Freud, Volume XII (1911–1913): Case History of Schreber, Papers on Technique and Other Works*. London: Hogarth Press. 1958; p. 152. (Original work published 1914)

7. Bion W. Notes on Memory and Desire. In *Melanie Klein Today*. Vol. 2. *Mainly Practice*. London: Routledge. 1988; 17–21.

8. Lemma A. Assessment and formulation. In *Introduction to the Practice of Psychoanalytic Psychotherapy*, 2nd ed. Chichester: John Wiley & Sons. 2016; pp. 128–68.

Appendix 3.1

Psychodynamic Psychotherapy Service: Guidelines for Referrers

These guidelines are to help you when thinking about whether or not to refer someone to the Psychotherapy Service (PS). If in doubt about whether or not to refer someone please contact the PS to discuss. Referrers are also welcome to seek an opinion about the management of complex cases rather than referring to us for treatment. From the point of view of NICE guidelines, psychoanalytic therapy should usually be viewed as a Step 3–4 specialist intervention. We operate a Stepped Care model for psychological therapies so most patients would have had some form of talking treatment prior to referral for psychotherapy.

A Psychotherapy Assessment is likely to be helpful for:

- **Complex cases/co-morbidity** – usually referrals to the PS meet criteria for at least 2 diagnostic categories within the context of long-standing personality or interpersonal problems
- **Longevity of difficulties** – for brief episodes of difficulty or for episodes clearly reactive to specific external circumstances, counselling or psychology services are likely to be preferable as an initial intervention
- **Difficulties seriously affecting capacity to work, function and to maintain relationships**
- **History of treatment in other modalities** with only partial success, leading to a realisation of the more complex or ingrained nature of the patient's difficulties. **These treatments should be completed before referral to psychotherapy and the referral should** not be made as part of the ending process of another psychological treatment
- **Patient recognition** that the problem is psychological and **preference** for longer term, exploratory therapy
- **Commitment to psychological development and growth with recognition of some perhaps unconscious contribution to their difficulties**
- **Sufficient resilience/ego strength/ coping strategies to commit to and manage a potentially challenging treatment without resorting to self destructive behaviours**

Exclusion Criteria (We are happy to discuss cases if you are in doubt)

- Current major drug/alcohol abuse/ unable to maintaining abstinence for a **minimum of six months**
- Actively psychotic/diagnosis of chronic psychotic illness
- Organic brain disorder as central to presentation
- History of violence or recurrent major self-harm when stressed
- Undergoing an acute crisis or court proceedings about child custody
- History of previous long-term NHS psychotherapy with no significant benefit
- Having ongoing, well-recognised psychotherapy elsewhere

Criteria for Treatment (assessed at consultation within PS)

- Ability to make use of psychotherapy as evidenced during consultation
- Capacity to commit to treatment (practical issues as well as motivation)
- Benefit likely to outweigh risk – not likely to significantly increase dangerous acting out
- Likely to promote some change

Contact details of service

Psychodynamic Psychotherapy: The Consultation Process

Jo O'Reilly

Nothing ever becomes real 'til it is experienced
Keats [1]

The consultation for psychodynamic psychotherapy is a unique encounter, quite unlike any other form of interview. This chapter will outline an approach to carrying out a psychodynamic consultation from the perspective of an NHS psychodynamic psychotherapy service. Chapter 3 discusses factors to consider in progressing referrals, including the potential impact of the consultation upon the patient. The setting and structure for the consultation and the importance of the emerging process between the therapist and patient will be described, with clinical examples.

Assessment or Consultation?

As with all therapeutic encounters, the approach of the therapist plays a central role. Key to this is the therapist's perception of the task and their role. The term 'assessment for psychodynamic psychotherapy' is commonly used to describe the interview. There is some risk that this sets up the meeting on the basis of some form of test that may be passed or failed. The patient is allocated a rather passive role, deemed as suitable or unsuitable for this form of therapy. The therapist could then be seen as holding all the expertise and agency, and as making decisions on the patient's behalf.

The term consultation seems to better capture a process that involves two participants working actively together to better understand the patient's situation. In reality, both parties will to an extent be assessing each other, both at conscious and unconscious levels. Transference and countertransference responses exert pressures on any interaction between two people and these are likely to be intensified by the specific nature of this meeting. The discussions that have led to the referral, completion of the self-report questionnaire and the wait will amplify the anticipation of an emotionally meaningful experience. The patient's transference responses become activated and the therapist is likely to have already become a significant figure. Attending to these processes, how they shape the encounter, how they can be glimpsed and understood is a fundamental component of the consultation.

The consultation is experiential, without the use of psychological measures or data. It concerns the process in the room. A detailed and particular focus upon unconscious aspects of the patient's mental life offers an opportunity to consider the difficulties more deeply. The task is therefore broader than an assessment for a specific treatment and may lead to new ways to understand the presentation, in a way that is helpful to both the patient and the referrer.

I am conducting a psychoanalytically informed interview with someone so that I can get as good a picture as possible in the limited time, of their inner world and the way it functions, and try to understand the nature of the distress they are presenting with. This will then help me to comment to the patient and referrer about a number of things, only one of which is their so-called suitability for psychotherapy Milton [2]

The style and approach will vary considerably between different therapists and services. There is considerable debate about the extent to which the therapist should put the patient at ease. A stance of strict analytic neutrality, which resists any pressure to relieve the patient's distress, may enable the assessor to rapidly access the deeper layers of anxiety and more primitive fears in the patient's internal world. Some therapists may see this as unacceptably intrusive or potentially harmful in a consultation and may offer some relief from anxiety during the meeting; this may be more easily acceptable to the patient but may avoid making direct contact with their disturbance.

As Keats described in the opening quote, unless one has direct contact with an experience it can feel unreal or detached. The same is true for a psychoanalytic consultation, in which the patient's main emotional difficulties may be described rather than actually experienced. The nature of the disturbance can only be felt in reality if it can be brought to life in the room. It is likely to require a degree of anxiety and emotional tension for the disturbance to become manifest, with an avoidance of any unconscious pressure to reassure or collude with the patient's habitual defences against this happening. An example of this type of collusion may be an overly intellectual discussion of their difficulties, or the therapist adopting an explanatory approach as if to nullify rather than explore an emerging discomfort, frustration or negative transference. Unless there is some challenge, it remains unknown how the patient's defensive organisation will respond to stress.

At the same time it is important to take into account the particular patient and their ability to tolerate anxiety and manage a degree of scrutiny. The capacity to reflect about thoughts and feelings requires an ability to think symbolically; if anxiety levels become unbearably high the capacity for symbolic functioning may collapse and concrete or paranoid function can take over. The therapist will need to make a judgement about how much to intervene to steady things should the patient become more distressed or disturbed during the meeting. Many of us who conduct psychoanalytic consultations will have experiences of patients who may have left the meeting prematurely in a vulnerable or disturbed state, perhaps even making accusations or complaints. Although it can be tempting to attribute this outcome to 'unsuitability' on the patient's part, it may be the case that the therapist has not made a sufficiently sensitive assessment of the patient's fragility. The example of the surgeon whose technique was described as perfect but the patient died can also be applied to the psychodynamic consultation; a premature or overly challenging interpretation can also lead to a patient lost in terms of the opportunity to understand something more clearly. If a patient becomes unduly distressed it also raises the question as to what has been gained from the consultation, other than contributing to a painful, humiliating or traumatic experience of an already vulnerable patient. While there is some evidence that increased anxiety allows paranoid-schizoid functioning to be observed more clearly, there is little to substantiate this as increasing the predictive power of the consultation [3].

Mr M started the consultation with a series of what felt like quite aggressive questions about waiting times, the therapist's (Dr E's) qualifications and experience, who was employed in the service and how they were vetted. Dr E didn't answer these questions but instead made an interpretation about Mr M's wish to control their interaction, to get him to talk in response to Mr M's questions and fear that he may be insufficiently qualified to help. Mr M snorted with contempt and abruptly left the room, never to return.

In this example, although there may have been some accuracy in Dr D's interpretation, it seems it had been made without sufficient recognition of the intense fear and the fragility behind Mr M's bravado and interrogative style. In supervision Dr D recognised how he had felt defensive in the countertransference and his interpretation had been premature.

The balance to strike between the need to mobilise a degree of anxiety sufficient to allow contact with the disturbance while also establishing a containing frame for the task can be illustrated by the possible difference in outcomes this may achieve.

When invited to talk about her family Ms F launched a tirade against both her parents and her sisters, outlining in detail all the efforts she had made to get them to respond to her in the way she needed them to. She conveyed how grievously she felt they had all let her down and rejected her, describing her family members as self-obsessed and toxic. The therapist, Dr G, was struck by the power of the accusations and the blistering nature of her attacks upon them. She was aware also of her own mounting anxiety about becoming the focus of such a hostile attack herself, and another figure perceived as letting her down. It was unclear whether Ms F was able to consider her own potential contribution to the relationship difficulties she described.

Possible responses and risks:

1. Dr G takes primarily a reassuring approach, asking questions about the history and taking up how much Ms F has conveyed her efforts to improve relationships within her family to no avail. Ms F agrees, leaves the consultation saying she has never felt so well understood. The risk however is that she has rapidly formed an idealised transference to Dr G, her defensive organisation in which disturbance is projected into others has been supported and the underlying paranoia and pressure to 'take sides' has not been addressed. It remains unknown how Ms F will respond if these defensive structures are challenged. Furthermore, Ms F has not had sufficient experience of a psychodynamic approach from the consultation to make an informed decision about treatment

2. Dr G does not respond to Ms F's request for support but sits quietly. After a while she says it seems that Ms F feels all her family interactions have become toxic, and how much Ms F wants her to see it like this as well. Ms F nodded and seemed to agree with this. Based upon this response to the initial mild challenge, Dr G continues by saying that the problem with this is that it does not allow Dr G to help Ms F with the underlying feelings about herself, which perhaps is what Ms F is also wanting help with. In response Ms F become very tearful, openly sobbing and saying she feels like there is 'toxic waste' inside her and no one loves her as result. It became possible then to think together about this toxic part of her, which falls out with people, and how frightened she is of addressing it

Broadly speaking, a consultation can be described as a psychoanalytically informed conversation towards trying to arrive at some shared understanding of the issues behind the symptoms and difficulties the patient presents. This includes considering how experiences earlier in life may continue, through unconscious processes, to exert their influence in the present – including how they relate to the therapist in the consultation. This means that defences do need to be challenged to allow some direct engagement with the disturbed parts of themselves during the consultation. The patient's perceptions and responses to the therapist's presence and interventions when in a more disturbed and vulnerable state means they are better able to make an informed decision about how to proceed, based on a realistic experience of what ongoing therapy may entail.

Psychodynamic Psychotherapy Consultation: The Physical Setting

As with ongoing therapy, the physical frame provides the containing space within which consultation takes place. The features of this should include:

- Appointment offered clearly as a consultation to explore the difficulties and what form of psychological therapy may be helpful
- Private, uninterrupted room
- Up to 90 minutes for the initial meeting, some therapists prefer longer
- Option of a follow-up appointment
- Parameters of the meeting clearly explained at the outset

Psychodynamic Psychotherapy Consultation: The Process

Consultation is a skilled craft, achieving lucid understanding of what the trouble is, past and family history, some formulation as to the unconscious aetiology and the meaning of the symptoms.
Coltart [4]

The frame and setting for the consultation provides the containing space necessary for the 'skilled task' of the consultation. It is important to start with a brief description of the purpose and parameters of the meeting. For example, the therapist may give an outline as below:

> *As you know you have been referred to the psychotherapy service by Dr . . .. This appointment is a consultation for us to think together about the difficulties you have been experiencing and to see if we can together find a way to understand them better. This will then help us to think about what may be helpful as a next step for you. There are a range of forms of psychological therapy as you may already know, this service offers psychodynamic psychotherapy and sometimes we recommend a different approach if we think this may be more helpful. We will be discussing this together and if it seems therapy in this service may be helpful this will involve time on one of our waiting lists, and treatment with a different therapist than myself. Although this isn't the start of ongoing therapy with me the more freely you feel able to talk to me the better able we are to understand the issues and to see how best to help. If we need more time we can arrange a follow-up appointment. Once we've agreed a way forwards I would usually write a brief letter back to Dr . . . letting them know the outcome of what's been decided. Do you have any questions about his and is it in line with what you have been expecting?*

This introduction draws attention to one of the central issues during the consultation process; most psychodynamic psychotherapy services offer a consultation service with a different clinician to the therapist who would be allocated the case for ongoing work. In addition, having started this process, if ongoing therapy is recommended there will likely be a wait for treatment. The patient is being asked to speak openly about some of their most intimate and painful experiences with someone they have not met before and with the knowledge this is not going to be an ongoing therapeutic relationship. The consultation can powerfully evoke previous experiences of abandonments, rejection or other brief and intimate encounters with others and this needs to be attended to and worked with throughout.

> Mr T had grown up with a single mother after his father suddenly left the family. At the end of the consultation, during which he had spoken openly about his early life and sensitivity to feeling rejected in adult relationships, he became very distressed and seemed to realise for the first time that this was the end of the consultation and not the start of therapy. The therapist was confident that he had explained this at the beginning of the meeting and also referred back to this difficult reality several times during the meeting. It seemed that this had not registered at all with Mr T and was experienced as a sudden abandonment and a terrible shock. There seemed to be something of a repetition compulsion that could then be explored, looking at how he tended to become immediately attached and then to feel abruptly rejected, as if unable to see any signs that indicated the limits of what the other could offer.

The Emerging Process of the Consultation

Once the parameters of the meeting have been described, the consultation then becomes a relatively unstructured space. Within this space a great deal of psychological work and detailed thinking will be carried out at a number of levels.

The therapist may start by encouraging the patient to tell them something about what has brought them here. The patient's response to this open invitation provides immediate material about their transference to the therapist and the nature of their anxieties; a glimpse from the outset into their internal object relationships. Fear, silence, automatic trust, indifference, subtle flirtation and other responses all make available important material for understanding.

During the patient's narrative account, gaps, shifts in affect, points of anxiety, psychic pain and deployment of defences will occur. These all convey meaningful aspects of their mental life. The therapist generally resists the urge to ask direct questions (which are likely to simply provide a factual answer), commenting instead in a way that draws attention to the unfolding relationship between the two participants. For example the therapist might say 'I've noticed you've hardly mentioned your father', rather than asking direct questions about the father. During this process a great deal of conscious and unconscious assessment of each other is likely to be occurring – and the therapist shows their deep commitment to taking seriously all that is described and communicated by the patient.

The neutral stance of the therapist, revealing little about their own views or agenda, allows observation of how the patient relates towards them in the absence of cues or encouragement. For example, suspicion, compliance or challenge may emerge. Under these conditions it becomes possible to see how habitual patterns of perceiving and relating to others are unconsciously recreated. The therapist also aims to be consistently alert to their countertransference responses. This is a kind of dual listening process; attending to both the patient's account and emotional state as well as the therapist's own internal responses. For example, anxiety, detachment, curiosity and issues of control may become unconsciously communicated through projective processes for the therapist to notice and to think about.

At the same time the therapist will be considering a range of factors such as whether the patient is likely to be able to tolerate anxiety, and frustration without decompensating in a manner harmful to them ('ego strength'), if they are able to see their difficulties as psychological in origin and to reflect about themselves ('psychological mindedness') and to maintain some ability to think under the pressure of intense anxiety ('mentalization'). It is important not to confuse a neutral stance with an absence of compassion or empathy; the therapist needs to act with kindness and acknowledge distress. Specific to the psycho-dynamic consultation however is trying to understand the underlying reasons explaining why the patient may have become so distressed, angry or agitated at that point in the meeting.

The judicious use of questions such as asking the patient to describe their mother or father, or how others would describe the patient, gives an indication of their ability to observe and to reflect about themselves in relation to another. Asking for the patient's earliest memory, described by Freud as a screen memory in its depiction of meaning rather than an actual event, also provides access to the early object relations world of the patient. This also assists with the task of determining the internal resources that may be available to support the process of psychotherapy.

> When asked for her earliest memory Ms P said she thought she could remember playing alone in her cot after her brother was born. No one else was there but she really liked looking after her dolls and it was a happy memory. She added that she was always a good child, which was fortunate as her mother was busy. This memory draws attention to early experiences of separation and how she defended herself perhaps through identification with her mother as a provider of care and projection of need into the dolls who she cared for. This defensive organisation may also have contributed to her choice of career as a nurse. Issues to consider in the consultation include the extent to which she is able to be vulnerable herself as a patient, and how psychotherapy will likely uncover aspects of herself which may not fit with a perception of herself as 'always good'.

As with any clinical encounter, concern about risk should be followed up and a management plan put in place in open discussion with the patient.

The Role of Dreams in the Consultation

It is often very illuminating to ask the patient to describe a dream in the consultation. In addition to providing access to their internal world and unconscious phantasies, the patient's response provides information about their attitude towards their unconscious mental life. As in a psychotherapy session, it is helpful to obtain as much detail as possible about the dream and the patient's own associations in order to jointly explore its meaning, which may be closely linked to anxiety about the consultation.

> Ms H spoke freely about her difficulties in a rather superficial manner, relating to the therapist as if she already understood herself well and knew the answers to her problems. The therapist felt rather controlled, helpless and detached. After a while she asked Ms H if she could describe a dream. Ms H responded positively, saying she dreamt a great deal and was very interested in her dreams. In fact only the night before she had dreamt she travelled to a strange country thinking she knew where she was going but found her maps were inadequate. She found herself

confused and completely lost in a paddy field. The dream had puzzled her and she had told her flat mate about it who had said 'you're going to see that paddy (Colloquial term for Irish) doctor today aren't you?' This association made sense to Ms H and further exploration in the consultation led to material emerging about her intense fear of becoming engulfed by her mother's crazy mind as she put it. Her need to create and try to control a degree of distance between herself and her objects was helpful to Dr R in understanding her countertransference response; early object relationships becoming repeated in the consultation.

Trial Interpretations and the Consultation

By the time the therapist and patient meet curiosity and anxiety are likely to have intensified and provoked ideas and unconscious phantasies about the therapist in the patient's mind. The emotional charge and significance of the encounter means the therapist may have already become a powerful transference figure for the patient. The interpretation is an opportunity to explore this phenomenon, directly addressing the activity of unconscious processes in the interaction between them. If no interpretations are made the risk is that the therapist becomes fixed in the patient's mind as having particular characteristics without any exploration of this. An opportunity to think about how unconscious expectations shape the patient's perceptions and responses to others may be lost. In addition, the therapist may unconsciously respond to the patient's projections and the two may start to fit together in an unconscious re-enactment of past dynamics, in an unexplored way.

As the interview progressed the therapist felt increasingly aware of how cooperative Ms H was being, agreeing with her every comment and eliciting a countertransference that she was being a very good therapist able to fully understand and meet the needs of her patient. She interpreted to Ms H that she thought she was showing her what a very good girl she was being here, and wondered if she was anxious not to place any demands upon the therapist, or to show any feelings that may be more difficult to think about. This seemed to free Ms H up to consider the therapist as having more resources available for her than she had assumed through the transference relationship, and she started to speak about her long-standing self-harm.

There are different levels of interpretation. At the simplest level an interpretation invites the patient to reflect about themselves, perhaps by making a link between biographical experience and their current predicament and relationship patterns. A more challenging interpretation may address how the patient seems to be relating to the therapist, directly addressing the power of their unconscious processes in the present. It is important to try to titrate the level of the challenge to the capacity of the patient to be able to think about it, as opposed to becoming too threatened or anxious. A patient who functions in a very concrete way, or whose presentation suggests an easily mobilised paranoia may not be well served by an interpretation that stresses them beyond their capacity to mentalize.

The case of Ms F, who forcefully projected into her family as described earlier, shows how Dr G proceeded cautiously with an interpretation. He was then able to access deeper fears in MS F's internal world through his sensitive approach. A more challenging interpretation may have been to say something along the lines of 'I think you are telling me that you are frightened of the angry part of yourself, and want me to side with you in how you see your family to avoid this rage becoming directed at me.' This would be a considerable challenge to Ms F's defensive projection and Dr G recognised this as too anxiety provoking an interpretation to make at this early stage of Ms F's contact with the service.

Ending the Consultation

As the initial meeting draws to a close, there is some clarification of what has been agreed and an acknowledgement of what has been uncovered and explored. It is often helpful to ask how the patient has experienced the consultation and the therapist. A wide range of responses may emerge, giving some indication of the reflective capacity and defences against the contact. Comments may include *'you've been very strict but given me new things I need to think about'* (a hopeful and realistic sounding response), to *'you have understood me completely'* (suggesting a rapid idealisation which needs addressing) or *'I've gained nothing new from this I didn't already know'* (a degree of dismissal/omnipotence). Consultation is a two-way process and the patient's assessment of the therapist allows them to discover if they wish to further engage in this kind of process. Commonly patients may be surprised by how distressed they have become while also discovering new ways of understanding themselves. There is often some recognition that this has been a significant event.

The Follow-Up Appointment

It is common practice to offer a follow-up appointment, sometimes two, after an interval of one to three weeks from the original consultation. This allows both patient and therapist to digest the experience of the initial encounter, and to reflect on what course of action may be helpful. The impact of the initial consultation upon the patient can also be observed as an indicator of their likely response to ongoing therapy. In a few cases the patient may not return to the follow-up appointment, or express ambivalence through lateness or repeated requests to change the appointment. It can feel an opportunity has been missed to better understand a patient who drops out at this point, but does at least prevent them being prematurely placed upon a waiting list for a treatment they may never take up. For some patients their defensive organisations may have become more mobilised, increasing troublesome symptoms such as obsessional behaviours or somatisation. Others report difficulties containing their distress, may have put the initial consultation completely out of their mind or appear in a more disturbed or paranoid state. These are all issues to take seriously as they may indicate some of the potential risks of a psychodynamic approach.

Signs that psychodynamic psychotherapy may be of benefit include a patient who returns having thought a great deal about the initial meeting, perhaps wanting to ask further questions or to share a dream they have had since. It can seem that a door has become opened in their mind which they wish to explore further. As with the initial consultation, attention should be paid to the ending of the contact between the therapist and the patient and how this may fit with previous experiences of attachment and loss.

Outcomes of the Consultation

The consultation will hopefully have arrived at a shared understanding of the patient's difficulties and a formulation that can provide the basis of a decision about how to proceed (see Chapter 5). Importantly this is a discussion in which the therapist is able to share their perspective to assist the patient in making an informed choice. While it is always difficult to predict the longer-term outcome of therapy, there are helpful indicators. These include:

- The patient has engaged in the consultation process
- The potential risks and benefits of treatment have been realistically considered
- Practical issues have been addressed such as the ability to attend regularly for the duration of treatment
- A process of inward reflection has developed without harmfully mobilising unhelpful defences or self-destructive behaviours
- An understanding that the origin of difficulties may lie beyond conscious awareness
- An openness to exploration of unconscious processes as evidenced by the experience of the consultation

The consultation is not an exact science and is made up of both the objective assessment of the history and the qualitative experience between patient and therapist. There are a range of treatment options and potential outcomes both within and external to the psychotherapy service which may include:

Consultation only – this may help to relieve and to clarify issues sufficiently for the patient and referrer. Equally a decision may be made that this form of therapy does not feel helpful or may not be in the patient's best interest currently.

Individual psychotherapy – this is frequently on a once weekly time-limited basis in NHS services although some may provide more intensive treatment (see Chapter 6).

Group psychotherapy (see Chapter 11)

Extended consultation/brief intervention – complex cases may require a short intervention which may inform the decision about whether longer-term treatment is likely to be helpful.

Intermittent therapy – less frequent sessions on a longer-term basis may be offered by some services for patients with chronic difficulties. This allows the slow development of a therapeutic alliance and an opportunity to see if more reflective capacity can be gradually developed. Patients may be able to progress in time for more intensive treatment.

Referral to alternative therapy services – for treatment such as psychoanalysis on a three, four or five times a week basis if indicated. This usually requires access to local training organisations offering reduced fee schemes.

Couple or family therapy – if the consultation reveals underlying relational dynamics, which mean the symptoms or distress has become entrenched and maintained within the couple or family system, any intervention on an individual level is unlikely to lead to any change.

Referral to other specialist psychological therapy services – personality disorder services, cognitive behavioural therapy or trauma services where the psychological therapy offered can focus upon specific difficulties. Such onward referrals are best carried out in liaison with these services to ensure a coherent approach to treatment.

Conclusion

A psychodynamic consultation is often a crucial encounter for patients – a 'crossing of the Rubicon' as they recognise for the first time the impact of their developmental experiences on their emotional life. This chapter has outlined an approach to conducting this crucial encounter.

The psychodynamic consultation is a unique intervention, with specific tasks and techniques and is quite unlike any other interview [5]. It is a necessarily challenging experience where anxiety acts as a stimulus that reveals the nature of the patient's disturbance and their habitual defences. This offers to both the therapist and the patient a realistic experience of an exploratory approach as the basis of deciding about treatment. The therapist has a responsibility to be sufficiently sensitive to the patient's fragility while assessing their ability to maintain a reflective position when their pre-existing ways of understanding themselves are challenged. This reduces the risk of the consultation becoming unbearably exposing and provoking an unhelpful decompensation. A broad approach offering a psychodynamic understanding of the underlying issues and their unconscious origins can be extremely helpful for referrers and potentially life changing for patients.

References

1. Keats J. Letter to George and Georgiana Keats Feb 14–May 3, 1819.

2. Milton J. Why Assess? Psychoanalytic assessment in the NHS. *Psychoanal Psychother* 1997; 11: 47–58.

3. Hobson P. *Consultations in Dynamic Psychotherapy. Tavistock Clinic Series*. London: Karnac Books, 2013.

4. Coltart N. Diagnosis and assessment for suitability for psychoanalytic psychotherapy. *Br J Psychother* 1988; 4: 127–34.

5. Garelick A. Psychotherapy assessment: theory and practice. *Psychoanal Psychother* 1994; 8: 101–16.

Psychological Models for Case Formulation

Rachel Gibbons

Introduction

The capacity to formulate a case is at the heart of all psychiatric and psychotherapeutic work and is a core competency in training. So what do we mean by formulation? There is a summary and organisation of a patient's case into a concise hypothesis that explains, describes and predicts. For any individual case, the formulation evolves with growing experience and understanding of the patient and their situation. The skill and expertise developed over time by the clinician comes into practice. The formulation can be used by the psychiatrist, therapist, treating team and patient, and when constructed, at times it can be similar to a piece of art or poetry – capturing the essence of the patient's difficulties and providing a deep insight in a condensed form.

Models of Formulation

There are different methods of formulating specific to different theoretical models, but the core principles are similar. In this part of the chapter three different but related and interlinking models of formulation currently used in mental health will be described.

1. The Biopsychosocial Model
2. The Presenting, Predisposing, Precipitating, Perpetuating and Protective (five Ps) Model
3. Psychodynamic Formulation

The first two, the biopsychosocial and the 'five Ps', are descriptive. These models identify different contributory aetiological factors in the history and current situation. The psychodynamic model aims to integrate the history with the current situation to identify patterns repeated from childhood and acted out in the patient's present relationships.

Information Required for Formulation

Formulation requires information about the patient. The more data gathered, the more accurate and helpful the formulation is likely to be. The information required includes:

- A personal history as a pathway or timeline from before birth to the present
- A transgenerational and family history
- Relationships with caregivers and others
- Significant events, including separations, losses and trauma, and the emotional responses to these experiences
- Description of psychological problems and symptoms and how they have emerged and developed, including circumstances and events leading up to current crisis or illness

- Countertransference responses and relationships created with caregivers and teams. How this is demonstrated in the therapeutic encounter

Theoretical Background

Two areas of theory important in formulation are:
- Symptoms and symptom formation
- The repetition compulsion

Symptoms and Symptom Formation

What one sees, the presenting problem is often only the marker for the real problem which lies buried in time, concealed by the patient shame, secrecy and sometimes amnesia – and frequently clinician discomfort
Felitti [1]

In this model symptoms are not seen as the problem but important signifiers of the underlying difficulty which needs attending to. They represent the mechanisms the mind uses to contain anxiety when it cannot be easily escaped or avoided. Anxiety is the body's alarm system. Danger posed by either an external event, or an internal source that jeopardises the psychic status quo, raises anxiety. In both situations the body's physiological response is flight, fight or freeze [2]. This response is more easily seen with external danger where an avoidance, escape or fight response is visible. This response is more complex when the threat is internal. In this case flight is accomplished by the creation of symptoms that contain and transform the anxiety. This maintains the equilibrium but does not address the underlying cause of the anxiety. Symptoms therefore, while often distressing, are important, meaningful and containing. Why and when they arose is of utmost importance.

Case Example

Ellen, an 18-year-old young woman, was seen by the psychiatric liaison team on a medical ward where she had presented with a sudden inability to move her left arm. She said she had been looking forward to starting university that summer but because of these symptoms this had to be postponed until the following September. She had been investigated by the neurology team and no organic cause for this difficulty was found. Angela, one of the nurses from the psychiatric team, sat with Ellen and took a full history. In this history Ellen described how her mother had developed multiple sclerosis when she was transferring from primary to secondary school. Ellen had spent a lot of time at home caring for her mother and missing school. Ellen was not sure her mother would cope when she went to university. Angela asked about the first symptoms of her mother's illness. Ellen looked a bit shocked and said that the first sign of this was the loss of use of her left arm and she started crying. She engaged with her feelings of loss over the next few days and gradually started to move her arm again. After attending weekly therapy for a few months she was able to leave home and start at university.

In this case the symptom Ellen developed had meaning. The fear about separating from her mother was not consciously known and the anxiety transformed into dissociative symptoms that expressed both her fear that separation was dangerous, and the identification with her mother. The symptom itself also served to prevent her leaving home.

The Repetition of Historical Trauma

. . . the patient does not remember *anything of what he has forgotten and repressed, but* acts *it out. He reproduces it not as a memory but as an action: he repeats it, without, of course, knowing that he's repeating it. . . . in the end we understand that this is his way of remembering . . . the patient yields to the compulsion to repeat, which now replaces the compulsion to remember, not only in his personal attitude to the doctor but also in every other activity and relationship which may occupy his life . . .*
Freud [3]

In his very accessible book, *The Body Keeps the Score*, the psychiatrist Bessel van der Kolk describes profound differences in the storage and processing of traumatic and non-traumatic memories [2]. These disparities have been discovered through neuroimaging and provide a coherent explanation for the long-term physiological and psychological effects of developmental disturbance. When traumatic memories are triggered later in life there is a regression to early behavioural responses that in turn elicit powerful reciprocal responses in others. This leads to the repetition of the early dysfunction. The seminal Adverse Childhood Experience Study (ACE 3) conducted in the USA between 1995 and 1997 showed that abused girls were seven times more likely, than those who had not been mistreated, to be raped in later relationships, and boys who witnessed domestic violence were more than seven times more likely to abuse their partners [1].

This neurobiology provides the physiological and biological background to the 'repetition compulsion' described by Freud and considered important in contemporary psychoanalytic thinking [3]. This postulates that disturbed and traumatic memories that cannot be symbolically represented are repeated throughout life. It is only through becoming cognisant of these patterns and transforming them into words that gradually over time there is an attenuation of pain and an escape from this repetition. Therapy provides a safe environment for these patterns to emerge in the transference, allowing the therapists to help the patient translate them into words in a suitably containing environment. These patterns are very important to identify and key to formulating and predicting the progress of future treatment. What has happened before will happen again. There is more discussion of the effect of trauma in Chapter 16.

Biopsychosocial Model

The average physician today completes his formal education with impressive capabilities to deal with the more technical aspects of bodily disease, yet when it comes to dealing with the human side of illness and patient care, he displays little more than the native ability and personal qualities with which he entered medical school. The considerable body of knowledge about human behaviour which has accumulated since the turn of the century and how this may be applied to achieve more effective patient care and health maintenance remain largely unknown to him. Neglect of this important dimension of the physician's education lies at the root of frequently voiced complaints by patients that physicians are insensitive, callous, neglectful, arrogant, and mechanical in their approaches. There undoubtedly are many reasons for this situation, but the most important is the pervasive influence of the biomedical model of disease . . .

Engle [4]

For many years the biomedical model was the predominant framework for understanding illness in Western medicine. This changed in 1977 when challenged by George Engle and John Romano. George Engle, a psychiatrist and psychoanalyst, and his colleague John Romano worked at Rochester University in New York State. They developed an interest in psychosomatics and recognised the inadequacy of the biomedical model to helpfully formulate the difficulties of their patients. They proposed the biopsychosocial model which subsequently quietly revolutionised thinking about illness and health and gained popularity over time. This is now the predominant accepted overarching model for mental health formulation. The importance of psychosocial factors has been experimentally demonstrated both in the formation of the brain, and through epigenetically changing DNA which is passed on to future generations. We now know that there is constant interplay between biological, psychological and social factors and their relative influences on mental and physical health. The biopsychosocial model is now used as the basis for diagnosis and formulation in one of the two diagnostic manuals used in psychiatry (DSM).

The biopsychosocial model is holistic and systematically considers: the biological, the psychological and the social. It conceptualises illness as multifactorial, contributed to by a complex interaction between these three factors (see Table 5.1).

The 'Five P's' Model

The biopsychosocial model has been further developed over time and currently the 'Five Ps' model is used in many different mental health environments (Table 5.2). Freud's description of the repetition compulsion provides the psychological mechanism explaining why psychological symptoms and breakdown may be predictable and be in response to specific precipitating factors on an individual basis. The 'Five P' model takes the biological, psychological and social factors and considers them in a temporal manner, further subdividing them into:

1. Presenting problem: the presenting problem itself and how the person's life is broadly affected at the time of presentation
2. Predisposing factors: vulnerability factors from the longitudinal history
3. Precipitating factors: the significant events preceding and triggering the onset of the difficulties
4. Perpetuating factors: those factors that are currently maintaining and contributing to the difficulties and their lack of resolution
5. Protective factors: strengths and resilience factors that mitigate the effect of the disorder and contribute to improving prognosis and recovery

Psychodynamic Model

The psychodynamic model integrates information from the previous two models, the countertransference relationships, and repeated patterns of behaviour, into a narrative which considers the role of unconscious factors underpinning the emotional distress and attempts to understand the meaning of the symptoms at a deeper level. The description of

Table 5.1 Summary and examples of the biopsychosocial model

Group	Description	Example of areas included	Examples in individual case
Biological	• Physically or genetically related • Relatively fixed	1. Genetics 2. Injury 3. Organic illness 4. Medication, drugs	1. Family history of bipolar affective disorder and alcohol dependency 2. Alcohol use 3. Cannabis use 4. Previous heart surgery
Psychological	• Facing inwards, personal, individually based	1. Loss events 2. Head injury 3. Illness 4. Relationships 5. Personality style	1. Early loss of brother 2. Emotional deprivation 3. Anxious attachment
Social	• Outward facing, to society	1. Culture 2. Social standing 3. Living environment 4. Social connections and support 5. Stigma 6. Lifestyle 7. Poverty and wealth	1. Homelessness 2. Social support 3. Unemployed 4. Mental health difficulties denied in religious/cultural community environment 5. Isolation

Table 5.2 Summary and example of the 'Five Ps' model

P	Summary	Description	Examples in individual case
Presenting problem	• Current	1. Diagnosis 2. Symptoms 3. Social situation	1. Becoming socially isolated 2. Poor self-care 3. Problematic displays of anger 4. Inability to work
Predisposing	• From the past	1. Genetics 2. Early relationships 3. Hardship 4. Abuse	1. Family history of mental illness 2. Father absent 3. Mother alcohol and drug use
Precipitating	• From the recent past	1. Loss events 2. Injury or illness 3. Illness 4. Current relationships 5. Finance	1. Relationship breakdown 2. Eviction 3. Substance use
Perpetuating	• Ongoing and into the future	1. Relationships 2. Housing 3. Finance	1. Divorce proceedings 2. Not being able to see children 3. Homelessness 4. Ongoing substance dependency 5. Dependency in relationship with health services
Protective	• Contribute to resilience	1. Finance 2. Work 3. Relationships 4. Family	1. Children 2. Friendship group 3. Fitness behaviour 4. Supportive relationship

this model varies in psychodynamic/psychoanalytic literature. A simple structure for psychodynamic formulation is suggested in Table 5.3 with two brief illustrative case examples.

Table 5.3 Summary and example of a psychodynamic formulation model

Summary	Age
	Sex
	Relationship status
	Employment
	Economic
	Cultural
	Mental health history
Presenting problem and their meaning	How presented
	Symptoms
	Effect on life
	Why now?
Early object relationship and attachment pattern	Mother
	Father
	Attachment pattern
	Relationship history
Major life events	Losses external and internal
	Abuse and neglect
Defences	Used predominantly
Countertransference	In assessment and treatment
Repetition pattern	From early history throughout development into the present
Prediction for the future	Where there may be problems in treatment

Psychodynamic Formulation Example 1

Delilah is a 28-year-old single schoolteacher brought up in Wales with no previous mental health history. She presented to her GP having become withdrawn and developing depression. Prior to this she had ended a relationship with a partner whom had become controlling and violent. She was fearful of having another relationship not trusting herself to find someone who cared for her. Her parents' relationship was abusive. Her father was violent and her mother passive. She did not enjoy school where she was bullied. At work she feels picked on by the other teachers. Her therapist feels trapped and provoked in the sessions and finds it difficult to say the right thing. When he challenges Delilah, she retreats as though confronted by a sadistic bully. Delilah projects her aggression into others, controlling them through projective identification resulting in repeated re-enactments of her childhood trauma. Delilah may find it hard to take back projections and own her own aggression allowing her to give up her perception of herself as a victim, losing the protection she perceives this role gives her.

Psychodynamic Formulation Example 2

James is a 58-year-old single English man, with no known mental health history. He was found wandering unkempt in the street after the death of his mother, and was sectioned under the Mental Health Act. He had lived his whole life with his wealthy mother and had never worked himself. When assessed he said that his mother was being experimented on at the local hospital. James has no siblings and his father left in his early childhood. James suffered from separation anxiety early in his life and his mother allowed him to remain at home with her. He had a dependent attachment with his mother who remained the primary attachment figure throughout his life. She did not provide the containment necessary for him to develop the ability to separate and individuate and therefore he has a limited capacity to mourn. His primary psychological defences are immature and consist of splitting, projection and denial. When his mother died he relied on these primitive psychotic defences to manage the distress of the loss. The result was a psychotic episode which allowed him to believe his mother was still alive. James may be very resistant to treatment because he lacks the capacity to mourn the momentous loss of his mother.

Conclusion

Formulation is a very important, but often neglected, part of clinical work. It involves the recognition of patterns and repetitions, and the impact of the past in the present. Understanding the unconscious mechanisms really assists in the formulation process, adding a *how*, and a *why*, to what we see in everyday clinical practice. To spend time thinking about, and developing, a coherent formulation provides a stable base for both clinical thinking, and the therapeutic work with patients.

References

1. Felitti VJ. Adverse childhood experiences and adult health. *Acad Paediatr* 2009; 9(3): 131–2.

2. van der Kolk B. *The Body Keeps the Score: Mind, Brain and Body in the Transformation of Trauma.* London: Penguin UK, 2015.

3. Freud S. Remembering repeating and working through (further recommendations on the technique of psycho-analysis II). In J Strachey, ed., *The Standard Edition of the Complete Psychological Works of Sigmund Freud, Volume XII (1911–1913): Case History of Schreber, Papers on Technique and Other Works.* London: Hogarth Press. 1958; p. 147. (Original work published 1914)

4. Engle GL. The biopsychosocial model and the education of health professionals. *Gen Hosp Psychiatry* 1979; 1(2): 156–65.

Further Reading

Cabaniss DL, Cherry S, Douglas CJ, Graver R, Schwartz AR. *Psychodynamic Formulation.* Chichester: John Wiley & Sons, 2013.

Ghaffari K, Caparrotta L. *The Function of Assessment Within Psychological Therapies: A Psychodynamic View.* London; New York: Taylor & Francis. 2018; p. 62. Kindle Edition.

Hinshelwood RD. Psychodynamic formulation in assessment for psychotherapy. *Br J Psychother* 1991; 8(2): 166–74.

Macneil CA, Hasty MK, Conus P, Berk M. Is diagnosis enough to guide interventions in mental health? Using case formulation in clinical practice. *BMC Med* 2012; 10: 111.

Psychodynamic Psychotherapy Practice: An Introduction

Rachel Gibbons

Introduction

This chapter is designed as an introduction to psychodynamic psychotherapy practice for psychiatrists, training therapists, and for those who are interested in this work. This is an extensive area and this chapter is intended as a summary of its aim and process. The cases reported are composites of those presented in supervision by those in training, the majority of whom were seeing their patients once weekly for one year in NHS settings. The description is intended as a general guideline and is simplified from a broad heterogeneous theoretical area. Psychodynamic terms in italics are defined in the glossary.

Aim of Therapy

Where Id was there Ego shall be

Freud [1]

Psychodynamic therapy aims to help the patient make conscious what is unconscious. This is achieved by providing a **containing** space where feelings, or **affects**, that have been unknowingly hidden, or **repressed,** because they would cause too much conflict with the conscious mind, can emerge and be gently confronted. These feelings then pass and through the process, patients gain **ego** strength and resilience.

Why Patients Seek Therapy

Patients tend to present with a range of psychological or psychiatric difficulties. They may have the feeling that 'something is not right' with some awareness that this is beyond rational or conscious explanation. They can be seeking a deeper exploration of themselves and wishing to resolve profound difficulty in securing or maintaining nurturing intimate relationships. They may be struggling with a stage of development, for example wanting a relationship or children, but fear commitment. In many cases there has been a painful loss that may not be fully recognised.

The Importance of Psychic Defences in Managing the Conflict between the Unconscious and Conscious Mind

. . . if life is going to exist in a Universe of this size, then the one thing it cannot afford to have is a sense of proportion.

Douglas Adams – Restaurant at the End of the Universe *[2]*

Psychic defences manage the permeability of the boundary between the unconscious and the conscious mind, keeping feelings and urges thought unacceptable out of awareness. Titration of the relationship with internal and external reality is necessary in normal functioning for many reasons some of which include:

1. To be aware on a daily basis of one's global insignificance is likely to result in feelings of hopelessness and lack of motivation

   a. This is entertainingly illustrated by Douglas Adams in the Hitchhikers Guide to the Galaxy series quoted above. In this book a philosopher, Tin Tragula, built the Total Perspective Vortex to annoy his wife who kept telling him to get a 'sense of proportion' and 'into one end he plugged the whole of reality as extrapolated from a piece of fairy cake, and into the other end he plugged his wife: so that when he turned it on she saw in one instant the whole infinity of creation and herself in relation to it. To Tin Tragula's horror, the shock totally annihilated her brain.'

2. To maintain one's sense of self

   a. For example, an individual may have a deeply held conviction that they are a 'happy go lucky' person and not an angry or jealous person. Angry or jealous feelings will therefore threaten self-identity and may cause a **narcissistic injury**

3. To resist or postpone change

   a. The acceptance of feelings of unhappiness in a job or relationship might trigger a major life change that would cause upheaval and pain that would better be postponed

Case: James

James came to therapy in his early fifties. His last child had just left home to go to University and he had become aware he wanted to leave his wife. He told his therapist that he had probably been unhappy in his marriage for the last 10 years but had not realised this until now. He thought he might have delayed acknowledging this because the thought of separation from his children was unbearable.

4. A loss can be too large or too painful to face

   a. Frequently patients will express concern that if they really faced their pain they might start crying and never stop

5. Habitual behaviour

   a. In early stages of life, it can be helpful for a child's survival to hide feelings that could destabilise an unpredictable or easily hurt caregiver. This frequently becomes dysfunctional later in development. The following case example illustrate this

Case: Barbara

Barbara was in her fifties when she started psychotherapy. During her childhood her mother had been emotionally overwhelmed and angry a lot of the time. Barbara had learnt to hide her angry feelings, because they would trigger maternal violence. Barbara achieved well and became a nurse. In retrospect she thought that she began suffering with depression in her twenties. She did not manage to form any long-term relationships or have children. She put all her energy into work which she said became her 'family'. When a new manager, an older woman, was appointed Barbara could not get on with her and six months after her arrival a patient died on the ward. The manager implied that Barbara was responsible for the death through poor supervision of a junior nurse. Barbara became depressed and stopped work for the first time in her life. She lost weight, her mood became very low, she became very self-critical, couldn't sleep and had suicidal thoughts. At this point Barbara started psychotherapy and gradually recovered over the next two years. She told her therapist that one of the most helpful elements in her recovery was the realisation that she was full of anger and hatred for her mother. The new manager reminded Barbara of her mother. She felt angry at what she perceived as unfair treatment and this anger was turned back onto herself. This resulted in depression.

This case illustrates a number of key themes in psychodynamic psychotherapy. Through excessive use of **repression** Barbara's own anger was turned inwards causing her intense self-hatred and self-criticism. There had been unconscious patterns of relating throughout her life that had been reactivated by her experiencing at work. This is an example of how feelings about our self and others are linked with key formative relationships and are powerfully active throughout our lives. For further discussion of defences see Chapter 1.

Process of Therapy

The therapist's role is to tune into communications from the unconscious of the patient and gently, where appropriate, feed these messages back in a digestible form through **interpretation**. Over the passage of time the unconscious gradually becomes conscious, the patients develop a deeper understanding of themselves and their unconscious contributions to the difficulties they are experiencing. Sometimes patients can come to therapy wanting a large amount of change in a short space of time. They might not be aware that addressing long-standing beliefs about themselves and others requires commitment and their distress and anxiety might get worse before it gets better. The emotional challenge of the therapeutic process is often rewarded and by the end of therapy their symptoms of psychological distress have receded, and significant gains are made in the capacity for intimacy, work, creativity and pleasure.

Therapeutic Relationship

The relationship is the key tool in therapy. Both therapist and patient are involved in co-creating the therapeutic experience. The therapist's role is to accompany the patient in emotional exploration that can, at times, be painful for both participants. Unconscious patterns can be explored in this confidential and containing setting.

Transference and Countertransference

The unconscious communication from the patient is received by the therapist through **transference** and **countertransference**. Transference is the name given to the emotional residue of the patient's past attachments brought live into the therapeutic relationship. These patterns of relating affect the patient's other relationships and when seen clearly in therapy, where dysfunctional, they can be worked with and gradually changed.

The therapist's countertransference response is formed by their emotional reaction to the patient's transference, and their own past history. Sometimes these two aspects of countertransference are difficult to identify and separate, this is one reason why therapists need their own therapy and supervision.

A very common example of transference in therapy is that a patient can treat their therapist as they would one of their parents. This then can elicit an emotional counter-transference response in the therapist whereby they experience the patient as childlike. They can then be pulled into behaving in a maternal or paternal manner. Supervision is important in helping the therapist identify their countertransference response and work with it in a productive way.

Countertransference is a 'whole body' experience and affects the therapist physically, emotionally and psychically. It requires open, honest and compassionate self-attention to be used effectively. The therapist can have angry or disturbed countertransference feelings. They can, at times, feel physically sick, in pain or restless. The following example illustrates a somatic countertransference response.

Case: Nelly

Amina was becoming preoccupied. Every time she was in a session with her patient, Nelly, she found she was thirsty. She tried drinking before each session but that did not help. As soon as Nelly left the room at the end of the session, Amina would rush to the kitchen to have a drink. It gradually emerged in therapy that Nelly had an alcohol dependency earlier in her life and the emotions emerging in therapy were stimulating her 'need for a drink'. Once this was recognised and discussed in the sessions, Amina's feeling of thirst subsided. There then was the opportunity to address Nelly's underlying feeling of deprivation and dependency.

These somatic experiences can be very powerful. The mind and body are interlinked, and the body is a potent tool that resonates with others.

Case: Zeynep

Pardeep's patient Zeynep had been suffering with chronic pain for five years since her mother's death from cancer whom she had nursed through the final years of her life. Zeynep had been struggling with increasing pain in her legs, back and head since her loss. Pardeep found that he too started to feel pain in his head during the sessions which would build until Zeynep began crying about her mother's death. When she started active mourning Pradeep's headache evaporated. Pradeep realised that Zeynep was projecting her pain at the loss of her mother into her body, so that her psychic pain became physical pain, which Pradeep then identified and resonated with.

During a session a therapist can find their mind going to their own early memories, creative internal images, or to an event or conversation they had the day before the session. They can have primitive **phantasies** related to sex or aggression. These experiences are helpful if the therapist recognises them as part of their countertransference pointing them in the direction of the unconscious of their patient.

Case: Annabel

Asim's patient Annabel had been struggling with anorexia. While she was talking an image formed in Asim's mind of a small girl holding a bunch of balloons. The girl was being lifted up off the ground and drifting off into the sky. Asim linked this to the dissociated state of his patient who was not in contact with the ground, or reality, about the seriousness of her condition. She also talked later of 'drifting off' somewhere where she would no longer feel pain.

Another example of a more challenging but frequent countertransference response follows.

Case: Desmond

Andy found that he was starting to feel bored with his patient Desmond. It was hard to concentrate, and he started making a shopping list for his dinner. He felt guilty about this and was concerned that he was not attending to Desmond. When this continued to happen, he wondered if this was a countertransference response. He asked Desmond how he was experiencing the therapy; he said that he dreaded it, feeling exposed and he tried to hide what he was feeling. Andy realised this feeling of boredom was related to the sense of dread that Desmond felt where he hid everything creative from Andy. Once acknowledged, Andy felt more connected to his patient and more alive as a therapist.

Therapists' countertransference responses occur largely through identification with their patients' **projected** feelings. Patients may or may not be aware of these feelings themselves.

Projections and Projective Identification

Projection is a powerful primitive defence where feelings that cannot be digested are propelled out of the internal world into the external environment in either an attempt to get rid of them for good, or as a primitive attempt to communicate. These projections may penetrate the therapist's mind triggering an amplification of their own emotional state. This is called **projective identification**. There is a risk that the therapist misallocates these projections through identification, takes ownership and acts based upon them. They then lose their usefulness and they can be harmful to the therapeutic relationship.

In the two cases illustrating projection that follow, Mary, the patient in the first case, is aware of her emotional state and Robert, in the second case, is not.

Case: Mary

*Hannah's patient Mary has been coming to therapy for six months and they had developed a good **therapeutic alliance**. Mary had started talking about the miscarriages she had suffered when younger. When she cried about her loss Hannah also felt very sad and sometimes she could feel her eyes fill with tears. She found herself thinking about the loss of a friend the previous year. In this case she could share and identify with Mary's pain and Mary's sadness could be addressed in the session.*

Case: Robert

Serina's patient Robert had been coming to therapy punctually but full of complaint for three months. He didn't miss a moment of his allocated time where he complained about the uselessness of the therapy and Serina's inexperience. He repeatedly stated that he felt fine, didn't need any help, and really didn't know why he continued to attend. Serina felt inadequate and didn't know how to approach Robert. This was her first therapy case and she found herself comparing herself to an imagined expert therapist whom would know exactly what to do. Serina found these feelings difficult to discuss in supervision because she was embarrassed by them. Her supervisor wondered if this inadequacy was a projected communication from Robert that Serina was over-identifying with. In the next session Serina asked Robert whether he could feel inadequate at times. This resulted in a sudden and surprising change of mood. Robert told her that is exactly how he felt. He recently lost his job and over the subsequent sessions was able to talk about this. Sadness started to emerge and Serina's countertransference changed. She regained her competence and started to enjoy the work.

Containment

In therapy containment is provided for the patient. This means a safe, receptive and non-judgemental space. If a patient feels contained they are more able to relax conscious control of their thoughts and **free associate**. This allows the unconscious to emerge and be identified by the therapist, who, when the time is right, can feedback their under-standing of the unconscious communication in a digestible form, through interpretation, to the patient.

Interpretation

It is through the interpretive process that there is a gradual change from feeling, or taking action, to thinking. Interpretation can be as straightforward as saying 'you seem upset'.
Interpretation can include:

- Clarification, making links, encouragement, comment on observation, empathic validation and affirmation

  ○ 'It seems difficult for you to say more about that?'

- Identifying emotions as they arise

  ○ 'I can imagine you might feel very angry about that?' A patient can feel very inhibited about revealing their feelings which they may fear could be experienced as terrible or shocking. For the therapist to receive these feelings in a non-judgemental way can be a profound relief

- Here and now transference interpretations

  ○ This is where the therapist identifies past patterns of relating that come into the present. 'I wonder if you expected me to feel angry with you or to criticise you for that ...?'

- Reconstructive interpretation

  ○ Actively relating the past history to the patient's current experience. 'As we have discussed your relationship with your father was one where you were constantly trying to please him and gain his approval ... do you feel that you may be reproducing this in your relationships with men ... and with me, as your therapist, as well?'

Supervision

Supervision is an important part of any therapy and it provides containment for what can be very challenging work. When a therapist is in training they have supervision on a weekly basis, and when qualified generally monthly or bimonthly. The supervisor accompanies the therapist, providing reflective space where countertransference can be worked on effectively. This increases potency of the therapy itself and reduces the chance of boundary violations (see below) and **enactments**.

Patient Discontinuation

Research has shown that between 20 per cent and 50 per cent of patients end therapy early or drop out, many in the first few months [3]. It is important for the therapist not to take this too personally. It can be a painful experience and the therapist is often left uncertain as to the reason and can feel that they have 'done something wrong'. It is important to remember that this is unlikely to be the case. Patients respond to therapy in different ways and leave for variety of different reasons.

These include:

- They feel better

  ○ Some patients approach therapy when they feel bad but as soon as they feel better their defences re-establish themselves and further painful work is avoided

- It is too painful

  ○ It takes commitment and stamina to accept and withstand the painful thoughts and feelings that emerge in therapy

- Feelings of destabilisation due to normal defences being challenged
- Relapse

  ○ If dependency on drugs or alcohol has been used to regulate emotions, the disturbance caused by therapy can trigger to move back to this habitual response. This is why many services do not accept patients for therapy when they are in the early stages of recovery

- Intimacy and commitment difficulties

  ○ Therapy may feel too claustrophobic for some patients

- The negative therapeutic reaction

  ○ Counter to logic, patients can leave because they feel that they have been helped and understood by the therapist (see Chapter 2)

If the patient can be encouraged to return and work with their therapist their flight from treatment can provide important information, and an invaluable opportunity to learn about themselves.

Boundaries of Therapy

"I do not know where you end and I begin"
Father to son during a family therapy session

Boundaries are the physical and psychological manifestation of the difference between patient and therapist. They are needed for therapy to be effective.

Boundaries might initially seem straightforward, but they can become the most challenging aspect of the therapy. Powerful feelings emerge as a normal part of the therapeutic process and can pull the therapist to act and cross a boundary, an enactment. This is normal and happens at different times and in different ways. In most cases it provides important information helpful for the therapy. On occasion it can put a pressure on the relationship and stop the therapist functioning. In extreme cases it can lead to serious boundary violation. Supervision provides a space for these enactments to be recognised and worked with.

Boundaries are managed by both implicit and explicit rules. It is the therapist's role to manage the boundaries, and not the patient's. It is up to the therapist to recognise when boundaries have been crossed, and to restore them.

Case: Noreen

Demetri had been seeing his patient Noreen for five months. She was unpredictable and would surprise him repeatedly catching him on the 'back foot'. She was often late and would phone and email him repeatedly. She found things out about him and surprised him with information about where he had been or where he worked. She frequently tried to get the session started with him while they were walking to the therapy room and to engage him in general 'chit chat'. She would launch into long emotional stories just as Demetri was bringing the session to a close. On several occasions she reached over and turned the clock away from him so he couldn't see the time and didn't know when the session was ending. The effect was that Demetri often felt 'off balance' and had to think on his feet in each session to work out when a boundary had been crossed and how to rectify it. On one occasion Noreen brought her four-year-old daughter to the session. On this occasion Demetri said how sorry he was, but it would not be appropriate to have the session today. He understood that it was difficult for her, but this was her confidential space. He said he looked forward to seeing her the following week. Noreen was upset and angry and Demetri worried she would not return. In fact, this marked a significant shift in the therapeutic process and relationship. Noreen returned the next week for the first time on time. She engaged well and seemed to become more settled and trusting.

Boundaries can be physically manifest in the following areas that will be discussed below:

(i)   The structure of the setting
(ii) Emotionally manifest in the therapeutic role and stance
(iii) Clinically manifest in the therapeutic commitment

Structure and Setting

The structure and setting of the therapy are concrete manifestations of boundaries which need to be maintained as stable and predictable as possible.

The therapist needs to clarify in their own mind the structure of the therapy before they meet their patient for the first time where it can be discussed openly and clearly. This reduces the chances of misunderstanding or enactment later and becomes part of the therapeutic commitment discussed later in this chapter.

The key areas of the structure are:

- Time
  - The length of a session is 50 minutes.
  - If the patient is late, the session is rarely extended. If the patient is early the session is not started prematurely

- Consistency
  - The sessions are at the same time and same place each week
  - It is important for therapists to notify patients about breaks, and changes to session times well before they occur. Six weeks is a reasonable length of time to accommodate changes and to allow the emotional effect to be digested within the therapeutic setting. Occasionally sessions need to be changed at short notice by the therapist. On these occasions alternative sessions may be offered
  - If the patient does not attend or cancels a session this is usually not replaced. However, this is negotiable depending on the reason, and how long in advance a patient notifies their therapist
  - Change can bring up feelings, such as insecurity and anger, that are very useful and helpful to work with

- Duration
  - The therapist keeps in mind the timeline of the therapeutic work which is discussed regularly and keeps both patient and therapist engaged with the reality of their relationship. In the NHS patients tend to be offered a year of therapy with breaks
  - The end of the therapy is in focus from the beginning and is actively brought into the treatment to be thought about around three months before the end date
  - The ending of the therapy is likely to bring up the patient's previous experiences of loss, abandonments and rejection. This is very useful and allows work on these challenging areas

  The key areas of the setting are:
- Consistency
  - The setting of the therapy remains as constant as is practicable. Little changes can be disturbing for patients and therapists alike once the therapy has started. The therapist aims to have the same room, at the same time, with the same physical appearance each week. Thought is given to the therapeutic appearance of the room, which may need to be softened for the session if the room has other uses. It is important the patient feels safe and relaxed. Sometimes therapists bring in cushions, lights, a small carpet or table

- Security
  - Therapists take steps to ensure that there is no disturbance of the session. For example, using an engaged sign on the door and letting others in the environment know that there is therapy happening at that time so they can be quiet during the session

- Pleasant and relaxing decor

  o In general, the therapeutic setting has: two chairs facing towards each other, or slightly turned at an angle so therapist and patient can look to other parts of the room and manage the intensity of eye contact. The analytic couch generally is not used for once weekly work

  o Pens and paper are not used because the therapist's body and mind are their tools. The therapist will write up the session notes after the meeting with the patient. This delay allows their unconscious to work on the material that has been presented. What is, and is not, remembered is important and can be thought about in supervision

- A small table with a box of tissues
- A clock placed where the therapist can see it easily

Therapeutic Role and Stance

Exclusion of memory and desire

Bion [4]

The therapeutic role is a particular one, like no other. A therapist is not a friend, colleague, mentor or expert. The role is serious, important and unique, allowing highly privileged access into the internal world of another person. It is clearly boundaried and receptive. The patient is the focus and it is important for the therapist to not bring into the therapy aspects of their life and personality that may disrupt the therapeutic process.

Psychotherapy is an activity where attention is focussed on the present moment. It is about attending to the 'here and now'. This means not having any clear expectations about where the therapy is going or what the outcome is going to be. The therapist lets go of their other roles, feelings and wishes before starting the session. It can be difficult to remain in the therapeutic role particularly when anxious. So, for example psychiatrists can be pulled into the psychiatric role where they feel more assured and competent.

To get into the therapeutic frame of mind can takes some preparation. It can help to:

- Have time to relax before the session to mentally calm and settle

  o The therapist may be full of feelings that will block their capacity to listen and be emotionally present for their patient. It is important for them to attend to their countertransference, before the session, how it changes during the session, and what remains afterwards

- Keep to the boundaries of the session

  o The therapeutic discussion doesn't start until therapist and patient are in the therapy room

- Have a professional and well-cared-for appearance

  o This is an outward expression of self-esteem and conveys respect for the role of therapist and patient

- Neutrality

  ○ It is rare for a therapist to answer direct questions or give reasons for breaks or cancellations. Their aim is to explore the unconscious **phantasies** that underly the patient's enquiries and emerge in these periods of uncertainty

- Patient-focussed and -led

  ○ The therapist watches, feels and listens actively to their patient noting when and where defences are used, and which emotions are emerging

- Affect focus

  ○ This means following the feeling in the session. This can feel very difficult because there may be a lot of pressure for the therapist to not mention the 'elephant in the room' and it is invariably this 'elephant' that needs to be talked about. Real therapeutic skill lies in how communication around these challenging areas occurs

- Tolerance of silence and anxiety

  ○ Silence is a challenging but important part of any therapy. Both therapist and patient can feel anxious in silence and can be pulled to 'fill' it. This can block the unconscious, which needs space to emerge. Titrating the amount of silence in a session is part of the art of therapy. Too much and the patient may feel persecuted and too little may obstruct the process. The most important and instructive emotions can emerge as a gift for this patience

- Free-floating attention

  ○ The unconscious communications from the patient can be identified by what happens in the therapist's mind during a session. The therapist relaxes control of their own thoughts and attends with interest to what emerges. Thoughts take time to form and there is often a period of preceding anxiety and uncertainty before they materialise

- Compassion for oneself and the patient

  ○ Which does not mean feeling compassionate all the time. The therapist needs to be open to really scrutinise and think about their countertransference which may contain some very difficult feelings such as disgust, coldness, boredom, hatred etc. It is important the therapist feels compassionate about their own responses and aims to try to really understand this in a way which is helpful. Patients are very sensitive to the emotional communication from their therapist. The most challenging communication can be received and tolerated if expressed by the therapist with care

Therapeutic Commitment

The therapy commitment is the conscious and unconscious agreement that patient and therapist enter into together. Both are working on a shared task and need to be aware that they enter into this with uncertainty about the outcome. The therapy might not help, the patient, or therapist, might not tolerate the intimacy of the therapeutic relationship.

Therapists and therapy services tend to manage this commitment in different ways. In some cases, it is in a written contract and in others it is only verbally discussed. This is an area of discussion and controversy within different services. The discussion around this commitment is usually in the assessment and/or the first meeting.

Commitments Required of the Therapist
- To be responsible and reliable
- To try to think about how their patient stays on their mind in between sessions
  - ○ This important period allows the therapist to mentally digest the therapeutic experience. Supervision helps with this. If the therapist finds their patient difficult to hold in mind and think about, this isn't necessarily a problem. It may represent an important unconscious communication that once thought about can be used helpfully in the therapy
- To commit to the length of therapy
  - ○ Of course, life events do intervene, but it can be very disturbing to have a therapy end prematurely. It is important for the therapist to ensure that they are starting the therapy at a time where they have a period of reasonable stability and are not planning to move far away or change career
- Confidentiality
  - ○ The therapist does not share anything their patient brings outside the clinical environment. It is very important that this is stated explicitly to the patient. It is also important for the patient to be aware that confidentiality will be broken if there is good reason to be concerned about their, or someone else's, safety. This is rare and if it occurs the therapist's supervisor and other colleagues are there to help them think about what to do
- To treat all aspect of their patient presentation as requiring careful attention and thought
- To try to challenge and confront the difficult emotions in the sessions as sensitively, compassionately and truthfully as possible

Commitments Required of the Patient
- To commit to the process as far as possible
- To attend the sessions offered on time
- To be open and honest as possible about what is in their mind, including an attempt to free associate

Glossary
- **Affects:** feeling or emotion.
- **Containing:** first described by Bion [5]. The mother's soothing through mental digestion, or alpha function, of the baby's projections of beta elements.
- **Countertransference:** the therapist's emotional response to the transference.

- **Ego:** part of the mind that mediates between the conscious and unconscious. It engages with reality and is where self-identity is located.
- **Enactment:** non-reflective acting out of both therapist and patient of the unconscious content in the therapy.
- **Free associate:** the expression of thoughts that come to mind without conscious censorship. Allows for access to unconscious processes.
- **Interpretation:** attempting to put the unconscious emotional communication of the patient into words in the session.
- **Narcissistic injury:** challenge to one's ego, view of oneself and self-worth.
- **Phantasies:** unconscious fantasies.
- **Projection:** unwanted emotional states ejected from the internal world into external space or objects.
- **Projective identification:** emotional amplification of projections that have penetrated the mind.
- **Repression:** repression has different meanings in psychoanalytic literature. It can be used broadly to cover the process of defending the conscious mind. It can also be thought about as a particular defence mechanism. In this chapter the former definition is used. 'The essence of repression lies simply in turning something away, and keeping it at a distance, from the conscious' [6].
- **Therapeutic alliance:** the relationship between the patient and the therapist where both engaged in the therapeutic task.
- **Transference:** Feelings from relationships earlier in the patient's life brought into the 'here and now' of the therapeutic relationship.

References

1. Freud S. On narcissism: an introduction. In J Strachey, ed., *The Standard Edition of the Complete Psychological Works of Sigmund Freud, Volume XIV (1914–1916): On the History of the Psycho-Analytic Movement, Papers on Metapsychology and Other Works.* London: Hogarth Press. 1957; pp. 67–102. (Original work published 1914)

2. Adams D. *The Restaurant at the End of the Universe (Hitchhiker's Guide to the Galaxy).* London: Pan Macmillan. 2009; p. 79. Kindle Edition.

3. Swift JK, Greenberg RP. Premature discontinuation in adult psychotherapy: a meta-analysis. *J Consult Clin Psychol* 2012; 80(4): 547–59.

4. Bion WR. Notes on memory and desire. In R Lang, ed., *Classics in Psychoanalytic Technique.* New York and London: Jason Aronson. 1967; pp. 259–60.

5. Bion WR. *Learning from Experience.* London: Tavistock. 1962; pp. 1–116.

6. Freud S. Repression. In J Strachey, ed., *The Standard Edition of the Complete Psychological Works of Sigmund Freud, Volume XIV (1914–1916): On the History of the Psycho-Analytic Movement, Papers on Metapsychology and Other Works.* London: Hogarth Press. 1957; pp. 141–58. (Original work published 1915)

Further Reading

Budd S, Rusbridger R. *Introducing Psychoanalysis: Essential Themes and Topics.* London: Routledge, 2005.

Lemma A. *Introduction to the Practice of Psychoanalytical Psychotherapy*, 2nd ed. Chichester: John Wiley & Sons. 2015; pp. 67–8.

Cognitive Behavioural Therapy and Dialectical Behavioural Therapy: An Introduction

P. J. Saju

Introduction

Cognitive behavioural therapy (CBT) is an umbrella term, including several related theoretical models each with its own approach and techniques. This chapter will give an overview of the history of CBT, its underlying principles, therapeutic models, treatments and applications. It will also include a brief outline of dialectical behavioural therapy (DBT).

The fundamental tenet of CBT is that the way we think affects the way we feel and act. This deceptively simple statement has profound implications in practice. It means our distress could be modified by changing the way we think, or changing the way we respond to our thoughts.

The roots of CBT lie in both behavioural and cognitive theories. The focus is on observable aspects of behaviour as distinct from therapies that seek to explore unconscious mechanisms.

First Wave: Behavioural Therapy

Early behaviour therapy was based on Pavlov's classical conditioning theory. Here, learning was seen as a process of forming association between stimuli and response. A series of famous experiments followed. In 1920, John Watson (known as the father of behaviourism) experimentally induced phobia in nine-month-old Little Albert. A loud bang was made whenever Albert touched a white rat. Eventually, Albert began to show persistent fear of the white rat and later, to other furry objects.

In 1924, Mary Cover Jones, an American psychologist referred to as the mother of behaviour therapy by Joseph Wolpe (his contribution is discussed below) for her pioneering contribution to the field, worked with a young child, Peter, who was afraid of rabbits. While Peter was having his favourite food, Mary brought the rabbit close to him. Through repeated pairing and by process of counter-conditioning, Peter's fear was gradually overcome, a process subsequently referred to as desensitisation. Interestingly, Peter's fear was less when he saw other children playing with the rabbit. It was also less when he was with a supportive adult. These early observations of observational learning and the role of therapeutic relationship would be further elaborated by Albert Bandura in his Social Learning Theory in the 1970s.

In the 1940s, B F Skinner, another American psychologist, formulated operant conditioning theory. He argued that all organisms were influenced by the consequences of their own behaviour. The environment (situation or event) acts as cue for a particular behavioural response. If the consequence of the behaviour is positive, there will be an increase in the behaviour. If the consequence is negative, the behaviour would reduce in frequency.

This means behaviour could be shaped through environmental manipulation and learning occurs by reinforcement.

The journal entry below is by a patient with symptoms of post-traumatic stress disorder (PTSD) following a car accident. Having had to undergo a number of operations for the injuries sustained, she developed a fear of hospitals, which impacted on her further treatment.

> At work: My new manager wears same perfume as Dr X used to wear when I was in hospital. As soon as I could smell it, my heart started racing and then I became restless. I logged off the computer, grabbed my belongings and left the office. I went for a coffee and kept thinking to myself how 'stupid' I was being. I was scared of the smell of somebody's perfume!
> I was angry with myself for being so stupid, so I went to the gym to release my frustration.

Here, the smell of perfume elicits severe anxiety through classical conditioning. Leaving the situation resulted in reduced fear, which is a positive consequence. This consequence reinforces further avoidance behaviour through operant conditioning.

Functional Analysis of Behaviour: The ABC Model

Within a behaviour therapy approach detailed analysis of antecedents (A), behaviour (B) and consequences (C) is necessary to identify the cause–effect links, which may be hidden. Information can be gained from interview, self-monitoring and behavioural observations.

Problems and Goals

In behaviour therapy, problems have to be defined clearly. This will help to set specific, measurable, achievable, realistic and time bound goals.

Antecedents: Where did this happen? Who was around? When? What was happening before the problem? What were the external triggers? Any internal triggers such as thoughts, mood or bodily symptoms?

Behaviours: Get a step by step account. What did you do? How long this behaviour continue? When did it stop? What made it stop?

Consequences: What was the outcome? Did it cause further difficulties? Was there anything slightly good? Did it give you any benefits at all? What did others do? How did it feel afterwards? Did it help with your problems?

Functional Analysis, which seeks to establish the relationship between stimuli and responses, can inform understanding of behaviour and lead to interventions, by changing antecedents, behaviour and/or consequences as the examples below illustrate.

Changing Antecedents

When we can identify the antecedents to behaviour (Table 7.1), then these could be avoided, reduced or modified.

Changing Behaviour

When antecedents could not be changed, we can choose to behave differently with an alternate response which is pleasant (e.g. going for a walk, talk to someone, exercise,

Table 7.1 Antecedents to behaviour

Condition	External triggers	Internal triggers
Alcohol use	Drinking partners, weekends, pay day	Boredom Depression Anger Frustration
Binge eating	No regular eating Advertisements of food Interpersonal conflict	Hunger Tiredness Low self-esteem

relaxation, hot bath) or necessary (cleaning etc.). Delaying problematic behaviour through different activities often reduces the urge to do it.

Changing Consequences

Changing consequences may involve rewarding positive behaviour, or adding a negative consequence, when undesired behaviour occurs. For example, using Star Charts (giving a star for positive behaviour) in children encourages further positive behaviour. Time out (placing in a low stimulus unrewarding environment, when the child misbehaves) reduces frequency of misbehaviour.

When used in therapy, the consequences are set by the therapist and clearly explained to the patient as in contingency management.

Contingency Management is used to shape adaptive behaviour or reduce problematic behaviour. These take the form: 'If you do action X, then consequence Y would follow'. For example, making a behavioural contract between patient and therapist and following it consistently – such as if the patient phones over x times inappropriately, they lose the right to call the therapist in the next week. The therapist would reinforce adaptive or desired behaviours. The most powerful positive reinforcers are often expressions of the therapist's approval, care and concern. Treatment developed from some of these ideas include:

- Token Economy: in the 1950s patients with negative symptoms of schizophrenia in state hospital settings were rewarded with tokens when they engaged in 'desired behaviours' such as improved self-care. The tokens could be exchanged for rewards, mostly cigarettes
- Aversion therapy: painful stimuli such as electric shocks or emetic medications were paired with undesirable behaviour (alcohol, drugs or deviant sexual interests). The expectation, based on classical conditioning theory, was to create an aversive conditioned response

Long-term effectiveness of Token Economy and Aversion therapy was poor and ethical considerations also led to its withdrawal.

Interestingly, alcohol consumption on disulfiram treatment creates an unpleasant and aversive physical reaction and the patients stop drinking to avoid the negative consequence. This can be seen as pharmacological aversion therapy.

Behavioural Interventions for Anxiety

Systematic Desensitisation (SD) was developed by Joseph Wolpe, a South African psychiatrist in the 1950s, based on reciprocal inhibition theory. For example, relaxation and fear could not co-exist at the same time due to the relaxation response inhibiting the anxiety response.

SD involves three phases: relaxation training, constructing anxiety hierarchy and desensitisation proper. A hierarchy of fearful scenes from minimum to maximum on a 0–100 scale will be constructed with the patient. Desensitisation is carried out by the patient visualising the least anxiety-provoking scene while deeply relaxed. When the patient can do this without anxiety, the patient moves to the next item in the hierarchy and proceeds ultimately to the top item of hierarchy.

SD is not used now as it is very time-consuming and more effective techniques such as Gradual Exposure (GE) became available. SD was done in imagination through visualisation, but in GE, exposure in visualisation and real situations is done. In GE, anxiety hierarchy is used, but relaxation is not used (see Table 7.2).

Implosive therapy and Flooding were used in the 1960s and 1970s. This involved exposure to extreme fear-provoking imagery or situation for an extended period, without hierarchy or relaxation. It was difficult for most patients to do due to intense fear and is no longer recommended. For example, in flooding, a person with fear of heights may be brought to the top of the building and asked to remain there till anxiety subsides over time.

Gradual Exposure involves provoking anxiety in a graded manner and allows it to decrease naturally, without avoidance, distraction, neutralisation, relaxation or other safety-seeking behaviours. Reduction in anxiety is through the process of repeated exposure (habituation) where gradually the anxiety is totally dissipated (extinction).

Exposure can be in imagination or in real situations (exposure in vivo). The sessions are planned in advance collaboratively and controlled with regard to difficulty or distress levels. Patients are asked to rate their subjective anxiety on a scale of 0–100 at 15-minute intervals. Typically, sessions last 30–60 minutes at a time. Prolonged exposure sessions are better.

Table 7.2 Example of anxiety hierarchy in two patients

Example 1 Fear of contamination in obsessive compulsive disorder	Estimated Subjective Units of Distress (SUDS) Rate 0–100	Example 2 Fear of hospital
Using a public toilet in a hospital	100	Attending hospital appointment
Using a public toilet	80	Inside the hospital – not attending appointment
	60	In hospital grounds
	50	Hospital car park
Using toilet at friends	40	Thought of going into hospital
	30	Hospital appointment letter
Using toilet at home	20	Picture of local hospital

Exposure is terminated when anxiety is decreased to a mild to moderate level (30–50/100), that is, when 'extinction' has occurred. The exposure has to be repeated in between sessions, through homework assignments.

A single session of prolonged exposure can dramatically reduce phobias of small animals, snakes, injections etc. In panic disorder, exposure to the patient's own interoceptive cues, or bodily signals of anxiety, is a key component of treatment. Physical symptoms of panic are deliberately provoked, such as exercise to increase heart rate or spinning in a chair to provoke dizziness. The exposure in obsessive compulsive disorder (OCD) is to the intrusive thought, object or action that triggers obsession. Exposure is combined with response prevention, that is the patient is not allowed to do any compulsion, neutralisation or compensatory action to defuse anxiety for 30–60 minutes. In PTSD, the patient's detailed verbal narrative of trauma itself is the exposure. Retelling and re-experiencing help to desensitise the fear evoked by the memories and flashbacks.

Behavioural Therapy for Depression

Early behavioural theories in the 1970s conceptualised depression as a behavioural response to aversive events or the absence of pleasant events. In therapy, patients were encouraged to generally increase activities believed to be positive or enjoyable. This generalised approach was less effective, as it ignored the reinforcement value of specific activities for the person, such as avoidance of the aversive stimulus.

Behavioural Activation (BA) is an evidence-based treatment for depression, based on behavioural theory. Depression often leads to inactivity and rumination which leads to further depressed mood. The main goal is to change avoidant coping and behavioural patterns that maintain depression.

An increase in pleasurable activities is not the main goal in BA, but it is often a consequence of BA. The first step is to monitor activities on an hourly basis. This helps to educate the patient about links between inactivity and depressed mood. The next step is to schedule activities. Once completed, rate whether activities brought a sense of achievement or pleasure. The third step would be to develop a hierarchy of activities in a systematic manner, based on the person's values, ranked from easy to difficult. The activities should be tangible and measurable, for example going for a walk for 30 minutes in the park, rather than abstract or cognitively oriented, for example thinking about a happy time in life. Scheduling valued activities and monitoring the outcome are important to keep the momentum. Progress is monitored systematically through objective measurements, for example keeping a record of positive activities.

Second Wave: Cognitive Therapy (CT)

Early behaviour therapists focussed on specific, measurable behaviour and the environmental reinforcements of the behaviour. Early behavioural therapists were suspicious of mentalistic concepts, such as the one used by psychoanalysts (e.g. ego, superego etc.) and this suspicion extended to patients' explanations about their own behaviour, which were thought to be unreliable and unverifiable. However, the 'cognitive revolution' in psychology in the late 1960s brought about evidence of cognitive processes in human behaviour. The paradigm shifted from a reinforcement model to an information processing model. In addition, early proponents of combined cognitive behaviour techniques reported success through cognitive techniques.

The philosophical origins of CT can be traced to Stoic philosophy and Buddhism. Both regarded role of thought as fundamental in creating negative emotional states.

In the late 1950s and early 1960s, Albert Ellis's Rational Emotive Therapy (RET) and his ABC model (Antecedents–Beliefs–Consequences) focussed on the central role of irrational thinking in needless human suffering. Ellis posited a general model of psychopathology, by listing a set of common irrational ideas (example – one should be thoroughly competent, adequate and perfect to be worthwhile). In therapy, Ellis challenged and confronted the patient's illogical beliefs robustly.

In the late 1960s, Aaron Beck, a trained psychoanalyst became more interested in the conscious thoughts that lead to emotional distress. The cognitive model proposed by Beck states incorrect maladaptive beliefs and/or biased information processing are central in maintaining emotional distress. Systematic biases in thinking results in inaccurate perceptions of objective reality. Beck's model identified specific and idiosyncratic thoughts rather than general irrational beliefs, as posited by Ellis.

Beck described three levels of thoughts.

Core Beliefs: deeply held, dominant beliefs about self, others and the world (e.g. I am worthless, I am unlovable, people are cruel, life has no meaning). They develop from significant life experiences, often from childhood. They may remain dormant, until they get activated by significant events.

Intermediate Beliefs: these are silent underlying assumptions, attitudes and rules that guide life. These rules (I must be perfect) and conditional statements (If I am not perfect, then I would not be respected) operate to overcome the pain of negative core beliefs. But in the long term, these beliefs are maladaptive because they are rigid, extreme and inflexible.

Negative Automatic Thoughts: they are experienced in a specific situation as seemingly plausible ideas, but in reality, they are exaggerated or false. They may reflect underlying core beliefs. For example, a woman with a core belief (I am unlovable), encounters her old class mate who does not smile at her (activating event) and then thinks 'She does not like me', 'I can't live like this' and experiences sadness.

Key Aspects of CBT

Socratic dialogue is a distinctive method of CT to encourage learning through self-discovery. The therapist would ask questions about how the patient has come to a particular thought or belief, their reasons to think it is true and whether they could find anything that does not fit their belief. At the initial stage, there should be no prejudgement about thoughts being irrational or dysfunctional. Instead the focus is to discover the person's 'database' or evidence for their beliefs and assumptions. Questions to expand the perspectives can be used later to generate alternative meanings.

Collaborative empiricism is a central principle in CBT. This involves collaborative understanding of the patient's beliefs and then systematically testing their subjective hypothesis through questions and experiments. The process is transparent and open. Assumptions would be seen as hypothesis to be tested, rather than an established fact. By working jointly as an investigative team, the therapist and patient tests the accuracy and usefulness of the thoughts, beliefs and assumptions. If the thoughts were not accurate or useful, the therapist is encouraged to revise them, using more valid facts.

Table 7.3 Behavioural interventions

Technique	Conditions in which it is used
Behavioural monitoring	Useful as baseline and outcome monitoring of behaviour of interest (bingeing, alcohol, aggression, avoidance etc.)
Positive data logs	In low self-esteem – to collect disconfirming data
Graded exposure	All anxiety disorders, where there is avoidance behaviour
Activity schedules	Depression, lack of structure
Graded task assignments	Depression, procrastination, amotivation
Mastery and pleasure rating	Depression

Cognitive behavioural integration: cognitive therapists combine cognitive and behavioural interventions in therapy (Table 7.3). They add a cognitive perspective to behavioural interventions such as exposure. For example, in behavioural experiment (BE), the patient's specific prediction about an exposure task is written down in advance (e.g. People will laugh at me if I go out). The patient is encouraged to test the prediction through an appropriate experiment. Once completed, the actual outcome would be compared with the original prediction. In most cases, the patient's predictions would be different to the actual outcome. The patient would be invited to think about the difference between prediction and outcome. Thus in CT, the exposure task (anxiety about being with people) was transformed to an opportunity to test underlying beliefs.

Therapeutic Relationship in CBT: CBT therapists believe Carl Roger's core conditions of therapy (accurate empathy, genuineness, warmth and being non-judgemental) are important and necessary, but they are not sufficient by itself to effect change. Beck emphasised the need to have specific interventions to change thinking and behaviour.

Therapists are seen as having expertise in the theory and method of change, and the client has expertise in applying new learning. Therapists are active and appropriately directive when necessary, while maintaining their collaborative stance. If disagreements occur, it is acknowledged and resolved early to maintain the positive working alliance. Issues related to the transference are usually not directly addressed.

A CBT formulation synthesises information to provide an understanding about the origin and continuation of the problem. Collaborative formulations help to create a joint understanding of the problem, and increase the patient's commitment to address it through appropriate interventions. CBT formulation can be constructed at different levels of complexity as the examples below illustrate.

1. Cross-sectional formulation links thought, mood and behaviour in a specific context. This 'here and now' formulation is useful to explain a particular symptom. For example, in the presence of crowds, Mary thinks she will be seen as an idiot and notes that she begins to shake and feel dizzy and has to run away

2. Disorder-based formulations are generic, standardised, readymade, 'off the shelf' formulations for specific disorders. They are useful but often unfairly criticised for being formulaic, mechanistic and not person centred. The manualised approach is popular for the purposes of randomised control trials

3. Person-based formulations are individualised, 'tailored', idiographic formulations based on the person's life experiences, personality and core beliefs. There is greater appreciation of the strengths and vulnerabilities of the person. Proponents of disorder-based formulation would argue this is labour-intensive and with poor interrater reliability. For an example, see Table 7.4
4. Transdiagnostic formulation focusses on the various processes (attention, imagery, memory, self-focus) rather than the content of thoughts

Table 7.4 Person-based cognitive formulation

Significant experiences	• Highly independent young woman, ambitious and successful • Road traffic accident with long-term need for long-term medical interventions • PTSD flashbacks
Core beliefs Self	I am damaged; I am a burden to others
Others	Others will pity me, but they will not care!
Life and the world	Life is unfair; future is gone; nothing will bring back my old life
Intermediate beliefs	I should have been more careful I cannot and will not forgive myself If I don't have the old me back, then there is no point If I accept what happened, I worry I would give up If I go to hospital, I will never come out I need to be in control Others should not have to care for me It is terrible if you depend on others If I get close to anyone, I will mess up their life I will be better off alone
Compensatory strategies	Work harder, leave no time to think/reflect Hide vulnerability; project strength Do not get close to people, keep your distance
Strengths	No previous psychological difficulty; no drugs or alcohol Wants to feel better, would attend sessions Can access thoughts and feelings (but blocks them usually) Willing to tolerate distress
Goals	Would like to manage flashbacks and anxiety
Therapy plan	Damaged self-esteem, guilt, hopelessness – address this first May leave therapy if feeling more vulnerable Requires grounding (work needed to stabilise anxiety, through calm breathing, focussing attention on colour, or sounds) before starting trauma work Patient worries about not in control, pace to be negotiated

In the presence of crowds, Mary's attention is focussed on herself, rather than outside and she can see her own image as a little trembling woman with flushed face. She remembers, previous situations, where she did not cope well.

In therapy, the therapist initially validated the patient's thoughts and feelings. There was a deep sense of loss, self-blame and criticism regarding their role in the accident. Interventions to reduce criticism through self-compassion and acceptance were chosen as the most appropriate strategy. Later, gradual exposure to hospital settings were undertaken, for example by visiting departments within a hospital. In the final phase, grounding techniques were used to prepare the patient to undertake trauma-focussed CBT where the narrative of the trauma was discussed in order to process trauma memory and flashbacks.

Cognitive Interventions

Thought diary: a thought diary can be used in any condition but is commonly used in people with depression. The thought diary shows the link between thought and emotion to patients clearly. Initially this is done by the patient and therapists together in the session; later this is set as a homework. More importantly, it identifies recurrent themes and unhelpful thinking styles. The thinking styles process information in a biased and prejudiced manner.

Table 7.5 Format of thought diary

Date	Situation	Thoughts, image, memory, interpretations and meaning	Mood	Action

Cognitive Restructuring: a thought diary is used to reflect on the thinking and identify the problems in accuracy of usefulness of specific thoughts. Cognitive restructuring is the process of actively changing problematic thought patterns and beliefs to more constructive beliefs. CBT therapists use five broad approaches to question negative thoughts.

1. Accuracy:

   Is my belief based on facts/evidence?

   Is only based on personal opinion/emotions?

   Would my friends agree with my interpretation?

2. Alternative:

   Could there be other explanations?

3. Usefulness:

   What is the usefulness of this belief?

   Could I find more helpful belief?

4. Thinking styles:

   Am I thinking in habitually biased patterns?

5. Action:

   What can I do about it differently?

Box 7.1 Unhelpful thinking styles

Selective abstraction: focussing on a detail, ignoring other salient factors
Arbitrary inference: conclusions drawn from inadequate information
Personalisation: everything is my fault and I am responsible
Overgeneralisation: general conclusion based on a single event
Dichotomous thinking: black and white without the middle grey area
Magnification and minimisation: of the importance of particular events
Mental filter: believe negative things about self, disregard any positives
Labelling: name calling self or others (He is rubbish)
Catastrophisation: the worst possible outcome is going to happen
'Should/Must' thinking: unrelenting standards for self or others to behave
Emotional reasoning: if I feel this, then it is unquestionably true

Table 7.6 Additional cognitive interventions

Other cognitive interventions	
Cost benefit analysis	– List advantages and disadvantages of a belief or behaviour – After weighing up the above, decide what is best
Decatastrophisation	What would be the worst scenario? How would you cope then?
Behavioural experiments	Testing negative predictions in real life, followed by reflection and learning
Reattribution: responsibility pie for guilt	Apart from your contribution, do you think anyone, or any other factors played a part?
Mindfulness	Awareness in the present with full acceptance, without judgement and expectation
Imagery interventions	Imagining a safe place, a compassionate person or a rescripting of trauma images
Continuums/Scaling questions	Antidote to dichotomous thinking. On a scale of 1–10 rate your sense of having failed … What action would make you less of a failure?
Definition/Semantic method	When you say you are a failure, how do you define it? What would be the criteria?
Metaphors and stories	Helps to bring a different perspective and meaning
Time projection	How will you feel about this in 6 hours/days/months? What would you do differently in future?

Suitability for CBT

Though CBT is used in a wide variety of conditions, the evidence is strongest for depression, panic disorder, generalised anxiety disorder, PTSD, OCD and social phobia. In considering CBT as a treatment and after a brief explanation of the model, the individual should have some capacity to identify their own thoughts and be willing to examine their accuracy and usefulness. The individual should be seeking to change unhelpful beliefs and behaviour to the best of their ability.

Cognitive Therapy for Generalised Anxiety

Underestimation of self-efficacy and overestimation of risks is common in anxiety disorders. The primary focus in therapy is on the patient's incorrect or biased appraisals. The aim would be to form an appraisal that fits with reality of the situation. This often requires a shift from affect-based appraisals (I feel anxious, so it must be true!) to evidence-based appraisals (Despite my feelings, evidence shows actual risk is low). Philosophically, the therapist has to emphasise the universality of threat, while promoting acceptance and tolerance of uncertainty.

- Overestimated probability appraisals: Am I exaggerating the likelihood of X happening?
- Exaggerated severity appraisals: Am I overly focussed on the worst possible outcome?
- What effect is this thinking style having on my anxiety?
- What are the benefits of my thinking?
- What are the disadvantages of my thinking?

Decatastrophising of core fears: this should be planned carefully. This involves three stages: (1) preparation, (2) exploration of the imagined catastrophe and its impact on life and relationships (this could be emotionally distressing and uncover more deeper worries) and (3) problem solving: behavioural experiments are an excellent way to test anxious predictions.

Metacognitive Therapy (MCT) was developed by Adrian Wells, a psychologist based in Newcastle in the UK, for anxiety disorders and depression. Therapy is based on an information processing model of psychological disorder.

Metacognitive theory focusses on how the thought is processed rather than the content of thought. While CBT tries to change the content of illogical thoughts, MCT changes unhelpful processing of thought, such as rumination and thought control strategies.

Direct challenge of positive beliefs about worry ('It is as if you believe worry helps me to be prepared.' 'What would happen if you decided to do nothing with your worries?') and developing new plans for information processing are key interventions. Detached mindfulness is cultivated to attend to the process of worrying, rather than getting trapped in it. Experiential exercises such as attention training technique and worry postponement exercises are used in MCT.

CBT Models for Specific Problems

A range of applications of CBT techniques have been developed for specific psychological and psychiatric conditions such as CBT for PTSD, social phobia, OCD, body dysmorphic disorder which are beyond the scope of this chapter. All the models use exposure techniques, but will also have additional techniques, for example video feedback in social phobia. Clark and Beck [1] is recommended for reference. For CBT in psychosis see Chapter 14.

Changing Core Beliefs: Personality Disorders and Complex Trauma

Negative core beliefs are highly emotion laden and strongly held in personality disorders and in complex trauma (I am utterly worthless, I can never trust others, life would never get better). Rather than challenging these strongly held beliefs, it would be more appropriate to use empathy and validation, initially ('Given what experiences you had, it makes good sense to think that way'). In validation, you acknowledge the persons views, but also keeps the option of reviewing and revising them later. A safe, trusting therapeutic relationship characterised by empathy and validation is essential to change the emotion laden negative core beliefs.

With regard to cognitive interventions, instead of challenging negative core beliefs (this may be perceived as invalidating), developing new core beliefs based on their interests, values and hopes is more useful. Developing a different version of self (new core belief) can be a creative and liberating process, and taps on to unidentified strengths. Intermediate beliefs (if–then predictions) can be tested through behavioural experiments. Recognising and recording positive events (positive data log) would be helpful to track positives in life and helps to create a new narrative. Practising new strategies would strengthen the new emerging self.

Schema Therapy was developed by Jeffrey Young in the 1990s as a variant of CBT for people with personality disorders. Schema therapy addresses five core childhood emotional needs:

1. Secure attachment which includes basic needs
2. Autonomy/sense of identity
3. Freedom to express valid needs
4. Spontaneity and play
5. Realistic limits and self-control

If these needs are not met the child will develop a maladaptive schema which refers to an abnormal response to triggers.

Schema therapy has developed the concept of *modes* which are seen as emotional states arising out of responses to stimuli based on the underlying schema. For example, child modes: angry child, vulnerable child. There is an aim to strengthen what is referred to as the healthy adult mode, to change schema-driven life patterns and eventually for the patient to get their core emotional needs met in everyday life.

Schema therapy employs more experiential interventions, such as chair work and imagery. It may require the therapist to go beyond normal therapeutic limits, 'limited reparenting' is used by therapists in an attempt to repair the patient's unmet needs of childhood. Empathic confrontation is used to challenge and set limits. Randomised controlled trials show good results in borderline and narcissistic personality disorder.

Third Wave of CBT

The central focus of second wave CBT was in content of cognition (thoughts, beliefs, imagery etc.). But over time, attention shifted to the process of cognition itself.

The third wave of CBT includes DBT, Mindfulness-Based Cognitive Therapy (MBCT) and Acceptance and Commitment Therapy (ACT). In these models, goals are broader than simply changing a behaviour or thought; it is a new way of interacting with the world. In the second wave of CBT, the emphasis is on changing meaning through changing unhelpful thoughts or behaviour. This can be termed as first order change, as it is based on logic and hence the direction of change is predictable. For example: repeated handwashing in OCD is unnecessary, as the fear is based on faulty appraisals about contamination. OCD is seen as a problem that needs to be defeated using recommended treatment protocols.

In third wave CBT, the focus is on **second order change.** Here change in thinking comes from being aware of the process of thinking itself, rather than the content. This metacognitive process is often based on mindfulness, which allows to look at thoughts in a different way. This perspective changes our relationship to our thoughts and problems.

Interestingly these models have been drawn upon by Buddhist philosophy to varying levels. In Buddhist philosophy, the three fundamentals of existence are Dukkha (unsatisfactoriness), Annica (impermanence) and Anatma (selflessness). Everything, including the Self is seen as a process, established in a network of relationships within a particular context. Everything is impermanent and changeable in the long run. Those with wisdom can radically accept positive and negative changes with equanimity. Such profound re-orientation of life is not expected in third wave therapies, but therapy brings about a different view about life problems.

Buddhists mention four interlinked infinite and boundless good qualities. These are Metta (friendliness), Karuna (compassion), Mudita (empathetic joy) and Upekkha (equanimity, even mindedness). These qualities are developed through various meditative practices. These qualities are important in relating to self and others, and third wave therapies encourage developing these qualities, particularly compassion.

Dialectical Behavioural Therapy (DBT) integrates Buddhist mindfulness with behaviour therapy. In addition, dialectical philosophy of synthesising the opposite view is an important part of the wise mind.

Acceptance and Commitment Therapy (ACT) is derived from functional contextualism; the theory underpinning it is called relational frame theory. Experiential avoidance and psychological inflexibility are the fundamental cause of emotional problems.

The six core principles help to develop psychological flexibility.

1. Acceptance
2. Diffusion – getting past 'language traps'
3. Self in context and as a process
4. Being present
5. Connecting with values
6. Committed action

Mindfulness skills help to develop the first four core principles. The last two principles lead towards a meaningful life.

ACT focusses on the function of thinking rather than truth value of thoughts. Diffusion is like having a decentred and deconstructed view about own thoughts, but the ACT therapist does not work to challenge thoughts as in traditional CBT.

Mindfulness-Based Cognitive Therapy: Jon Kabat Zinn developed Mindfulness Based-Stress Reduction (MBSR) working with patients with physical problems in 1979. Zindel Segal, Mark Williams and John Teasdale adapted MBSR to develop MBCT. The central idea is to practise mindfulness skills to focus on the present, and observing the sensations, thoughts and emotions in a non-judgemental manner. The attention is decentred, and this helps to look at our internal processes with curiosity and equanimity. The attitude is one of allowing (instead of suppressing) and also letting go (instead of rumination). Thoughts are seen as merely impressions, rather than incontrovertible facts. Distressing thoughts and emotions come and go and one does not always need to engage with it.

MBCT for recurrent depression is delivered in a group setting, when patients are in remission. It has shown to reduce relapse. The structured modules are led by a professional, who regularly practises mindfulness.

Compassion-Focussed Therapy: Paul Gilbert, a psychologist from the UK, developed this, influenced by various theories (CBT, Buddhism, evolutionary theory, attachment and affect regulation). Consequently, he uses techniques from various theoretical models to address a patient's deep-rooted self-criticism, shame and guilt. Self-compassion is necessary to develop a sense of safety and satisfaction in life.

Gilbert postulated three interacting emotion regulation systems [2]: threat and self-protection system, incentive and resource seeking system and soothing and contentment system. Deficits in the soothing and contentment system leave one with distressing emotions, self-criticism, depression, guilt and shame. Using mindfulness and experiential imagery exercises people are helped to generate compassion for self.

In therapy, diaries and journals are used to addresses deep-rooted self-hatred, guilt and shame issues. In contrast to MBCT and ACT, the therapist engages with the content of negative thoughts, similar to CBT. In contrast to CBT, the focus is on being compassionate to self when reflecting on the negative thoughts and accepting the imperfect nature of self. Similar to Schema therapy, attachment patterns, childhood developmental and traumatic experiences are explored in detail.

CBT in the NHS

Improving Access to Psychological Therapy (IAPT) was developed in 2008 as a systematic way to organise the delivery of, and access to, evidence-based psychological therapies for depression and anxiety within the NHS. Though IAPT uses other modalities, CBT is the main modality as there is more evidence for CBT for depression and anxiety disorders.

By mid-2017 IAPT was seeing over 950,000 patients per year, with around 60 per cent having a course of treatment, and others having an assessment, advice and signposting. Disorder-specific CBT formulation and interventions backed by evidence are delivered by adequately trained therapists, with routine outcome monitoring session by session. Clinically and organisationally, this has been an impressive achievement. IAPT has expanded its scope to include long-term medical conditions and medically unexplained symptoms recently. The NHS has committed to further expanding IAPT services so 1.5 million people per year will be seen by 2020/21.

IAPT is based on a stepped care model, and if the problems are complex or pose high risk or require multi professional input, people can be stepped up to secondary care services, where CBT based on more individual based formulations, or other forms of psychotherapy such as psychodynamic psychotherapy may be offered in combination with psychiatric interventions. CBT interventions for psychosis, eating disorders and neurodevelopmental disorders are typically offered within secondary care services.

Evidence Base of CBT

CBT has a large evidence base for a wide variety of disorders. Dobson et al. review the evidence base [3], but also highlight the need for comparative efficacy of different active treatments, and long-term efficacy of CBT.

Training is widely available in the UK, and the website www.babcp.com gives information about short and long courses in CBT.

Dialectical Behavioural Therapy

DBT was originally developed by Marsha Linehan, a psychologist in the 1980s, for suicidal and self-injuring patients with borderline personality disorder (BPD). Originally trained in behaviour therapy, she was one of the first therapists to systematically introduce Buddhist concepts such as acceptance and mindfulness skills into Western therapy. She was able to construct a highly structured and replicable modular therapy model that was rigorously tested in randomised trials.

Linehan stated that a dialectical perspective on the nature of reality and human behaviour has three primary characteristics [4].

1. Interrelatedness or wholeness: a dialectic world view looks at life as a complex whole with interconnections. Identity formation is best understood as a process connecting biology, important relationships and the broader sociocultural context; that is, identity develops within a system rather than as an isolated entity
2. Polarity: reality is not static but composed of opposing forces referred to as thesis and antithesis. A dialectical perspective on polarity means within darkness there is light and within light, there is darkness. Or we can state, within the dysfunction of BPD, there would also be function. Thus, Linehan believes in the construct of 'wise mind', the inherent wisdom within all patients
3. Continuous change: even when a synthesis of opposing forces is achieved, it will not be a permanent state, and out of this synthesis, further polarities will emerge. Thus, the process of change, rather than structure or content, is the essential nature of life

The best way to represent these three aspects pictorially would be the Chinese symbol of Yin and Yang, where seemingly opposing black and white forces are in fact complementary, interconnected, and interdependent, influencing each other moment to moment.

BPD is viewed as a difficulty in effectively resolving the dialectic tensions that characterise the human mind, relationships and life more generally (dialectic failure). The goal of treatment is to help patients to engage in their dialectic dilemmas and transcend them through synthesis.

In therapy, there are three dialectic challenges.

1. Dialectics of acceptance and change
2. Dialectics of unwavering goal centredness and compassionate flexibility
3. Dialectics of nurturing and benevolent demanding

These dialectics of therapy make the therapy highly structured, yet flexible. There is a behavioural focus, yet a compassionate, respectful and irreverent style.

Despite the value-based philosophical stance, DBT is also a biopsychosocial theory, with a robust evidence base. People with emotional dysregulation may have a biological predisposition to this such as genetics, temperament etc. These combine with psychological and

Table 7.7 Overview of DBT strategies

Five areas of dysregulation	DBT skill modules and strategies	Dialectic strategies	Case management strategies	Behavioural strategies
Emotional dysregulation	**Emotion regulation** Understand, observe, describe, modulate and change emotions	**Core strategies** 1. Validation 2. Problem solving	Environmental interventions Therapist supervision and consultation strategies Consultation to the patient	Behavioural chain analysis Behavioural formulation based on antecedents, behaviours and consequences
Relationship dysregulation	**Interpersonal effectiveness** Reducing conflict – GIVE: (be Gentle, act Interested, Validate, use Easy manner) Maintain self-respect: FAST (be Fair, no Apologies, Stick to your values, be Truthful) Getting what you want and saying No to unwanted requests and demands	**Dialectical strategies** 1. Entering the paradox 2. Use of metaphor 3. Devil's advocate 4. Extending 5. Activating the wise mind 6. Making lemonade out of lemons 7. Allowing natural change		Solution analysis Didactic strategies: Teaching, coaching Activities to increase positive emotions Contingency management Observing limits
Behavioural dysregulation	**Distress tolerance** Ability to tolerate and survive crisis situations without making them worse. 1. Crisis survival skills 2. Reality acceptance skills		**Other strategies** Commitment strategies Crisis strategies Suicidal behaviour strategies Telephone strategies Termination strategies	Positive reinforcement Negative reinforcement Shaping Extinction
Self dysregulation	**Core mindfulness** Observing, describing, and attending to the present moment without judgement.			
Cognitive dysregulation	Walking the middle path			

social factors, such as difficulties in early nurturing and containment such as an invalidating environment.

An understanding of the biological basis of emotional dysregulation [5] helps to appreciate the difficulty involved in changing behaviour. Behavioural problems are 'hard wired 'in the brain and not merely wilful misbehaviour. Behavioural theory can help to assess and formulate about both the antecedents and reinforcing factors of problematic behaviour. Behavioural change is achieved through a synthesis of change approaches based on new skills and acceptance strategies, which in turn are built on the inherent wisdom of the self. The therapeutic relationship is characterised by validation, acceptance, warmth and spontaneity. The Buddhist philosophy and mindfulness practice integral to the model helps to develop a tolerant and realistic stance in resolving the personal suffering of the patients.

The DBT model for BPD describes five areas of dysregulation that lead to clinical difficulties: emotional, interpersonal, self, behavioural and cognitive. Throughout therapy, there is an emphasis on dialectical reasoning, moving the patient from an 'either–or' to 'both–and' perspective, helping the patient to achieve a synthesis of opposing views. **Validation and problem-solving strategies** are two core strategies. Validation is not always agreeing with the patient, but finding the kernel of truth in another person's perspective or situation. This is essential before using problem-solving or change strategies.

Table 7.7 shows a broad map of DBT in terms of domains of dysregulation and different strategies to address symptoms.

Linehan was able to make use of the theory and practice of mindfulness to develop a set of skills that can be taught to patients who experience high levels of distress. DBT is delivered through a programme of individual and group therapy weekly over a year to 18-month period. In the pretreatment stage, orientation, commitment and agreement in goals are clearly explained and sought. Therapy progresses through clearly defined stages, and goals are set and prioritised in a hierarchy. For example, an emphasis on increasing safety and reducing behavioural dyscontrol that interfers with therapy is addressed from the beginning.

Though originally developed for patients with self-harm, DBT has been adapted for various disorders such as trauma and PTSD, substance use, depression, anger and eating disorders. In many disorders the core feature of emotional dysregulation is common. There is an evidence base that DBT is a useful treatment and is a primary model for treatment in some personality disorder services.

References

1. Clark DA, Beck AT. *Cognitive Therapy for Anxiety Disorders: Science and Practice.* New York: Guilford Press, 2010.

2. Gilbert P. *Compassion Focused Therapy.* London: Routledge, 2010.

3. Dobson KS, McEppalan AM, Dobson D. Empirical validation and cognitive-behavioural therapies. In KS Dobson, DJA Dozois, eds., *Handbook of Cognitive-Behavioral Therapies*, 4th ed.

New York: Guilford Press. 2019; pp. 32–63.

4. Linehan M. *Cognitive Behaviour Treatment of Borderline Personality Disorder.* New York: Guilford Press, 1993.

5. Niedtfeld I, Bohus M. Understanding the bio in biosocial theory of BPD: recent developments and implications for treatment. In M Swales, ed., *The Oxford Handbook of Dialectical Behaviour Therapy.* Oxford: Oxford University Press. 2019; pp. 23–46.

Further Reading

Beck J. *Cognitive Therapy Basics and Beyond.* New York: Guilford Press, 2011.

Beck AT, Emery G. *Anxiety Disorders and Phobias.* New York: Basic Books, 1985.

Beck AT, Rush A, Shaw BF, Emery G. *Cognitive Therapy of Depression.* New York: Guilford Press, 1979.

Kennerley H, Kirk J, Westbrook D. *An Introduction to Cognitive Behaviour Therapy: Skills and Applications*, 3rd ed. London: SAGE, 2016.

Koerner K. *Doing Dialectical Behavior Therapy: A Practical Guide.* New York: Guilford Press, 2012.

Rizvi S. *Chain Analysis in Dialectical Behavior Therapy.* New York: Guilford Press, 2019.

Brief Psychodynamic Psychotherapies

Frank Margison

Brief models of psychotherapy have been discussed for nearly a century but there is still considerable ambiguity about what exactly is meant by a brief therapy and what constitutes an effective brief intervention.

The focus in this chapter is on the brief therapies that are drawn from a broad set of psychodynamic and relational approaches, and emphasising those with evidence of effectiveness. It will look in more detail at some examples of well-established models of psychotherapy which work from this stance such as Dynamic Interpersonal Therapy (DIT) [1] and Psychodynamic Interpersonal Therapy (PIT) [2]. Initially, some of the basic concepts involved in brief therapy will be explored.

How Do We Choose Which Therapy?

The plurality of methods available makes it difficult to decide what approach is best for an individual patient. There is very little evidence that demonstrates that a particular therapy is superior to any other for a particular condition. That position has barely changed since Luborsky and colleagues commented about the Dodo bird effect – 'all have won and all shall have prizes' – citing Alice in Wonderland [3]. This is perhaps not surprising as the sample size of a study having enough statistical power to differentiate between two therapies would be enormous. It is generally considered, however, that the lack of differences relates to 'common therapeutic factors' [4] which contribute a lot of the variance in comparison studies.

Common Therapeutic Factors

Different methods of psychotherapy and counselling are thought to share *common factors* that account for much of the effectiveness of a psychological treatment. The empirical evidence for common factors is strong and refers back to writers from half a century ago who tried to describe the key factors. Jerome Frank described these common themes [5, p. 350]:

> *Common to all psychotherapies are (a) an emotionally charged, confiding relationship; (b) a therapeutic rationale accepted by patient and therapist; (c) provision of new information by precept, example and self-discovery; (d) strengthening of the patient's expectation of help; (e) providing the patient with success experiences; and (f) facilitation of emotional arousal.*

There is more that unites different approaches to therapy than separates them. The Centre for Outcomes Research and Evaluation (CORE at University College London) has developed a competence framework that provides a map describing common features down to specific details of particular models across these psychological approaches [6, 7]. This has allowed similarities and differences for most models of therapy to be described in very practical ways, including generic and specific areas of competence in different models of therapy including brief dynamic/analytic models such as DIT.

The *generic therapeutic competences for brief therapy* include relatively non-specific skills and knowledge, such as

- engaging the patient
- assessing and managing risk of self-harm

The next level of competence covers *basic psychodynamic skills* which are pertinent to brief therapy such as

- deriving a psychodynamic formulation
- managing therapeutic frame and boundaries
- maintaining an agreed focus

The next level covers skills specified in a *psychoanalytic way of working* with unconscious communication such as

- helping the patient become aware of unexpressed or unconscious feelings
- making psychodynamic interpretations
- working with countertransference
- recognizing and working with defences
- working through the termination phase of therapy

There are also a set of overarching '*generic meta-competences*' to support therapeutic flexibility concerning

- use of clinical judgement and adapting interventions in the light of patient feedback
- making use of the therapeutic relationship as a vehicle for change
- maintaining an appropriate balance between interpretive and supportive work
- applying the model flexibly and in context
- identifying and using the most appropriate among the analytic/dynamic approaches

After all of these shared aspects for the psychodynamic therapies there can then be specified techniques that delineate a very specific model, such as the specific competences for DIT or PIT.

What Do We Mean by Brief?

There is a somewhat arbitrary definition of less than 25 sessions in the psychotherapy research literature constituting brief therapy [8, p. 666], so in practice up to around six months of weekly therapy.

Initially brief and time-limited were seen as broadly synonymous as they were being contrasted with the mainstream psychoanalytic practice of an open-ended therapy, usually occurring several times a week, whereas brief psychodynamic therapies were typically weekly and over a much shorter period. Gradually the concept was refined through a multitude of research studies defining brief interventions as anything from 2 sessions [9] to around 24 sessions, with most clustering around 8, or 16 sessions [10].

Built into the concept of all brief therapies were gradually assimilated ideas that

(a) there is an inherent structure (even if only beginning, middle phase and ending phase)
(b) the intervention can be compared and contrasted with other therapies (usually through a treatment manual and fidelity measure)

(c) there should be some agreement about the desired result of the therapy (ultimately leading to ways of assessing outcome and setting agreed goals)

(d) the therapist is active, meaning that the therapist provides structure, intervenes more often than is common in psychoanalytic practice and often co-constructs meaning as part of the therapy

(e) there is a focus on maintaining and if necessary repairing a secure, positive therapeutic alliance

History of Brief Psychodynamic Approaches

The main purpose of Short-Term Dynamic Psychotherapy (STDP) was described by Michael Hobbs, previously consultant psychiatrist and psychotherapist in Oxford [11, p. 115], as

> ... to engage the patient in active examination of his difficulties, including how these impact on the therapeutic relationship, and thereby to liberate adaptive capacities and develop mental potential.

This idea is based on the assumption that individuals are blocked in their psychological development and that by gaining greater understanding of the origins and current manifestations of difficulties they can become freer to develop their potential.

The Therapy Is Time-Limited and Focusses on Ending

James Mann, a former professor of psychiatry in Boston and psychoanalyst [12], developed the idea that limiting the length of a therapy, usually 10 sessions in his model, was not just a practical aid to efficiency, but allowed a sharp focus on core anxieties about loss and separation. Mann's Time-Limited Therapy became a popular approach in its own right, but its lasting legacy was on having an agreed ending date at the outset and constantly keeping issues of ending in mind as a practical way of focussing on themes of loss. These principles have been incorporated into most forms of brief psychodynamic therapy.

The Therapist Is Active

A common feature of early brief psychodynamic models was in the therapist being active. This means that the therapist may be more directive about the structure and works with the client in understanding meaning, rather than commenting as if from outside. Typically, the therapist will say more and be more 'transparent' about his or her own thoughts and responses.

The disadvantage of greater therapist activity from a psychoanalytic perspective is that the therapist can become intrusive and foreclose options for the patient to imagine the therapist having qualities belonging to key figures from the past. Initially, this was seen as a 'trade-off' with brief psychodynamic approaches in effect being 'weaker' versions of psychoanalysis. There was criticism of these newer active methods for 'gratifying' the patient and losing valuable information by not holding to an 'abstinent' approach.

The current view is that psychoanalysis and brief psychodynamic psychotherapy are within the same broad family, but are essentially different in their methods and aims. STDPs have now evolved to the point that they can stand alone as distinct therapies in their own right, rather than diluted forms of psychoanalysis.

So, for example, in short-term psychodynamic therapies the therapist is less likely to leave long silences. There is likely to be greater collaborative effort in finding shared meaning, and the therapist is more likely to bring in to the conversation more information based on his or her own reactions.

These features are not absolute and different models and different therapists will fall on a spectrum of how comfortable they feel about being active. In some therapies, for example PIT, an active conversation between therapist and patient is seen as central to therapeutic change. This collaborative approach is also seen as central in other approaches to therapy (see Chapter 10 on cognitive analytic therapy), whereas some models expect the therapist to be less active and rely more on interpretation rather than jointly co-constructing meaning.

Inner Representations of Key Figures or Relationships

All psychodynamic therapies have in common ways in which key figures from the past continue to shape perceptions in the present, through unconscious psychological processes. Some approaches to therapy are based on psychoanalytic theory. For example, Brief Psychoanalytic Therapy developed by R Peter Hobson, a British psychoanalyst, psychiatrist and researcher in developmental psychology [13], works with a revised and updated model of transference and countertransference drawing on Object Relations theory based on the work of Melanie Klein and her followers.

Another powerful way of understanding these inner representations is from Attachment Theory. This theoretical approach began with John Bowlby [14] (see Chapter 1) but has become an underpinning concept for many psychodynamic and relational therapies and has developed its own specific school of therapy. Holmes and Slade [15] describe an Attachment-based psychotherapy based on the work of John Bowlby and colleagues reiterating the key emphasis on modifying internalised models of attachment figures.

Another influential approach came from Lester Luborsky, a prominent US researcher into psychotherapy effectiveness [16], who described the *Core Conflictual Relationship Theme* (CCRT). This approach is characterised by three components: a wished-for state, a typical response from the Other and a response of the Self.

This has been developed into a full coding system for relationship themes in his symptom-context method [17], and an example is given below.

> Wish: I wish to be loved and positively responded to and to avoid the recurrent experiences of rejection.
> Response from Other: Rejects and dominates me
> Response from Self: I am self-critical, self-destructive, helpless, and sometimes oppositional (for example by cancelling the session to get back at my therapist)   Luborsky [17, p. 9]

Other psychotherapy researchers developed similar models of repetitive conflicts in relationships as the core of the work in brief therapies. Hans Strupp, another prominent US psychotherapy researcher, and colleagues developed *Time-Limited Dynamic Psychotherapy* (TLDP). The patterns are called Cyclical Maladaptive Patterns (CMPs) [18]. The key themes are similar to those in the CCRT in including

- Acts of the Self
- Expectations of the reactions of others and
- Acts of others towards the self with an additional category of

- Acts of the self towards the self

The additional category is helpful in unpicking the damaging internal relationships with overwhelming self-criticism that is difficult to access without understanding the self-to-self aspects of object relations. Self-to-self relationships are often experienced as part of an inner dialogue – usually critical in nature, for example, 'I despise myself'. They are often hard to access because both aspects ('I and me') are experienced as part of the self.

At around the same time, in the United Kingdom, there was a similar growing emphasis on researchable, succinct models to understand repeated patterns in relating. Anthony Ryle (as described in Chapter 10) was developing a model of internalised *Reciprocal Role Procedures* as the templates of similar ways of habitually relating to the self and to others.

Robert Hobson [19, pp. 169–73] in his Conversational Model (later described as Psychodynamic Interpersonal Therapy (PIT)) described *'Explanatory Hypotheses'* to summarise these interpersonal conflicts that led to recurrent symptoms and relationship difficulties. In this model, the word hypothesis was used to emphasise the tentative, collaborative co-construction of the meaning of a symptom [2, pp. 167–8].

David Malan, a British psychoanalytic psychotherapist, made a major contribution to the development of brief dynamic psychotherapy in his seminal text *Brief Dynamic Psychotherapy* [20]. He provided an integrative summary described as the overlapping Triangles of Person and of Conflict. This highly influential model involved a pattern of a feeling or impulse leading to anxiety, and in turn to psychological defences that block the person's development. The same triangle of conflict can be traced in relationships (especially parents) in the past; others in the outside present; and in the (transference) relationship with the therapist [20, p. 80]. These triangles are still widely used in drawing up a psychodynamic formulation to help maintain the therapeutic focus.

An example Malan uses to demonstrate this triangle concerns a young man who has a repetitive pattern of backing off and being unable to feel as his relationships with women develop. The inability to feel is suggested as a *defence*, against the *anxiety* of something happening if he becomes more deeply involved. The deeper, hidden *feeling* is of overwhelming loss and grief. Initially this triangle is explored about his current relationship *outside (other relationship)*, but then further links are made to the same triangle in relation to his mother's death (*past or parental relationship*). After a period of resistance to change, a breakthrough occurs when the patient is made aware of a similar constellation in relation to the *therapist (transference relationship)*. The triangles act as a form of scaffolding to help the therapist build up links, eventually allowing change to occur [20, pp. 80–91]. What is most striking about reading Malan's example is the gradual, patient piecing together of links until the whole rich picture emerges. This is similar to Hobson's Conversational model which also gradually builds up hypotheses of increasing depth [19, pp. 197–8].

More recently, in *Dynamic Interpersonal Therapy* (DIT) the underlying pattern is described as an *Interpersonal Affective Focus* (IPAF) [1, p. 106].

This approach takes the same basic elements but describes them in terms that Otto Kernberg, a psychoanalyst and professor of psychiatry [21], had developed. The IPAF dimensions are described as:

- Self Representation (e.g. a demanding infant: *'I always ask for too much'*)
- An Object representation (e.g. a rejecting mother: *'No-one is there for me when I need them'*)

- An affect linking the two themes (e.g. terror: 'The worst moments are when I feel in pain and there is no-one to turn to.')
- The defensive function of this configuration (e.g. avoidance of own aggression – by maintaining the other in one's mind as 'always rejecting' the patient can remain in the victim position and avoid reflecting on his own tendency to reject.)

Focus

A common theme across the brief psychodynamic and relational therapies is an emphasis on *Focus*. The focus may be a restatement of a *formulation* as described using the methods described above, but expressed in practical ways and often linked to defined goals. Most brief therapies have an initial period of a few sessions agreeing such a *focus*.

It now seems obvious to focus the time available on some agreed aspects of the person's difficulties, but this was a contentious matter, and only after there was a clear consensus in the research literature did it become incorporated in routine practice:

> *The major technical error related to negative outcomes in brief therapy is the failure of the therapist to structure or focus the sessions* [22].

Setting Goals

How the therapist helps the patient to define their goals will determine how they work together. A goal may be very specific but limited in its depth of understanding. For example, an agreed goal may be to show reliable and clinically significant change on an agreed measure, say of depression. Reliable means that the change is more than measurement error, and clinically significant means that the person shifts from a score characteristic of an unwell population to the score typical of the general population – shown practically as falling below a threshold score [23].

. This way of setting goals is helpful in making sure a therapy stays 'on track' and in giving feedback on progress, but the goal is likely to lack any personal meaning. Some goals may be common and shared by most people, but more specific than a score on an outcome measure (e.g. feeling able to enjoy social events with friends), or something very specific and personal like being able to cry at the anniversary of the death of a child without feeling cut off and empty [24].

Length and Structure

Most brief therapies have an inherent structure embedded within an agreed length of therapy. DIT [1], for example, has 16 sessions as its standard length defining what they call a '*Trajectory of Therapy*', with an Initial Phase of Sessions 1–4 aimed at engagement, and identifying the focus. The Middle Phase of Sessions 5–12 is where the main intervention occurs using a variety of techniques including interpretation, focussing on affect, and mentalising interventions alongside more general interventions such as clarification. The final phase covers sessions 13–16 focussing on ending and paying full attention to loss. As with many brief therapies the ending is consolidated with a letter from the therapist to patient.

PIT [2, pp. 20–2] does not have a standard length but agrees a length as determined by the type of focus. At one extreme there has been a study of two-session therapy with one follow-up session [9] which showed that a skilled therapist can achieve substantial change after a very brief intervention in patients with mild depression. At the other extreme in Australian studies with patients with borderline disorders a therapy of one to two years has been evaluated [25]. However, the commonest lengths have been 8- and 16-session therapies with better results overall for the longer version in more severe depression, but no difference by length in less severe depression [2, p. 20; 26].

Key Factors in Encouraging Change in Brief Therapies

In brief psychodynamic and relational approaches, we discussed earlier the way in which a therapist is active, attentive to the therapeutic alliance, collaborative, and focussed on agreed goals, but the way in which change occurs needs further discussion.

Across models there are some common themes. In an effective therapy, patients learn new strategies for managing distressing experiences. This may be through learning new techniques such as mindfulness, distress tolerance, distraction or other active methods, or change may gradually occur as the individual learns new ways of relating to self and others. But we need a pan-theoretical model for how change occurs rather than ad hoc explanations. One such approach described below is the Assimilation Model [27].

Assimilation of Problems

The assimilation model provides such a pan-theoretical model of change. It sees the process of change in therapy as being focussed on particular problematic experiences as opposed to change in an abstract concept such as the personality of the person [2, pp. 47–50].

Different problematic experiences differ in how far they have already been assimilated. Problematic experiences vary considerably and include memories, wishes, feelings, attitudes and behaviours. In a successful therapy they gradually become less painful and the experience of success gradually becomes incorporated into the individual's self-schema. Prior to being assimilated, however, they are experienced as painful or jarring as they comprise, for example, threatening or painful events or difficult or destructive relationships.

The Assimilation model suggests that positive change is seen when patients follow a developmental sequence of initially *recognising*, then *reformulating, understanding* and eventually *resolving* problematic experiences. The way in which problems are assimilated will differ across models of therapy and Stiles and colleagues showed in some detail how the processes differ in two very different models (cognitive behavioural therapy (CBT) and PIT) [28]. This was summarised by Barkham and colleagues [2, p. 49]:

> *PIT is effective when the patient still has difficulty articulating the problem but experiences distress, whereas cognitive approaches may be preferable when the problem has already been clarified.*

While this particular research programme used PIT as the relational model, the findings are probably applicable to any therapy that is attempting to bring painful experience into awareness as a key element of the process.

Brief Dynamic Interpersonal Therapy (DIT) [1]

DIT, in common with many relational therapies, aims to help the patient to understand the connection between presenting symptoms and what is happening in relationships through identifying a core repetitive pattern of relating that can be traced back to childhood. It explicitly borrows from best practice across other brief dynamic therapies in terms of structure and approach. This approach was developed by Alessandra Lemma, Mary Target and Peter Fonagy, all professors of psychology in the UK, and describe in their authoritative account of DIT entitled *Brief Dynamic Interpersonal Therapy: A Clinician Guide* [1].

Once a problematic pattern is identified, it is used to make sense of current difficulties in relationships. It aims to relieve symptoms of distress, especially with symptoms related to relationship difficulties. When the relationship problem can be managed more effectively, psychological symptoms will often improve. DIT aims to help people recognise specific relationship patterns and to make changes to modify these relational patterns [1, p. 63].

The way that a problem is formulated in DIT follows the examples of Object Relations Theory discussed earlier [21] to develop an IPAF [1, p. 107].

A case example is given to illustrate this way of working [1, pp. 110–11]. This describes Carol, a 27-year-old woman with panic and binge-eating problems. The problems came to a head after the break-up of a relationship six months earlier when Carol was confronted with feelings of loneliness through her future. The formulation makes a link between anxious attachment in her adult relationships and the relationship with her mother. The clingy, rejection-fearing style of relationship was rapidly repeated with the therapist. Her mother was simultaneously presented as a perfect role model and emotionally unavailable and Carol coped with her mother's absences by not thinking about her. As the sessions developed, a theme about Carol describing her mother as cold and distant was also seen as a way of defending Carol against awareness of her own capacity to be aggressive to others.

This is formulated as a key object relation being:

> a needy, deprived self relating to a dismissive, unavailable other. The conscious affect with this was, in fact, a lack of affect: Carol described dissociating from her feelings, retreating into a 'nothing matters' state that she recreated in her binges.

The formulation goes on to describe Carol's core conscious fear as of 'loneliness', and this was recreated in the sessions as a need for 'a very intensive therapy'.

> [C]oming into therapy the internal model that was activated was one where Carol felt like a very needy, deprived child who needed to secure as many sessions as possible with her therapist as a way of controlling her because she anticipated in her mind an unavailable mother / therapist.

The case discussion leads into a summary of the key elements of formulation in DIT.

1. Describe the problem
2. Describe the psychic cost [restrictions] of the problem
3. Contextualise the problem from the history and relevant factors at the time of presentation
4. Describe the recurring self-other relationship patterns connected to the presenting symptoms

5. Identify the defensive function of the identified self-other representation

The book offers practical suggestions about staying focussed, working in the transference and working with defences, and then how to support attempts at changing patterns in relationships [1, pp. 140–2].

Psychodynamic Interpersonal Therapy (PIT) [2]

PIT began with a research project funded by the Medical Research Council to describe and define a model of psychotherapy to use in subsequent outcome studies. There is now a large research base supporting the effectiveness of PIT in various settings, especially for depression and in psychiatric liaison settings for upper and lower gastrointestinal tract disorders and self-harm. A longer form of the therapy has been developed in Australia for treatment of borderline disorders.

The outcome studies are described fully in a chapter in Barkham and colleagues' book *Psychodynamic Interpersonal Therapy: A Conversational Model* [2, pp. 15–32]. There is also an overview of the extensive research base using process-outcome methods to understand what is involved in delivering effective PIT therapy [2, pp. 32–50], and on the development of competence, including teaching methods to improve PIT skills [2, pp. 137–52] across several professional groups.

The Four Key Ideas in PIT

(1) Conversation

Robert ('Bob') Hobson developed the idea of a common 'feeling language' arising in a therapeutic conversation. The therapist and patient engage in creating a conversation in which shared understanding develops [19, pp. 247–54]. Some of the early research on the model showed that the conversational concept could be taught in some very practical ways by watching films of therapy sessions; practising basic skills; role plays; and eventually supervised practice [32].

The research on beginner psychiatrists showed that simple teaching could assist the trainees to shift substantially from an interrogatory style to something more collaborative and shared. By the time they were ready to see actual patients in a clinical setting they were safe and already reasonably competent in their practice [33]. At a practical level there was a marked shift after training from a series of questions to a more tentative, negotiated style with hypotheses in the form of statements rather than questions [34].

Over the last 30 years these initial findings have been replicated with several other professional groups (nurses, psychologists, social workers and counsellors) demonstrating how basic competence can be developed effectively for relatively inexperienced therapists. For example, Guthrie and colleagues showed that complex patients treated by primary care counsellors given additional training for one week in PIT plus weekly supervision could achieve clinically significant and reliable change in 50 per cent of complex long-term patients [35]. The counsellors gave positive feedback about feeling more able to manage the demands of seeing highly complex patients. A further study showed that PIT was effective and cost-effective in reducing admissions and other costs in a study of complex multi-diagnosis, long-term outpatients treated with short-term PIT [36], mainly through developing a conversation about symptoms such as depression, rather than taking a medical history.

These aspects of a therapeutic conversation can be assessed through a rating tool to check adherence to the model (Psychodynamic Interpersonal Therapy Rating Scale: PITRS) [2, pp. 157–75].

(2) Forms of Feeling

The notion of 'forms of feeling' is crucial to the conversational model approach found in PIT [2, pp. 192–3]. Hobson referred to a form of 'emotional knowing' which is very different to an intellectual way of thinking about problems. This alternative form of knowing requires a form of creative imagination or symbolic attitude which links together feeling states and associated symbols to produce greater coherence in the sense of self [37, pp. 84–92].

(3) Minute Particulars

Hobson used the term 'minute particulars' [19, pp. 161, 165–6] to refer to the ability of the therapist to pay especially close attention to the subtle nuances of a conversation. Paying attention to minimal changes in inflection or gaze, the therapist starts to share an understanding of the other's inner state through a series of tentative hypotheses (Box 8.1).

(4) Research and Practice Synergy

The minute details of how PIT therapists work with patients have been examined in a large number of process studies using the assimilation model, studies of impact and helpful aspects of therapy, repair of damage to the therapeutic alliance, therapist responsiveness, focus and style, attachment style, patient expectations and other process studies. These studies are summarised in detail elsewhere [2, pp. 33–50] with an overview of the implications for the practice of brief therapy.

Box 8.1 Core skills in PIT

Basic skills:
- Use of Statements rather than questions
- Picking up cues (verbal, vocal, non-verbal, and in the therapist)
- Negotiation
- Understanding hypotheses

Intermediate skills:
- Focussing on feelings (here and now)
- Metaphor (living symbols)
- Language of mutuality
- Linking hypotheses

Advanced skills:
- Explanatory hypotheses
- Rationale for exploratory therapy
- Sequencing interventions
- Relating interpersonal change to therapy
- Patterns in relationships

In brief, PIT therapists do what they say they do – they maintain a therapeutic focus; use a lot of reflection in the form of understanding hypotheses; focus on the 'here and now'; with attention to detail in the 'minute particulars'. They use a combination of collaboration and firmness in staying with difficult themes previously agreed through a shared understanding. These themes are exemplified in an initial session developed as part of a series of teaching films with Mary the therapist meeting Alex who has lost her child, Zoe:

> The session is dominated by unbearable feelings following the death of Zoe. The therapist helps her to stay with these feelings and powerful metaphors emerge about being frozen in time and feeling shattered into a thousand pieces.
>
> Alex is yearning and describes the loss as a bodily feeling. She is unable to move forward, and feels bewildered and stuck. The therapist then explores a link with an earlier loss as Alex had found her own mother dead after a stroke.
>
> Alex started to make links between the loss of her mother and the death of her daughter – feeling cheated as a child of her mother's love and now cheated of the chance to repair that loss by loving her own child. It becomes clear that the descriptions of the two losses mirror each other very closely, and Mary the therapist focusses on exploring the bewildering feelings of anger, sadness, fear and self-blame.
>
> They build on the extended metaphor of feeling shattered after what feels like a catastrophe and there are powerful moments about the coldness and stillness of her mother and finding her child Zoe also still and cold.
>
> At the end of the session Mary starts to pull these themes of loss together and the session ends with agreement to meet again to explore further.

Re-enactments of relationship problems from the past, or errors by the therapist, can lead to ruptures in the therapeutic alliance and the alliance is a key predictor of outcome, so several schools of brief therapy have developed methods of identifying and repairing the damaged therapeutic relationship. For example, in PIT, Agnew and colleagues [38] described the key stages: acknowledgement of the problem; negotiating; exploring the difficulties; reaching a new consensus; renegotiating; leading to deeper exploration and finally closure. Interestingly, Stiles and colleagues [39] showed that the outcome after a successful repair to the therapeutic alliance was *better* than if no disruption had occurred.

These findings were specifically from studies on PIT (or comparisons between PIT and CBT), but it is likely that many of these themes would apply equally to other brief relational therapies as they are so consistent with the findings about effective factors in brief psychotherapy from many reviews in the literature.

The theoretical underpinning of PIT [40] is not dissimilar in many ways to DIT and other psychodynamic models, but an important difference is in developing the model for practitioners who do not have wide experience and knowledge of psychodynamic principles, as seen in a recent development aimed to develop empathy skills in practitioners delivering basic CBT [41].

What Are the Fundamental Differences and Similarities between Models of Brief Psychotherapy?

There have been some specific differences highlighted earlier in this chapter, for example some therapies using specific theories such as object-relations and attachment theory. However, the main emphasis has been on what is common between the different models of dynamic and relational therapies, and the key points are summarised in Box 8.2.

Box 8.2 Key points in understanding brief therapies

1. Brief therapy covers a multitude of different approaches (see [42])
2. There is a structure with particular tasks linked to the different phases (see Lambert and Ogles for a fuller description [4]).
3. The length is conventionally defined as 25 sessions or less and commonly falls in the 8–16 session range (see [4])
4. There is a focus for the therapy – and this is typically agreed within the first 3–4 sessions (see [8–16])
5. The focus is usually linked to specific goals, ideally expressed in terms that are measurable but also meaningful and agreed with the patient (see [23, 24])
6. The focus is usually expressed in relation to areas of conflict, often linking the past, outside relationships and the relationship with the therapist (see [20])
7. These conflicts can be expressed in terms of repeating relationship patterns often expressed as internalised models of relationships (see [17–22])
8. The therapist will try to develop a secure therapeutic relationship within which conflict can be explored (see [37])
9. If there are ruptures in the therapeutic relationship (whether related to therapist errors or powerful past patterns intruding), the therapist will make specific efforts to repair the rupture [38] often with benefit to the eventual outcome if done skilfully [39]
10. Towards the end of the therapy there is typically a phase of consolidation, with particular attention to how what has been learned can influence future interactions. Commonly, though not in all models, a letter is given to the patient, or letters are exchanged, to support change [2, pp. 129–33]
11. Brief therapies tend to have active forms of supervision where close attention to detail is paid, often using audio or video recordings [2, pp. 149–52]
12. Active learning methods are commonly used to accelerate the learning of new psychotherapy skills, using role play, self-ratings, video feedback, teaching films, structured process notes [2, pp. 137–52]

References

1. Lemma A, Target M, Fonagy P. *Brief Dynamic Interpersonal Therapy: A Clinician's Guide.* Oxford: Oxford University Press, 2011.

2. Barkham M, Guthrie E, Hardy GE, Margison F. *Psychodynamic-Interpersonal Therapy: A Conversational Model.* London: SAGE, 2017.

3. Luborsky L, Singer B, Luborsky L. Is it true that 'everyone has won and all must have prizes'? *Arch Gen Psychiatry* 1975; 32(8): 995–1008.

4. Lambert MJ, Ogles BM. The efficacy and effectiveness of psychotherapy: common factors and outcome. In MJ Lambert, ed., *Bergin and Garfield's Handbook of Psychotherapy and Behaviour Change*, 5th ed. New York: John Wiley & Sons. 2004; pp. 139–93.

5. Frank JD. Therapeutic factors in psychotherapy. *Am J Psychother* 1971; 25(3): 350–61.

6. Lemma A, Roth AD, Pilling S. *The competences required to deliver effective psychoanalytic/psychodynamic therapy.* London: Research Department of Clinical, Educational and Health Psychology UCL, 2008. www.ucl.ac.uk/drupal/site_pals/sites/pals/files/migrated-files/PPC_Clinicians_Background_Paper.pdf [Accessed 22/03/2019]

7. www.ucl.ac.uk/pals/research/clinical-educational-and-health-psychology/research-groups/core/competence-frameworks [Accessed 22/03/2019]

8. Koss MP, Shiang J. Research on brief psychotherapy. In AE Bergin, SL Garfield, eds., *Handbook of Psychotherapy and Behaviour Change*, 4th ed. New York: Wiley. 1994; pp. 664–700.

9. Barkham M, Shapiro DA, Hardy GE, Rees A. Psychotherapy in two-plus-one sessions: outcomes of a randomized controlled trial of cognitive-behavioural and psychodynamic-interpersonal therapy for subsyndromal depression. *J Consult Clin Psychol* 1999; 67: 201–11.

10. Barkham M, Guthrie E, Hardy GE, Margison F . The efficacy and effectiveness of psychodynamic-interpersonal therapy: a 30-year overview. In: *Psychodynamic-Interpersonal Therapy: A Conversational Model*. London: SAGE. 2017; pp. 15–32.

11. Hobbs M. Short-term dynamic psychotherapy. In S Bloch, ed., *An Introduction to the Psychotherapies*, 4th ed. Oxford: Oxford University Press. 2006; pp. 111–40.

12. Mann J. *Time-Limited Psychotherapy*. Harvard: Harvard University Press, 1973.

13. Hobson RP. *Brief Psychoanalytic Therapy*. Oxford: Oxford University Press, 2016.

14. Holmes J. *John Bowlby and Attachment Theory*. New York: Routledge, 1993.

15. Holmes J, Slade A. *Attachment in Therapeutic Practice*. London: SAGE, 2018.

16. Luborsky L, Crits-Christoph P. *Understanding Transference: The CCRT Method*. New York: Basic Books, 1990.

17. Luborsky L. Documenting symptom formation during psychotherapy. In NE Miller, L Luborsky, JP Barber, J Dogherty, eds., *Psychodynamic Treatment Research: A Handbook for Clinical Practice*. New York: Basic Books. 1993; pp. 3–13.

18. Schacht TE, Binder JL, Strupp HH. The dynamic focus. In HH Strupp, JL Binder, eds., *Psychotherapy in a New Key: A Guide to Time-Limited Dynamic Psychotherapy*. New York: Basic Books. 1984; pp. 65–109.

19. Hobson RF. *Forms of Feeling: The Heart of Psychotherapy*. London: Routledge (Tavistock), 1985.

20. Malan DH. *Individual Psychotherapy and the Science of Psychodynamics*. London: Butterworths, 1979.

21. Kernberg O. *Internal World and External Reality: Object Relations Theory Applied*. New York: Jason Aronson, 1985.

22. Budman SH, Gurman AS. The practice of brief therapy. *Prof Psychol Res Pr* 1983; 14: 277–92. Cited in [8] p. 672.

23. Evans C, Margison F, Barkham M. The contribution of reliable and clinically-significant change methods to evidence-based mental health. *Evid Based Ment Health* 1998; 1(3): 70–2.

24. Feltham A, Martin K, Walker L. et al. Using goals in therapy: the perspective of people with lived experience. In M Cooper, D Law, eds., *Working with Goals in Psychotherapy and Counselling*. Oxford: Oxford University Press. 2018; pp. 73–86.

25. Meares R, Stevenson J, Comerford A. Psychotherapy with borderline patients: a comparison between treated and untreated cohorts. *Aust N Z J Psychiatry* 1999; 33: 467–72.

26. Shapiro DA, Barkham M, Rees A et al. Effect of treatment duration and severity of depression on the effectiveness of cognitive-behavioural and psychodynamic-interpersonal psychotherapy. *J Consult Clin Psychol* 1994; 62: 522–34.

27. Stiles WB. Assimilation of problematic experiences. In JC Norcross, ed., *Psychotherapy Relationships that Work: Therapist Contributions and Responsiveness to Patients*. Oxford: Oxford University Press. 2002; pp. 165–81.

28. Stiles WB, Elliott R, Llewelyn SP et al. Assimilation of problematic experiences by patient in psychotherapy. *Psychotherapy* 1990; 27: 411–20.

29. Stiles WB, Reynolds S, Hardy GE et al. Evaluation and description of psychotherapy sessions by patients using the Session Evaluation Questionnaire and

the Session Impacts Scale. *J Consult Clin Psychol* 1994; 41: 175–85.

30. *The Improving Access to Psychological Therapies Manual* [Gateway reference: 08101 Version number: 2] National Collaborating Centre for Mental Health: 2018. www.england.nhs.uk/wp-content/uploads/2019/02/improving-access-to-psychological-therapies-manual.pdf [Accessed 22/03/2018]

31. Lemma A, Target M, Fonagy P. The development of a brief psychodynamic protocol for depression: dynamic interpersonal therapy. *Psychoanal Psychother* 2010; 24(4): 329–46.

32. Margison FR. Psychotherapy: advances in training methods. *Adv Psychiatr Treat* 1999; 5: 329–37.

33. Shaw CM, Margison FR, Guthrie E et al. Psychodynamic-interpersonal therapy by inexperienced therapists in a naturalistic setting: a pilot study. *Eur J PsychotherCounsell Health* 2001; 4: 87–101.

34. Maguire GP, Goldberg DP, Hobson RF et al. Evaluating the teaching of a model of psychotherapy. *Br J Psychiatry* 1984; 144: 575–80.

35. Guthrie E, Margison FR, Mackay H et al. Effectiveness of psychodynamic-interpersonal therapy

training for primary care counsellors. *Psychother Res* 2004; **14**: 161–75.

36. Guthrie E, Moorey J, Margison F. et al. Cost-effectiveness of brief psychodynamic-interpersonal therapy in high utilizers of psychiatric services. *Arch Gen Psychiatry* 1994; 56: 519–26.

37. Meares R. *Intimacy & Alienation: Memory, Trauma and Personal Being.* London: Routledge, 2000.

38. Agnew RM, Harper H, Shapiro DA, et al. Resolving a challenge to the therapeutic relationship: a single case-study. *Br J Med Psychol* 1994; 67: 155–70.

39. Stiles WB, Glick MJ, Osatuke K et al. Patterns of alliance development and the rupture-repair hypothesis: are productive relationships U-shaped or V-shaped? *J Consult Clin Psychol* 2004; 51: 81–92.

40. Guthrie E, Moorey J. The theoretical basis of the Conversational Model of Therapy. *Psychoanal Psychother* 2018; 32(3): 282–300.

41. Guthrie E, Hughes R, Brown RJ. Pi-E: an empathy skills training package to enhance therapeutic skills of IAPT and other therapists. *Br J Psychother* 2018; 34(3): 408–27.

42. Parry S. *The Handbook of Brief Therapies.* London: SAGE Publications, 2019.

Systemic Family Therapy

P. J. Saju

Chapter 9

Introduction

Family therapy represents a major conceptual shift in the approach to understanding and treatment of psychological disturbance and mental illness. Within this approach symptoms are understood as the consequence of disturbance in the functioning of the family as a whole, expressed by the individual with the manifest difficulty. An understanding of how the identified patient and family affect each other both positively and negatively can lead to effective family interventions.

This chapter will introduce the development of key ideas and schools of thought within family therapy as a treatment approach. The history of family therapy provides a fascinating mirror for changes in society; the emergence of different theoretical models and treatment techniques within it reflects changes in attitudes towards what constitutes a family, with a greater recognition of diversity and cultural variation, as well as revealing assumptions and value systems which need to be challenged as society continues to evolve and to change.

The main theoretical framework is referred to as systemic theory. This is also applicable as a model in mental health care more widely, due to its focus on the system as the whole and its understanding of the wider context within which psychological disturbance occurs. This chapter will end with a consideration of how systemic thinking is helpfully applied within psychiatric practice.

The Origins of Family Therapy

In the 1930s **Alfred Adler**, an Austrian doctor and psychotherapist, whose ideas diverged from Freud developed Individual Psychology, and saw children with their parents for the first time. In the early stages of family therapy, the theoretical model was largely based on psychoanalytical approaches and was driven by ideas about families having potentially pathogenic influences on individual members. In the late 1950s, pathological family functioning was suspected to be linked to schizophrenia. This focus generated a body of research looking at family interactions, and communication.

A key contributor in the history of family therapy was Gregory Bateson, an anthropologist and social scientist. In 1956 Bateson introduced the term '**double blind**' communication, a term which refers to a contradiction between the different types of communications given out at the same time [1]. 'Digital' communication (verbal or written) may contradict with 'analogical' communication (non-verbal, gestures, tone of voice, facial expression etc.). A much-quoted example is of a mother who visits her son with schizophrenia in a hospital. He is glad to see her and puts his arm around her shoulders, in response to which she physically stiffens. Noticing this, he withdraws his arm at which point she asks, 'Don't you love me anymore?' When he then blushes, she says 'You must not get embarrassed and don't be afraid of your feelings.' The first bind in this example concerns the son's inability to confront his mother. The second bind is that the son is trapped by his dependence which prevents him from distancing himself from his mother. The contradictory nature of the mother's responses means that a coherent response or resolution is impossible. Prolonged exposure to this dilemma was considered to be associated with the development of psychosis.

A related idea was that of the schizophrenogenic mother [2], in which a mixture of maternal overprotectiveness and domination was seen as evidence of how the mother's own psychopathology could 'drive healthy children mad'. This also illustrated how these early theoreticians came to be seen as potentially blaming family members for the disturbance in their children.

A plethora of further ideas and new terms to describe them emerged; **Lyman Wynne** described **psuedomutuality** [3], that is families presenting with a facade of unity which ignored conflict and prohibited individual separation. **Psuedohostility** referred to a superficial alienation of family members that masked their needs of intimacy and affection. **Theodore and Ruth Lidz** in 1957 described '**marital schism**' where parents showed overt hostility but remained married because of pathological interdependence. In '**marital skew**', the conflicts and hostilities were hidden [4, 5].

Murray Bowen, a psychiatrist and major family theoretician in the 1970s, emphasised the importance of the **differentiation of self** from the '**families undifferentiated ego mass**' for psychological health and individual development. Excessive emotional interdependence, called **emotional fusion**, led to a poor differentiation of the self. Poorly differentiated parents raised poorly differentiated children. Bowen stated that unresolved problems were transmitted to the next generation through a process of **multigenerational transmission.** A person with a well-differentiated 'self' is able to have realistic dependence on others, and can handle conflict, criticism and rejection. Bowen also developed the idea of a **Genogram** representing three generations of family members and their relationship patterns pictorially (see below) [6, 7]. Genograms can show **triangles** (three person systems), historic and current **emotional cut-offs** and problematic patterns such as abuse, alcoholism over generations. Genograms continue to be used as helpful tools for mapping family relationships within a range of treatment approaches.

Systemic Family Therapies

In the 1960s families began to be conceptualised as complex systems. The term 'systems' refers to complex interrelated and interacting elements which are organised hierarchically. The system can vary from simple to very complex depending on the number of elements and their organisation.

To function in a coordinated way, the system needs to have control and feedback mechanisms. Cybernetics and general system theory help to understand the interactions. Cybernetics, a term coined by the mathematician Norbert Wiener, is the study of the self-corrective feedback mechanisms in complex systems including both mechanical and social systems. General System Theory (GST) was developed by the biologist, Ludwig von Bertalanffy to describe self-regulation through feedback in the living organism (e.g. levels of glucose, temperature control etc.) [8].

This idea that the family is a system governed by cybernetic principles was taken up by influential writings of Gregory Bateson. Some of the implications of Cybernetic/Systemic model are listed below.

1. The whole is more than the sum of its parts: each part can only be understood in the context of the whole and change in any part of the system will affect other parts

2. The family, as a cybernetic system is governed by its own organising rules and norms. The rules and norms are formed by all members based on their shared stories and beliefs about the family and not by any one individual. There is a tendency for stability and balance, that is, homeostasis, which requires interrelated dynamics to maintain stability

3. Systemic theory brought a paradigm shift in our thinking, from the focus on the individual to **interactions, patterns, connections, relationships and mutual influences** between people. While non-systemic theories are based on a linear model of causality (A causes B), in a cybernetic model, causation is circular with mutual influence (A influences B, and B influences A through feedback loops). This is why the therapist intervenes at the relational system, rather than an individual patient

4. Though the patterns may have been established over time, the therapist tends to focus on the ongoing interactions, that is, in the here and now. This was in part a reaction against the dominant psychoanalytic model of that time, drawing attention to current relationship patterns rather than analysing causes

First and Second Order Change

According to systemic family therapy there are two levels of change possible.

First order change occurs within the existing rules and structures and does not alter the operating system of the family. For example, when adolescent siblings fight the parents may use more or less punishment to control the fighting. The family's rule is that that power is used to control their children and therefore the children use physical power to control each other. The punishment may reduce the problematic behaviour (fight) by first order change, but underlying rule (one must obey or submit to those in power) remains unchanged.

Second order change involves fundamental changes in the rules and norms of the family. If the fight is reframed, with a positive connotation, such that siblings are learning to practice autonomy as developing adults, the meaning of the fighting is transformed, and the ways to respond to it will be different.

Early Models of Systemic Therapy: First Order Cybernetics (1950s to mid 1970s)

In first order cybernetics, the assumption is that the therapist could stand outside the family system as an independent, objective observer. The therapist believes they have the expertise and power to make judgements about what is normal and healthy and intervene to make changes.

The Mental Research Institute (MRI) in Palo Alto opened in 1959 and became a leading organisation in the development of family therapy. Gregory Bateson, and his colleagues Don Jackson, Jay Healy, John Wakeland and William Fry, developed a model of Brief Family

Therapy. In this model (MRI Brief Therapy), the problem was defined in clear, concrete terms and all previous attempted solutions were investigated. The therapist defined the desired changes in clear concrete terms and formulated and implemented a strategy for change. The MRI influenced the development of two schools of therapy, Structural Family Therapy and Strategic Family Therapy [9].

Virginia Satir, also working at the MRI, later developed Conjoint Family Therapy, which was firmly based on the family's innate capacity for growth. Communication skills and expression of emotions were important in her model, which was a forerunner of a 'strength-based approach' to family therapy, focussing on strengths and resources in the family, rather than their problems, pathologies and deficits [10].

Structural Family Therapy was developed by Salvatore Minuchin, an Argentinian child psychiatrist who also trained in psychoanalysis, worked closely with Jay Haley and introduced the use of a one-way mirror by which therapists could observe therapy sessions with families. The basic premise in this model is that a well-functioning family has an organisational structure with clear **hierarchies** between generations. An effective parental hierarchy refers to the parent's ability to set boundaries and limits while maintaining emotional closeness. Within the family structure are **subsystems** such as spousal, parental and sibling alliances. The **boundaries** of a subsystem are the rules defining who participates in a transaction and how. **Coalitions, alignments and alliances** between members are identified as contributing to the overall functioning and communication patterns within the family. Effective family boundaries are like the membrane of the cell: strong, but also remaining permeable. Healthy families are able to maintain an optimal balance between **connectedness and differentiation**, whereas less healthy family functioning is prone to either **disengagement or enmeshment**. In enmeshed families, boundaries are weak with low levels of individual differentiation and autonomy. In disengaged families, the boundaries are rigid and impermeable with low levels of nurturance or support to other members [11, 12].

In structural therapy, the therapist is active, like a stage director, setting up scenarios for enactments, and directing family members to interact in novel ways, to strengthen healthy and supportive structures within the family. An emphasis is placed upon 'Joining', the process by which therapists establish a working alliance with the family system. This is necessary before disrupting the pathological structures in treatment. **Crisis induction** forces the family to face a conflict that is typically avoided. In **unbalancing**, the therapist may deliberately create turbulence in the system by siding with one family member or ignoring a dominant member. These techniques as well as **restructuring interventions** challenge the rigid family hierarchy. **Family sculpting** is another way to enact the family dilemma.

Strategic Family Therapy was developed by Jay Haley and Chloe Madanes in the 1970s [13, 14]. The focus is on resolving presenting problems by disrupting sequences of behaviours and interactions which may maintain the difficulty and introducing alternatives to emerge. Gaining insight or understanding past influences are not emphasised in this model. Haley was influenced by Milton Erikson, a hypnotherapist who solved family problems through creative suggestions and paradoxes.

In strategic therapy, the first task of the therapist is to define a presenting problem in such a way that it can be solved. Again, the onus is on the therapist in his or her role as an expert to plan a strategy for solving the client's problems. Strategic Interventions includes

directives, paradoxical injunctions, and symptom prescription etc. An example of a directive from Haley, quoted by Madanes – 'a father who is siding with his small daughter may be required to wash the sheets when daughter wets the bed. This task will tend to disengage daughter and father or cure the bed wetting' [14]. Directives could be paradoxical, prescribing no change, which paradoxically triggers change.

Milan Systemic/Strategic Therapy (Mara Selvini Palazzoli, Guiliana Prata, Gianfranco Cecchin, Luigi Boscolo)

Further developments in family therapy were made through the contributions of a group of Italian psychiatrists and psychoanalysts who became known as the Milan research group. The fundamental principles of Milan therapy were stated in their classic paper in 1980: **Hypothesising, Circularity and Neutrality** [15].

Hypothesising: the purpose of a hypothesis is to connect family behaviours with meaning and to introduce a systemic view to the family to enable them to develop new views of their beliefs, behaviours and relationships. The Hypothesis is systemic in that it connects all components of the family; it is related to the family's concerns and useful in generating interventions.

Circularity: in the family, the patterns are circular and recursive (A triggers response B, and this triggers A and so on). Appreciation of the circular process helps the therapist to view the family members with a degree of neutrality and compassion. In linear thinking (A causes B), the tendency would have been to blame and judge one party.

Circular questioning is a style of interviewing where questions can help to transform the perceptions. For example, it can change a tendency for the family to blame an individual towards an interdependent and reciprocal view of causation. This is often through raising awareness of the different perceptions of family members and challenging the validity of their perceptions with regards to values, ideas and experiences (see Box 9.1).

Box 9.1 Examples of circular questions

Difference question: how does father's behaviour bother your sister differently than it bothers Mum?

Difference in perception of relationships: who is closer to your father, your daughter or your son?

Questions about the degree of difference: on a scale of 1–10, how bad do you think the fighting is? How bad do you think others feel about it?

Now/then difference: has this always been true? How was it different then?

Agreement and disagreement: who else agrees with this? Who is in disagreement? Who feels this way? Who doesn't?

Explanations: what is your explanation? How do you think an outsider explains this? If this happens how would you explain this?

Hypothetical future difference: if you were to divorce, which parent would the children stay with? Who will be closest to mother when you all grow up? What does mother need to do before your sister leaves home?

A **circular triadic question** does not ask about inner feelings of the respondent directly but is directed to another dyad in the family. For example, a question to the daughter might be 'What do you think your brother would feel when he sees father shouting at mother?' The answers help to connect with others in the family, while understanding similarities and differences.

Neutrality: this is a position of impartiality which allows multiple possible hypotheses to account for available information. A stance of neutrality also aligns the therapist with each family member and reflects the view of family as an organic whole. Neutrality can be viewed as a state of curiosity. The therapist's hypothesis is not taken as truth.

Reframing: as with strategic therapies, in reframing the meaning changes the way you perceive it. For example, **positive connotation** is the recognition of the usefulness of symptoms, encourages the family to think about the identified patient in a more positive way and avoids labelling and blaming of the individual.

Rituals are prescribed interventions to disrupt problem-maintaining interaction patterns. For example, on alternate days of the week, one parent decides alone how to deal with the child, while the other parent acts as if he or she were not there. This may create a new pattern of behaviour.

Second Phase of Systemic Therapy: Second Order Cybernetics (mid 1970s to mid 1980s)

Various criticisms of system theory, from feminism and postmodernism, emerged in the 1980s. The feminist criticism from people such as Rachel Hare-Mustin and Virginia Goldner [16, 17] included: ignoring the larger social context such as patriarchy, blaming mothers for family dysfunction, and the potential unethical practice of maintaining a neutral stance in circumstances of abuse or oppression. Existing models were challenged as privileging traditional masculine values such as autonomy, independence and control, while not recognising the values of relationships, nurturing and caring. System theory also failed to consider power relationships and sexism sufficiently. The extreme relativity view such as 'no objective truths or reality' was a problem when therapists had to deal with child abuse, domestic abuse etc.

These critiques heralded a move towards approaches in which therapists were called upon to see themselves, along with their own personal or theoretical biases, as part of the system. In what became known as **second order cybernetics** the therapists understand themselves to be part of the system they are studying and ongoing mutual reciprocal influences between the therapist and family are considered. Change is also considered to occur in all participants. Second order cybernetics is characteristic of social constructionist and postmodern schools of therapy.

Dallos states 'Second order cybernetics challenged expert's notions of "normal" or "healthy" families. The emphasis moved from behaviour to exploration of meanings, beliefs and stories. Multiple vantage points are inherent in any construction of reality. The aim was to see the situation differently and usefully. The therapist is not an expert, but a collaborative explorer who works with the family' [18].

The postmodern stance criticised the values behind the so-called normative well-functioning family. The models of well-functioning family did not include the social realities of single parents, stepfamilies, LGBT couples and parents, biracial families etc.

Family therapy had to change in order to meet the issue of culture, ethnicity and diversity in a respectful and validating way.

Lynn Hoffman summarised the characteristics of therapies influenced by **second order cybernetics** [19].

- An observing system stance and inclusion of the therapist's own context
- A collaborative rather than hierarchical structure
- Goals that emphasise setting a context for change, not specifying change
- Ways to guard against too much instrumentality (e.g. circular questioning being seen as the treatment in itself)
- A 'circular' assessment of the problem
- A non-pejorative and non-judgemental view

Solution-Focussed Therapy (SFT) was developed by **Steve de Shazer and Insoo Kim Berg** [20], arguably the most famous therapist couple in family therapy. In this model, there is no discussion of the problem or its causes. This radical perspective liberated therapists from searching for hypothetical causes. Problem-saturated conversations are seen as masking the ability to find solutions and in de Shazer's view the solution need not have any links to the problem or to its causation. Hence in SFT, the conversations are all about solutions and the work is based on releasing the innate strengths, resources and creativity of the clients. It takes a non-pathological view of people. Therapy is brief; the interventions are straight forward and therapists do not require lengthy training.

Based on their level of motivation and engagement, de Shazer divided clients to three groups, **visitors** (who are sent by others, but not interested in change), **complainants** (who complain about problems, but take little responsibility in change) and **customers** (who want to change for themselves). It is important to help clients find solutions, only when they want to change, that is, when they are customers.

The success of SFT depends on the client working towards well-articulated, achievable goals that are important to them. The goal should be positively framed (e.g. advice to stop overeating would be a negatively framed goal, spend more time exercising is a positively framed goal): the key question to turn a negatively framed goal to a positive goal is 'what would you like to do instead?'.

The most quoted intervention of SFT, is the **miracle question**, which encourages the patient to imagine a miracle, which would make the problem disappear. The therapist encourages the patient to give details of their consequent problem-free life, and then guides them to take small, incremental, behavioural steps to make this miracle come into their life. **Scaling questions** are used (What needs to happen for you to move from 3 to 4 on 0–10 scale of self-confidence?) and **coping questions** (How did you manage to prevent the situation from getting worse? What makes you not give up?) are used to elicit hidden strengths. The therapist asks **exception questions** (What is different when the problem does not happen? How did you manage that?) to promote learning about alternative strategies. The therapist elicits and **amplifies resilience, strengths and resources. Post-session message** includes **compliments** and homework, which is set collaboratively. From the second session onwards, the therapist asks 'What is better?' focussing on small and large changes from session to session. More recently, there is a shift from behavioural focus and homework to the role of emotions and cognitions in SFT [21].

Third Phase of Systemic Therapy: Influence of Postmodernism, Constructivism and Social Constructionism

The field of family therapy has continued to be significantly challenged and expanded by developments in society and challenges to re-existing beliefs and values, and in the 1980s the limits of models based upon cybernetic principles became increasingly apparent. Postmodernist thinking heralded the development of ideas about reality perception and the construction of value systems occurring through personal pre-existing belief systems and the medium of language. This brought with it the recognition that there are widely varying and equally valid ways to see ourselves or the world.

In social constructionism, beliefs are thought to be co-constructed within our sociocultural environment and knowledge of reality is constructed through language and cultural practices. These cultural discourses are not always conscious and establish norms and customs. Often, such dominant discourses serve the interests of powerful majority groups. For example, the ever-enlarging list of disorders in psychiatric classification systems such as DSM is the work of expert groups which are influenced by powerful political, pharmaceutical and professional interests. Postmodernism and social constructionism challenges grand narratives and truth claims of such systems, for example how biased evidence may be masked as science or objective truth.

In the field of family therapy, social constructionism has helped to form more radically open and transparent relationships and practices. No one can claim to be wholly neutral and we have to be constantly aware of the influences and biases that we bring into therapy. A number of therapeutic approaches developed reflecting postmodernist ideas such as narrative, social constructionist or solution-focussed therapy, all challenging notions of their being basic truths or theories known best by experts.

The Reflecting Team

Use of teams in family therapy occurs in Structural, Strategic and Milan approaches, but the style is different based on theoretical orientations. The Milan observing team passed instructions to the therapist working with the family through his/her earphone. The observing team sat behind the one-way mirror and acted as an expert resource, while maintaining distance from the family.

In contrast, the Reflecting Team approach, developed by the Norwegian psychiatrist and family therapist Tom Andersen in the 1980s [22], was influenced by social constructionism, and is more transparent regarding the power dynamics. The team interventions, particularly reflections, were open and transparent to the family. They eschewed interpretations and hypothesis.

In the first part of the session the therapist would converse with family members and would be observed by the therapists in the reflecting team, usually sitting behind a one-way mirror. In the second part, the therapist and family would observe the reflecting team having a conversation about what they observed in the family. The reflections are not expert interpretations; they are offered tentatively as possibilities worth exploring. The multiple perspectives of the team members stimulate the family to think about the issues from diverse perspectives.

In the third part, therapist and family will have a reflection about what they heard. The family could challenge the team's reflection, or they could take away something useful from the reflecting team's comments. Tom Andersen's reflective team approach has influenced later family therapy models such as narrative therapy and collaborative therapy.

Narrative Therapy

Narrative family therapy perceives problems as arising in the family when functioning does not fit in with socially dominant discourses, for example around class, ethnicity and sexuality. It takes a social justice approach and challenges these discourses that can shape someone's life in a destructive way [23].

Separating the problem from the person and the use of **externalising conversations** assist with this; examples of externalising questions about depression may include: *What made you vulnerable, for the Depression to take over your life? How does the Depression lead you to do things, you don't like?* This is different to thinking that problems are within the person, that *the person* is sad, anxious or angry. This can help to develop a different relationship to their problem.

Various metaphors can also be used (e.g. taming, disempowering or challenging the depression), and the therapist and patient together seek to develop a new narrative about themselves. Therapists ask about **unique outcomes** people want in their life, and often write **therapeutic letters** to patients, detailing the emerging story from an observer position. Narrative therapists may also take a playful approach, which helps to undermine the power of the dominant discourse on individuals, which may have caused guilt and shame.

Collaborative Therapy

This treatment approach seeks to develop a dialogue leading to positive change in which the therapist has a facilitatory role. Everyday language is used in session; there is no structure or preconceived plan in the conversations. A **non-expert, not knowing stance** is central. Not knowing does not mean you are ignorant; it means you remain curious. Rather than any technique, it is the attitude that matters. The underlying premise of the approach is that knowledge and language are social and communal processes and they are fluid and changeable. The therapist's focus is on how the clients construct meaning. A true dialogical conversation is also a mutually transforming experience. This exploration may lead to new connections, associations and understandings that help to move forward [24].

Other Models

Attachment and family therapy: Rudi Dallos and Arlene Vetere developed Attachment Narrative Therapy [25]. This is based on Bowlby's attachment theory (see Chapter 1) and comprises four key stages: (1) creation of a secure base for exploration, (2) exploration using genograms, stories and other methods to explore the family's experiences and relationships, (3) consider the alternatives or corrective steps and (4) maintain a therapeutic base. Progress through these phases is not linear by stage by stage.

Emotions and family therapy: ideas from attachment theory have also been drawn upon as an approach to couple therapy. In **Emotionally Focussed Couple Therapy** (EFCT) developed by Sue Johnson, people's attachment style is understood to influence the way they function within an intimate relationship. Understanding the roots of attachment patterns and responding to emotional needs of self and others is the central experiential learning in EFCT. For example:

- An insecure attachment can result in patterns of experiencing anxiety and avoidance
- A dismissive attachment style deactivates emotions and de-emphasises any need for connection to others [26]

- A preoccupied attachment style can lead to the use of hyperactivating strategies with open expression of emotions resulting in clingy and demanding behaviour. The primary emotions of sadness and anxiety can give rise to emotions of anger and hostility latterly

Cognitive and Behavioural Theory and Family Therapy

Albert Ellis has emphasised the role of irrational beliefs in marital conflict from 1960s. Early behaviour therapists based their interventions on behavioural exchange and operant theory and used positive reward systems to improve relationships.

Various models of integrated cognitive behavioural therapy (CBT) and family therapy approaches exist. Psychoeducation, problem solving, and communication skill training are commonly used in these approaches. Family interaction sequences often show biased cognitive processing, and hidden rewards of maladaptive behaviour (pay offs and secondary gains) maintains the family problem. Acceptance strategies would be appropriate for unchangeable aspects of relationships. Mindfulness-based approaches are helpful to develop empathy and compassion in family members.

Mindfulness and Acceptance in Family Therapy

Third wave CBT therapies use mindfulness approaches, as an intervention. From a philosophical and theoretical point of view, postmodernist and social constructionist family therapies have some interesting connections with Buddhist philosophy. Diane Gehart shows how family therapists have incorporated various Buddhist constructs such as emptiness, interdependence, impermanence and compassion in their work [27].

Other Models

Multisystemic therapy (MST) was specifically developed for treating chronic behavioural problems and emotional disturbances in adolescents. Interventions are well defined, action oriented and present focussed, to promote responsible behaviour. Therapy is time-limited, lasting four to six months. **Functional Family Therapy** (FFT) is another model of therapy addressing troubled adolescents. Both models have a large evidence base and disseminated in large scale projects.

The Evidence Base for Family Therapy

There is considerable evidence for family therapy in child and adolescent disorders as well as in adult disorders such as schizophrenia, depression, bulimia and drug and alcohol abuse. Please see reviews by Alan Carr for specific studies for specific conditions [28, 29].

Lucy Davies has summarised NICE recommendations for family interventions in various disorders, which is accessible through the link www.aft.org.uk/SpringboardWebA pp/userfiles/aft/file/NICE/NICE%20Clinical%20Guidelines%20recommending%20family %202016.pdf.

NICE guidelines for family intervention in schizophrenia recommend the intervention should include at least 10 sessions, between three months and one year, delivered either as a single-family intervention or multifamily intervention. The intervention should have a psychoeducational component, be delivered in a supportive manner and would often have skill components such as negotiated problem solving. Psychoeducational family therapy reduced relapse of psychosis by half when compared with routine treatment.

There is a serious criticism that a randomised controlled trial may not be an appropriate tool for establishing evidence in family therapy, where the change in the whole family system, rather than change in an individual's symptom, is the key outcome.

Family Therapy and Mental Health Services

This chapter has described the evolution of a range of theoretical approaches to family therapy, with consequent different techniques and treatment approaches. In ordinary clinical practice, however, most therapists use more than one model in their work and may draw upon techniques derived from a range of family-based approaches. Family therapy is a key approach taken in addressing disturbance in childhood and adolescence and family therapists form key members of child and adolescent mental health services (CAMHS).

As with all approaches to therapy, there are indications and contraindications for family therapy. Indications would include:

- difficulties in adjusting to key transitions, life events and crisis
- symptoms which seem closely linked to family dynamics or family dysfunction
- family responses which may maintain the problem and disencourage recovery

Contraindications may include:

- a family with very limited resource to reflect
- where there has been abuse and addressing this in a family context may be overwhelmingly difficult
- where exploration may increase risk to vulnerable family members, for example severe ongoing domestic abuse
- lack of family motivation to work together on the issues
- impossibility through death, estrangement or geography

Despite the evidence base, adult psychiatric services have been much slower to adopt family therapy as a treatment approach, for example in schizophrenia. Reasons for this can seem difficult to fathom given the high level of distress, relapse rates and impact of psychotic illness upon families.

A systemic approach to understanding mental illness and psychological distress and techniques derived from family therapy are however integrated to an extent within everyday psychiatric practice as described below.

Psychiatric Practice and Family Therapy

The psychiatric classification and intervention is dominated by focus on the individual, with less emphasis on the embedded relationship and contextual factors. To counteract this, a systemic perspective can and should be helpfully applied when working with patients. The examples below illustrate ways systemic thinking can be integrated in routine psychiatric practice.

A Systemic Perspective: Think Family

It is remarkable to see when people are given an opportunity to talk about their family and context, how they begin to make connections between their symptoms and the events and stress in the family system. Whenever possible, see a family member or carer with the patient, which allows different perspectives to be heard, interactional patterns to be observed and psychoeducational material to be offered.

Use of a Genogram

A genogram is a pictorial representation of family members with regard to their name, gender, age, occupation, death and other information such as substance abuse, critical life events, transitions, traumas, attachment, losses and relationship patterns to each other. Intergenerational patterns of difficulty and life cycle issues, as well as themes of resilience and strengths can often become clear during this exercise. McGoldrick gives a detailed guidance on constructing and using genograms [7].

Family Life Cycle

When assessing individuals, it is helpful to think about their stage in the family life cycle. The challenges faced by the family are different in different stages:

1. Leaving home – single adult: responsibility for self emotionally and financially
2. Marriage/Partnership: commitment to new system; new boundaries with family
3. Families with young children: adjustment in relationship with partner, child rearing tasks
4. Families with adolescent children: refocus on marriage and career
5. Launching children: developing adult to adult relationship with children
6. Family in the middle years: renegotiating relationship with ageing parents retirement, grandparenthood, own morbidity and losses
7. Family in later life: coping with loss of abilities, loss of partner, shift of generational goals

Family Formulation

Formulating an individual's difficulties in terms of family patterns of relating, communication, beliefs, roles and ability to adapt to changes and transitions offers an important way to conceptualise and to plan interventions. Attempts to treat an individual may be thwarted if they return to destructive patterns of family functioning and this should be considered routinely as part of psychiatric practice. Further information about formulation based upon systemic approaches can be found in Gehart [30] or Carr [31].

Training

There are various short and long training events. The full list can be accessed through the Association of Family Therapy (www.aft.org.uk). The best way to learn family therapy is through experience, through joining a family therapy team. This gives an experiential knowledge of various models in practice.

Conclusion

Family therapy covers a variety of approaches and schools. It has evolved in response to various challenges to it such as feminist criticism, social constructivism, postmodernism and social constructionism. The systemic perspective helps to balance the extreme focus on the individual and appreciate the need to harness the resources of relationships in responding to challenges in health and well-being.

References

1. Bateson G, Jackson DD, Haley J, Weakland J. Toward a theory of schizophrenia. *Behav Sci* 1956; 1(4): 251–4.

2. Fromm-Reichmann F. Notes on the development of treatment of schizophrenics by psychoanalytic psychotherapy. *Psychiatry* 1948; 11(3): 263–73.

3. Wynne LC, Ryckoff IM, Day J, Hirsh SI. Pseudo-mutuality in the family relations of schizophrenics. *Psychiatry* 1958; 21: 205–20.

4. Lidz RW, Lidz T. The family environment of schizophrenic patients. *J Psychiatry* 1949; 106: 332–45.

5. Lidz T, Cornelison A, Fleck S, Terry D. The intrafamilial environment of schizophrenic patients. II. Marital schism and marital skew. *Am J Psychiatry* 1957; 114: 241–8.

6. Bowen M. *Family Therapy in Clinical Practice.* New York: Jason Aaronson, 1978.

7. McGoldrick M. *Genograms: Assessment and Intervention.* New York: Norton Professional Books, 2008.

8. von Bertalanffy L. *General System Theory.* New York: George Braziller, 1968.

9. Segal L. Brief therapy: the MRI approach. In AS Gurman, DP Kniskern, eds., *Handbook of Family Therapy.* Vol. II. New York: Brunner/Mazel. 1991; pp. 171–99.

10. Satir V. *Conjoint Family Therapy.* Palo Alto, CA: Science & Behavioural Books, 1967.

11. Minuchin S, Fischman S. *Family Therapy Techniques.* Cambridge, MA: Harward University Press, 1981.

12. Colapinto J. Structural family therapy. In AS Gurman, DP Kniskern, eds., *Handbook of Family Therapy.* Vol. II. New York: Brunner/Mazel. 1991; pp. 417–43.

13. Haley J. *Problem Solving Therapy*, 2nd ed. San Francisco: Jossey-Bass/Pfeiffer, 1987.

14. Madanes C. *Strategic Family Therapy.* San Francisco: Jossey-Boss, 1981.

15. Selvini-Palazzoli M, Boscolo L, Cecchin G, Prata G. Hypothesizing–circularity–neutrality: three guidelines for the conductor of the session. *Fam Process* 1980; 19(1): 3–12.

16. Hines PM, Hare-Mustin RT. Ethical concerns in family therapy. *Prof Psychol* 1978; 165–71.

17. Goldner V. Feminism and family therapy. *Fam Process* 1985; 24(1): 2431–47.

18. Dallos R, Draper R. *An Introduction to Family Therapy*, 4th ed. Maidenhead: Open University Press, 2015.

19. Hoffman L. Beyond power and control: toward a 'second order' family systems therapy. *Fam Syst Med* 1985; 3(4): 381–96.

20. de Shazer S. *Keys to Solution in Brief Therapy.* New York: W. W. Norton & Company, 1985.

21. Lipchik E. *Beyond Technique in Solution Focused Therapy.* New York: Guilford Press, 2002.

22. Andersen T (ed.). *The Reflecting Team: Dialogues and Dialogues about the Dialogues.* New York: W. W. Norton & Company, 1991.

23. White M, Epston E. *Narrative Means to Therapeutic Ends.* New York: W. W. Norton & Company, 1990.

24. Anderson H, Goolishian HA. Human systems as linguistic systems: evolving ideas about implications for theory and practice. *Fam Process* 1988; 27: 371–93.

25. Dallos R. *Attachment Narrative Therapy: Integrating Systemic, Narrative and Attachment Approaches.* Maidenhead: Open University Press, 2006.

26. Johnson SM. *The Practice of Emotionally Focused Couple Therapy: Creating Connection*, 3rd ed. New York: Routledge, 2019.

27. Gehart D. *Mindfulness and Acceptance in Couple and Family Therapy*, New York: Springer, 2012.

28. Carr A. Family therapy and systemic interventions for child-focused problems: the current evidence base. *J Fam Ther* 2019; 41: 153–213.

29. Carr A. Couple therapy, family therapy and systemic interventions for adult-focused problems: the current evidence base. *J Fam Ther* 2019; 41: 492–536.

30. Gehart D. *Theory and Treatment Planning in Family Therapy: A Competency-Based Approach.* Pacific Grove: Brookes Cole, 2015.

31. Carr A. *Family Therapy Concepts Process and Practice*, 3rd ed. Chichester: Wiley Blackwell, 2012.

Further Reading

McGoldrick M. *The Genogram Casebook: A Clinical Companion to Genograms: Assessment and Intervention*. New York: Norton Professional Books, 2016.

Reiter MD. *Family Therapy, An Introduction to Process, Practice and Theory*. New York: Routledge, 2018.

Ritvo EC, Glick ID. *Marriage and Family Therapy*. Washington DC: American Psychiatric Publishing, 2002.

Cognitive Analytic Therapy (CAT):
Developing the Model and the Method

Jason Hepple

Introduction

This chapter introduces some recent developments in the application of Cognitive Analytic Therapy (CAT). After a brief, illustrated, overview of CAT; its theoretical base, its structure and its evidence base, it will concentrate on three more recent developments: eight-session CAT for anxiety and depression in non-specialist mental health psychological therapy services, CAT in groups and CAT reflective practice groups.

For an extended overview of CAT see [1, 2].

Overview of CAT

Theoretical Base

CAT, as its name implies, represents an integration of ideas from cognitive psychology and some elements of psychodynamic theory. Its originator, Dr Anthony Ryle, started out as a GP before developing his ideas in a university health service and then as a consultant psychotherapist at Guy's Hospital in London. He was struck by the volume of emotional and relational problems presenting in primary care and was interested in 'the non-revision of dysfunctional procedures'; essentially exploring the question: 'Why do people keep repeating the same relational patterns that take them back to where they started?' In a nutshell, he suggested that these patterns or 'procedures' are survival strategies developed earlier in life that are no longer helpful. He developed tools to describe these procedures in both narrative (reformulation letter) and visual forms (mapping) so facilitating recognition of the relational 're-enactments' of these procedures that can lead to subsequent revision and the discovery of 'exits'.

The main theoretical influences for Ryle's ideas include the object relations theorists Fairbairn, Guntrip, Winnicott and Ogden. On the cognitive side he drew upon the ideas of George Kelly and admired his collaborative exploration of the client's world using repertory grids. In essence, Ryle sought to 're-state object relations ideas in a cognitive language and to generate an approach compatible with observational studies of early development' [1]. Ryle also replaced the interpretation of unconscious process with a more collaborative and 'doing with' mapping out of relational sequences, including the relational 'enactments' that go on between client and therapist in the course of the therapy; a restatement of transference and countertransference.

Structure of the Model

CAT originated as a 16 weekly session model of individual therapy, designed to offer a time-limited, collaborative and focussed therapy that was affordable in public health services but that had the depth and interest in the past to help people with more complex personality-based problems resulting from abuse, neglect and trauma. CAT has always been more concerned with a jointly authored developmental formulation of the person's problems than in symptoms, diagnostic categories or an illness model of mental health. There is early negotiation of 'target problems'; the focus of the work of the therapy, and the linking of these to 'target problem procedures' that are subdivided into 'traps, dilemmas and snags'. These procedures are relational formulations of the 'survival strategies' mentioned above.

Typically at session four, the therapist reads out a prepared 'reformulation letter' to the client, which empathically retells the co-constructed client's story making links with the past and the target problems and their related procedures. It also tries to anticipate how these procedures may re-enact themselves in the therapeutic relationship (an anticipation of negative and positive transferences that may both help to understand the therapeutic alliance and may also threaten it). An example of a short, truncated, fictional reformulation letter:

Dear Jonathan,
(Introduction, context and target problems)

Now that we have reached session four of our sixteen sessions of CAT therapy, I am giving you this reformulation letter, as I said, where I am trying to link the problems you have brought to therapy with patterns that we have identified from your past experience. This letter is yours to keep but is only a draft and we can alter anything that is not right. You are welcome to write a reply to this letter if that would be helpful to you.

You came to therapy feeling very lonely and isolated. Since returning to your home town after college you have 'existed' in your flat and have not made any friends or found anything regular to engage in. You have suffered from depression and feeling like you would rather be dead but you say that you 'do not have the courage to kill myself.' You have tried antidepressants but they did not seem to help. You had a course of Cognitive Behavioural Therapy (CBT), but although you identified with the patterns identified by the therapist, you felt that this did not help you to make any changes in your life and you told me that you felt that the therapist was just 'going through the motions' and was not really interested in you; you were 'just another statistic'.

We identified two broad target problems: one connected to your 'minimal existence' that we framed as 'not being able to have anything for myself'. The second connected to your difficulty relating to other people that we framed as 'other people look down on me as a failure'. In the section below I will try to link these to the things that you have told me about your childhood.
(Reformulation of earlier life experiences)

Your childhood came across to me as very lonely. You told me that you were brought up on a farm as an only child. Your father was always out on the farm and when he did come home, was tired and withdrawn. He felt that children should be 'seen and not heard'. Your mother had lots of interests outside of the home and was active in the Women's Institute and local amateur dramatics. She was also out a lot and seemed to have no time for you. You learned to pass the time alone, sometimes just sitting in 'your tree' or lying on your bed staring at the cracks in the ceiling. I can feel how lonely and desolate this must have been for a child who needed love and encouragement. This makes me feel very sad for you.

As time went on your mother took to drinking and everything you did seemed to annoy her and be wrong. She told you that you needed to be 'self-sufficient' like she was and not be 'needy' and ask for attention or things. This is illustrated by the terrible story of what happened to Dasher, your dog. You were so pleased when you father brought Dasher home to keep you company. Dasher became your best friend but one day when you came back from school your mother had given Dasher away as she said he was a nuisance as he needed walking when you were at school and that she couldn't afford to feed him. You never found out where Dasher had gone. You were distraught but neither of your parents seemed to care and you made a resolution never to risk loving anything again.

At school you always felt that you did not fit in as the farm was a long way from any other kids' houses and you always had old clothes and shoes and were picked on for being 'the farm kid'. After a time you learned to keep yourself to yourself and the other kids just ignored you or sniggered at you as you set off on the long walk home. I can feel some anger in you about the way you were treated by them. Why would you want to mix with other people in the future when they are so cruel?

. . . .

Target problem: I can't seem to have anything for myself

Target problem procedure (Snag): because of my experiences as a child I learned that if I attached to something and loved it (like my dog Dasher) it could be taken away as a punishment, leaving me distraught and alone and feeling that nothing was fair. It seemed safer to invest no emotional currency in things for myself to appear self-sufficient. As I have grown up this has meant that I have nothing for myself and live in an empty flat. I am lonely and sad and left feeling that life has singled me out as a loner and a loser. Maybe it is as if I am now punishing myself?

Target problem: other people look down on me as a failure

Target problem procedure (trap/dilemma): because of the way that you were bullied and ostracised at school you learned to feel that other people look down on you for the way you look. You told me that you feel there is something in you that 'broadcasts failure'. This makes you more determined to be 'self-sufficient' and not need friends or a relationship as other people are cruel and uncaring. Sometimes you look down on them as 'morons' and 'breeders'. This confirms your alienation and leaves you lonely and isolated.

(Anticipation of re-enactments in the therapy relationship)

Jonathan, thank you for getting this far in therapy and for giving me a chance to get to know you. I can feel how hurt and angry you are because of how your life has ended up. I am hopeful that we can find a way forward but I am worried that you may not be able to risk having this therapy for yourself, or feel that I am just 'going through the motions' like your last therapist and that you may then feel angry with me and stop coming to our sessions to protect yourself from further disappointment. It will be good to talk about any of these feelings if they come up so that we can continue to work together on making your life better for yourself.

In the middle, or 'recognition' phase of a CAT therapy, the client and therapist work together on visual maps that are another way of gaining an overview or 'observing eye' on these procedures. At the heart of these maps are 'reciprocal roles', a simple restatement of cause and effect in relational templates from the client's past.

Figure 10.1 shows the visual representation of the example snag given above. The reciprocal role punishing / depriving to punished / hurting / unloved is called a 'self-state'. The Multiple Self States Model (MSSM) forms the basis of CAT's understanding of the survival of trauma and dissociation.

The final phase of a CAT therapy is called the 'revision' phase and the emphasis is on how these patterns from the past play out in day-to-day life. The client and therapist jointly work on recognising these re-enactments in recent events (including in the therapeutic relationship) and on the finding of 'exits' that take the client 'off the map'. In the final session there is the invited exchange of 'goodbye letters', where the therapist reflects on the therapeutic journey and the insights gained. An example of a brief fictional goodbye letter to Jonathan:

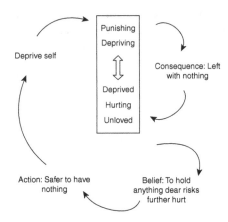

Figure 10.1 An example of a target problem reformulated as a CAT 'snag'.

Dear Jonathan,

I am writing to you as promised to mark the last regular session of our CAT therapy. I am pleased that we have got to the end together and I would like to thank you for sticking with me when you began to have doubts as to whether anything could really help. In session 12 you were able to express your anger to me and we were able to explore how you felt both inferior to me (as a professional) and in some ways superior to me, as part of you had written me off as a 'trumped up guru' who had no idea what it was like to have experienced the desolate childhood that you had told me about.

Following this session you were able to write the 'no-send' letters to your mother and father and we shared some of the anger and sadness and the realisation that they were unlikely to really change how that they have always related to you. We looked at some exits: we realised that 'self-sufficiency' was a good survival strategy for the child you were but that now the neglect and punishment has turned on yourself and that you have a choice to give the world another try. Perhaps our therapy relationship has shown you that someone else can see you as an interesting and bright young man who is yet to really venture from the tree you have been hiding in for so long. It was great that you managed to go to the appointment with Employment Support and are due to start voluntary work. I was pleased to see that you had bought some new jeans and trainers for the appointment too! Looking to the future I see no reason why you can't grow to have friends, a relationship and the family that you told me you would love but had given up on.

I wish you all the very best for the future and look forward to hearing how things have been going at our follow-up appointment.

There is typically one follow-up session after three months. CAT can be delivered over 24 sessions with three follow-ups for more complex clients.

The Evidence Base for CAT

For a detailed review of the small but encouraging evidence for CAT see the discussion in the review paper 'CAT at thirty'[2]. In this paper Steve Kellett comments that: '*This analysis suggests that there is evidence of the effectiveness of CAT under routine clinical practice and clinical trial conditions across a diverse range of presenting difficulties.*' The quoted weighted effect size (d+ = 0.83) indicates that: *'CAT for mental health problems has large effect on reducing psychiatric symptoms.'*

Noteworthy studies include a positive randomised controlled trial (RCT) of 24-session CAT with three follow-ups and some longer-term follow-up data, comparing CAT with treatment as usual in a population of clients with mixed personality disorder presentations in a clinical setting [3]. An Australian trial applied CAT to adolescents with features of borderline personality disorder, comparing CAT with a model of 'Good Clinical Care' and retrospectively with 'historic treatment as usual'. CAT produced the most marked improvement in 'externalising difficulties' and para-suicidal behaviour [4, 5] There is an encouraging pilot RCT of CAT with clients with bipolar disorder [6]. A randomised dismantling trial of eight-session CAT for anxiety and depression in a non-specialist service concludes that eight-session CAT has a large effect size in treating depression (d > 1.5, p < 0.01) [7]. Finally, there is published the first trial of Group CAT (GCAT) for woman survivors of sexual abuse [8].

CAT has also been applied clinically in a range of settings including later life [9], intellectual disability [10], working with mental health teams [11], offenders [12] and diabetes management [13].

Eight-Session CAT in Non-specialist Mental Health Services

CAT has developed a role in a number of non-specialist services (in the UK known as 'primary care'), often complementing CBT and other treatments for clients with anxiety and depression. CAT has tended to be targeted at clients with more identified relational problems or higher levels of risk, complexity and co-morbidity. It can be very hard to separate out, at assessment, clients with anxiety and depression from those with relational problems, formal personality disorder and histories of abuse and trauma, so CAT would appear to have face validity for working with this more complex group of clients. This use of CAT has been supported by the inclusion of CAT as a recommended psychological therapy for Serious Mental Illness – Personality Disorder at University College London (UCL-CORE).

In Somerset, UK, there are years of experience of applying eight-session CAT to anxiety and depression in a non-specialist service, with positive results. This database is currently undergoing analysis and benchmarking and will hopefully lead to publication that will provide quantitative evidence for eight-session CAT. The psychotherapist Stephen White has led the clinical development of the eight-session model that has been approved recently by the Association for Cognitive Analytic Therapy (ACAT).

CAT is a labour-intensive therapy for the therapist due to the amount of pre-session preparation needed to work on the reformulation letter, the maps and the goodbye letters. This is potentially problematic for therapists who typically see a very large volume of clients (sometimes dozens a week). Stephen found a pragmatic solution; forgo the formal reformulation letter and begin the mapping earlier in the therapy, while incorporating some of the narrative reformulation (or empathic retelling of the client's journey) into the goodbye letter. It is noteworthy that the dismantling trial of CAT in Improving Access to Psychological Therapy (IAPT) showed that this simplified model was equally effective in this particular setting [7]. Another development is the trialling of Cognitive Analytic Guided Self-Help (CAT-SH) for mild to moderate anxiety, designed for delivery by Psychological Wellbeing Practitioners [14].

CAT in Groups

CAT has been used in the group modality for many years and for a range of presentations. CAT, being a relational psychotherapy, would seem well suited to groups as it is likely that the relational procedures derived from the clients' past will be played out both in their relational enactments with the therapists and also with the other clients in the group; thus providing rich material for recognition and revision of dysfunctional procedures. For an overview of CAT in groups see [15, 16].

In the early development of CAT in groups, it was usual for the clients to have had a least four sessions of individual CAT prior to starting in a group, thus enabling them to bring and share their reformulation letters and maps in the group, allowing comparisons to be made with other clients' problems and the sharing of solutions or exits. In tertiary care, with clients who have had more severe experiences of abuse, neglect and trauma, it could be questioned whether it is beneficial to bring and share material from a previous therapy because of the level of exposure that this would involve. There is also a boundary issue when working in institutional settings; the therapist is party to a lot of clinical information about the client (from necessarily reviewing the case record and reading referral information etc.) and this also risks exposing the client in the group if this information is introduced by the therapist. It may be better to maintain the boundary that nothing about the client is brought into the group that has not been brought by the client his or herself: 'What is known to the group.' This allows that it is not necessary to have had prior individual CAT or to bring materials from previous therapies into the group unless the client chooses to do so. This makes joining the group less intimidating and allows the client to manage their own exposure and pace of disclosure. It is surprisingly easy, also, to self-monitor what information about the clients is discussed, so restricting material to that which has already been brought to the group by the client.

Another development is the move from a closed one-year group for around eight clients to an open group where clients join when there is a vacancy and stay for 52 sessions. This is much more desirable to referrers and managers as clients can be referred at any time and do not need to wait for the next cycle. It also makes the group more viable if there is a periodic higher dropout rate, as spaces can be filled, making the remaining clients more secure in thinking that the groups will survive.

So, how to adapt CAT to this open group format? In CAT the therapist is much more active than in psychodynamic or analytic approaches. There is an expectation to try to do CAT, and the three stages of CAT introduced above, namely, reformulation, recognition and revision, throughout the course of a CAT group. Sometimes this can be in an educational way, for example introducing the concept of target problems and target problem procedures and attempting to map out procedures in the group on an A3 pad. Some procedures will be related to one client who is bringing a lot of material to the group that day, or sometimes the mapping describes a commonality between clients, or an enactment between clients or between clients and therapists. Figure 10.2 illustrates the 'Can of Rage' that is often a common theme and describes the pressure of rage built up from earlier experience of abuse and neglect and how dangerous it feels when steam starts to leak from the can.

With the move to open groups, it has not been possible to continue with the writing of reformulation letters to each client in the group. This is similar to the adaptation made in the eight-session CAT model but for a different reason. Some clients will be very

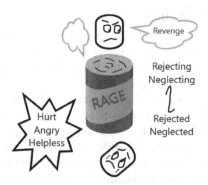

Figure 10.2 The 'Can of Rage'.

slow to bring difficult material from their past into the group and the idea of reformulating this at a fixed time does not work as well as in individual CAT. The day-to-day work of the group involves hearing from anyone in crisis and using verbal and mapped attempts to identify the relational patterns involved. There is an open invitation to talk about the past, write therapy 'no-send' letters and to share these with the group when the client is ready. There comes a point for each client when the story has been heard, reacted to and witnessed by the group. This 'witnessing' is one of the strengths of the group modality as it is very powerful to have empathic recognition from others who have been through similar struggles in their life. This process may be how CAT helps to reprocess emotional trauma in a containing environment [17]. The open group format lends itself to this as those towards the end of their group journey are often able to identify with and support those at the beginning of their journey. This is therapeutic both for the client receiving empathic recognition and for the client able to discover how their own life experience can be put to good use by providing responsive understanding for others.

As clients approach the end of their time in the group the emphasis is on procedural enactments in recent events and on obstacles to moving forward and exits from long-established patterns. There is explicit reflection on the future: where would you like to be living? Who do you want to spend your time with? What do you want to be doing? As each client leaves, the therapists write a joint goodbye letter and read it out with consent. The client is asked to read a letter they have prepared and other clients are invited to write a goodbye postcard to the person who is leaving that day. Sometimes there is also cake and tears! There is no follow-up in the group as, after a period of three months, the group would have different members and this would be more like a starting again than a reunion.

CAT groups can be explicitly named as a 'recovery/discharge group' for clients who have had extended periods of time in secondary care, allowing the majority of clients to move on from secondary care after the group experience, and it may be that the open CAT group format is more cost-effective and provides for clients, with more complex problems, a substantial, although time-limited, therapy experience. That is not to say that future CAT is prohibited as 'serial CAT' can be available for those who need more therapy over an extended period; the point about a brief therapy is that a lot of the movement tends to occur after the therapy is over and respecting the agreed ending is important to the method. This emphasises that CAT therapy is a 'manageable disappointment'.

CAT Reflective Practice Groups

For a discussion of the similarities and differences between a traditional Balint group and a CAT reflective practice group see [18]. Facilitation of a CAT reflective practice group is quite different to the traditional Balint method and reflects some of the overall differences between CAT and psychodynamic approaches.

As could be predicted, the role of the CAT facilitator is more active. The group starts with the usual question 'who has something to bring today?' and is clear that this could be a particular client or could be a contextual discussion of a work-related situation; team dynamics or how a client is experienced by different aspects of the service. After allowing the person who comes forward to describe the scenario or client there is peer-led questioning and reflection. Depending on how this goes the CAT facilitator may then go on to offer some CAT formulation and also some personal perspectives and experience. This is moving the role of facilitator more towards the role of supervisor and also teacher. This is particularly beneficial for trainees from a range of disciplines. Some trainees will be completely new to mental health comment in evaluations of these groups that they value some more concrete guidance and direction at times. Below are some of the types of intervention that can be made by the CAT facilitator.

Giving a CAT Perspective

Most commonly it is helpful to bring into the dialogue a relational, CAT, understanding. This will involve naming the reciprocal roles and sometimes procedures that can be picked up while listening to the peer-led discussion. To give a fictionalised example, a doctor new to psychiatry had had a difficult discussion with an inpatient about the nature of her restriction under the Mental Health Act. The group supported what the doctor had done and were clear that she had had no choice but to be clear about the boundary and that they would all have done the same. The patient had been distressed by being told that she could not leave the ward and later self-harmed in her room by cutting herself. When the doctor heard about this the next day, she had an intense feeling of guilt and the feeling that she had done something wrong and had to somehow make amends by going to see the patient and offer some comfort, although the patient did not want to speak to the doctor, leaving the doctor feeling more uncomfortable. This was reformulated as the doctor actually trying to seek reassurance from the patient in order to appease the horrible feeling that they had in some way abused the patient.

By using discussion and mapping, these feelings were linked to the patient's own history of sexual abuse and the reciprocal roles: abusing to abused and the compensatory roles of rescuing to rescued. Another way to think about this that was introduced was the idea of the 'abuser–victim–rescuer' triangle, which was a prominent part of the way that the patient tended to interact with services (and vice versa). The 'unmanageable feelings' experienced by the doctor were then located in the patient's history of abuse and the way this was being re-enacted in the relationship between doctor and patient. This 'observing eye' perspective helped the doctor take an overview of what had happened and they felt relieved. This was a very good introduction to the feelings that can be projected when working with clients with histories of abuse, trauma and neglect and the benefits of gaining support, supervision and reflection as a necessity rather than a luxury.

Reinforcing Boundaries and Managing Risk

Particularly with trainees who are new to mental health, it can sometimes be necessary to intervene to ensure that risk and safeguarding issues are being managed appropriately. This can involve talking about policies to do with clinical risk management, safeguarding of children and vulnerable adults and handling information relating to allegations of historic sexual abuse. As abuse is usually preceded by some form of neglect, it is a common enactment by those new to working with abuse and trauma to tend to want to not think about it or to assume that someone else will deal with it or, conversely, to intervene too heavy-handedly without thinking through the risks to, say, the adult survivor of abuse when the allegations are historic. These are the reciprocal roles neglecting / dismissing to neglected / dismissed, abusing to abused and rescuing to rescued again. These discussions are sometimes just about giving information to help with decision-making or being clear about a concrete next step such as discussing it with the senior doctor or psychotherapist or a dedicated safeguarding team. Occasionally, and with some thought, it may be necessary for the facilitator to ask for consent to take the issue forward in some way, for example by a discussion with the trainee's supervisor. Psychotherapists are used to working through the complexities of situations like this and it may be letting the participants and clients down not to use their experience to help them in this way.

Attending to Participants' Distress

Although it is necessary to be clear that the CAT reflective practice group is not a personal therapy group and that the material discussed should be work-related, there will be times when a participant is in distress and this needs empathic but boundaried handling in the group. A group like this is often seen by trainees as a place where others are interested in how they are feeling, so it is not surprising that sometimes a participant will bring a personal problem they are struggling with or some past experience of trauma that has surfaced following hearing some clinical material that has resonated with their own story. This is approaching the boundary between being a facilitator of a reflective practice group and being a psychotherapy supervisor. In CAT we recognise that there are always two real, unique people involved in an enactment; the client and the therapist, and that it is not always easy to separate out personal and elicited countertransference. The danger when a participant starts, unexpectedly, to explain their distress in the group is to enact the reciprocal role dismissing to dismissed, leaving the participant feeling unheard or guilty in some way for being unprofessional.

It may often be possible to manage this empathically by accepting that this has happened and that it is OK to be vulnerable and in need of support. With an emphasis on sign-posting the participant to the next step in getting the help that they need and trying to manage the level of disclosure in a peer group, the participant can feel heard and looked after. Sometimes it may even be necessary to speak to the participant outside of the group or meet with them and, say, the supervisor or line manager. This could be seen as a duty of care to the participant and sometimes, this would need to take precedence over the normal boundaries of a reflective practice group.

Conclusion

This chapter has served as a brief introduction to CAT as well as highlighting three areas of development of the model and the method that may be of interest to the reader. The references below offer a range of further reading; an interactive introductory module, a review paper and some of the major CAT trials and textbooks that illustrate CAT's application in specialist areas.

References

1. Hepple J. An introduction to cognitive analytic therapy (CAT). 2010 – revised 2012, 2015, 2016, 2018. www.psychiatrycpd.co.uk

2. Ryle A, Kellett S, Hepple J et al. Cognitive analytic therapy (CAT) at thirty. *Adv PsychiatrTreat* 2014; 20: 258–68.

3. Clarke S, Thomas P, James K. Cognitive analytic therapy for personality disorder: randomized controlled trial. *Br J Psychiatry* 2013; 202: 129–34.

4. Chanen AM, Jackson HJ, McCutcheon LK et al. Early intervention for adolescents with borderline personality disorder using cognitive analytic therapy: randomised controlled trial. *Br J Psychiatry* 2008; 193: 477–84.

5. Chanen AM, Jackson HJ, McCutcheon LK et al. Early intervention for adolescents with borderline personality disorder: quasi-experimental comparison with treatment as usual. *Aust N Z J Psychiatry* 2009; 43: 397–408.

6. Evans M, Kellett S, Heyland S et al. Cognitive analytic therapy for bipolar disorder: a pilot randomized controlled trial. *Clin Psychol Psychother* 2017; 24(1): 22–35.

7. Kellett S, Stockton C, Marshall H et al. Efficacy of narrative reformulation during cognitive analytic therapy for depression: randomized dismantling trial. *J Affect Disord* 2018; **239**: 37–47.

8. Calvert R, Kellett S, Hagan T. Group cognitive analytic therapy for female survivors of childhood sexual abuse. *Br J Clin Psychol* 2015; **28**: 1–23.

9. Hepple J, Sutton L (eds.). *Cognitive Analytic Therapy and Later Life. A New Perspective on Old Age*. Hove and New York: Brünner-Routledge, 2004.

10. Lloyd J, Clayton P (eds.). *Cognitive Analytic Therapy for People with Intellectual Disabilities and their Carers*. London and Philadelphia: Jessica Kingsley Publishers, 2014.

11. Kerr I, Dent-Brown K, Parry G. Psychotherapy and mental health teams. *Int Rev Psychiatry* 2007; 19: 63–80.

12. Pollock P, Stowell-Smith M, Göpfert M (eds.). *Cognitive Analytic Therapy for Offenders: A New Approach to Forensic Psychotherapy*, London: Routledge, 2006.

13. Fosbury JA, Bosley CM, Ryle A et al. A trial of cognitive analytic therapy in poorly controlled type I patients. *Diabetes Care* 1997; 20: 959–64.

14. Meadows J, Kellett S. Development and evaluation of Cognitive Analytic Guided Self-Help (CAT-SH) for use in IAPT services. *Behav Cogn Psychother* 2017; 45(3): 266–84.

15. Hepple J. Cognitive analytic therapy in a group. Reflections on a dialogic approach. *Br J Psychother* 2012; 28(4): 474–95.

16. Hepple J, Bowdrey S. Cognitive analytic therapy in an open dialogic group – adaptations and advantages. *Reformulation* 2015; 43: 16–19.

17. Hepple J. The witness and the judge. Cognitive analytic therapy in later life. The case of Maureen. *Br J Ther Integr* 2005; 2(2): 21–27.

18. Hepple J. CAT reflective practice groups. *Reformulation* 2019; 54:16–22.

Group Analytic Psychotherapy and the Group Analytic Model: A Clinician's Guide

Maria Papanastassiou

Introduction

You meet regularly with a group of people who also have problems and a psychotherapist. It is not provided because it is cheaper but because it is the best treatment for some people. It is particularly helpful if you have problems in relationships that happen again and again. It is actually powerful and encouraging to find that you aren't alone with your problem – and that you may even be able to help other people in the group [1]

Group analytic psychotherapy is an important psychotherapeutic treatment, both in the NHS and the private sector. Many patients seek help for difficulties in social relating and maintaining intimate and supportive relationships with families, colleagues, friends and partners. Relationships are key to how we live, function, develop and respond to adversity. Harmful patterns of relating and difficulties with intimacy predispose to mental health difficulties, and impact powerfully on the ability to recover. For many people presenting in distress and seeking psychotherapy, group analytic psychotherapy should be viewed as a treatment of choice.

In addition to being an important treatment option, group analytic psychotherapy has made a significant contribution to understanding how group processes influence and underlie human behaviour. This has implications for international relationships, sociocultural, political and organisational structures.

This chapter is divided in the following sections:

1. Historical context and emergence of group analysis in the UK
2. The group analytic treatment model
3. The role of the group therapist/conductor
4. Some important concepts in group analytic psychotherapy
5. Setting up a group: indications and contraindications
6. Setting up a group: practical considerations
7. Conclusion

Historical Context and Emergence of Group Analysis in the UK

The UK has led the way internationally in group psychotherapy with Foulkes and Bion being the two major contributors to the development of both theory and practice. In the USA Yalom has had a major impact and his views about therapeutic factors are widely used [2]. This chapter will mainly focus on the group analytic model which originated from Foulkes. In addition, it will briefly describe Bion's main group concepts.

S H Foulkes (1898–1976), a Jewish psychiatrist and psychoanalyst, arrived from Frankfurt, Germany to the UK in 1933. He developed ideas about treating patients therapeutically in groups having witnessed the utter destructiveness of War and how murderous processes can be enacted between groups. He worked as a psychiatrist at Northfield military hospital [3] introducing group methods as a method of treating soldiers who returned traumatised from the brutal experiences in battlefield [4]. Foulkes founded the Group Analytic Society in London in 1952. Group analysis is nowadays flourishing in many different countries under the auspices of the Group Analytic Society International (GASI).

W R Bion (1897–1979), a psychiatrist and psychoanalyst who was also based at the Northfield's Military Hospital, developed his own ideas about how people are affected by group processes around the same time as Foulkes. Bion was involved in the first 'Northfield experiment' but his approach was somewhat different to that of Foulkes and he left Northfield to further develop his ideas at the Tavistock Clinic in London. He introduced the term 'Work group' to describe a group which is functioning effectively in relation to its task, and the 'Basic assumption group' which functions more defensively in response to anxiety. According to Bion, groups can function both constructively and defensively, the balance between these forces can rapidly fluctuate and is influenced by powerful unconscious processes.

Bion described basic assumption groups as taking on three main forms;

1. Fight/flight – when the group acts as if its main task is self-preservation against extreme threat. The group then functions in an aggressive or hostile manner (fight mode) or takes flight from therapeutic work through avoidance strategies, for example lateness, social chat
2. Dependency – refers to an assumption that the group members' needs will be magically met by another, leading to passive behaviour by the group and the leader being seen as omnipotent or idealised. This is unstable and may lead to an attack and an unconscious wish to get rid of the leader
3. Pairing – when the defensive formation of 'couples' takes place in a group in light of extreme anxiety. A position of 'shared' understanding in the group then emerges and the 'couple' jointly takes on the work of the group through their interactions as a pair. The group may see the couple as if a sexualised pair and all creativity may become located within the couple

Group members vary in their tendencies towards these basic assumption positions and can oscillate between them, depending on the nature and intensity of the anxiety emerging in the group. These ideas describe universal processes in groups – be they therapeutic, social, political, organisational and so on. At times, these qualities may be necessary and desirable – for example the need for military discipline during conflict where dependency on the leaders to follow instructions may be vital. Bion's ideas have made a major contribution to the understanding of group processes, particularly in elucidating destructive forces. These ideas have informed the development of group consultancy for organisations, and group relations events such as the Leicester Conference, a highly regarded annual large group relations event in the UK [5].

In terms of group psychotherapy and overall clinical practice, the ideas of Foulkes and his group analytic approach have been widely spread across the UK and internationally, forming the primary group analytic treatment model.

The Group Analytic Treatment Model

The group analytic model embraces concepts from various disciplines such as psychoanalysis, sociology, systemic theory, and anthropology. Foulkes viewed the individual as a 'nodal point in a network of relationships' and the group as being 'larger than the sum of its parts'. He coined the term 'matrix' [6], which is a central concept in group analysis. The term refers to the hypothetical web of communication in the group that takes place both consciously and unconsciously during the group. He divided the matrix into the 'foundation' and the 'dynamic' matrix. A group member arrives in the group with the foundation matrix (his/her own history, culture, nationality, race, traumas, sex, gender, social status etc.) and this is quite a static position. What then occurs is an interweaving of processes and narratives between group members throughout the life of the group which forms the dynamic group matrix, which is an ever-changing, creative space between people that has a potential for transformation and change for its members. The group and its members co-create something similar to a piece of music produced by an orchestra, a 'creative intersubjective space between people' where each group member learns to adjust to the rhythm of the group [7] and each individual's contribution is understood in the context of the whole [8].

Foulkes was influenced by the sociologist Elias (1897–1990) and emphasised the fundamental need to *relate* and *belong*, as primary, and man's social instinct as an '*irreducible basic fact*' [9]. Humans cannot exist in isolation like a fish cannot live without water. They are interdependent, always part of one group or another, inseparable from their societies. According to Elias the individual is the singular, and the social is the plural of the same phenomenon [10, 11]. Each individual is both enabled and constrained by the expectations and demands of both themselves and others.

Mental health difficulties arise in the context of family and social groups. Within the therapy group, this complex web of family and interpersonal relationships becomes manifest through the transference relationships, between the therapist and the patient, the therapist and the group and between the patients themselves. New meaning is created through the group's common narrative which can be understood and offer new insights, allowing the possibility for different ways of perceiving and responding to others. The individual can then mature and grow through this process. The group as the 'environment mother' and the matrix of communication is the transformational object that in itself provides the basis and containment for psychological development.

While Foulkes has been criticised for neglecting the group's destructive forces in groups, several authors have further enriched group analytic theory [12–17] by paying attention to those processes. Nitsun for example, introduced the 'anti-group' concept which incorporates the destructive processes that take place during the group experience [15]. He suggested that the therapist must hold both creative and destructive processes in mind for the group's transformative potential to be reached. Without the therapist's awareness of these destructive processes, there is a danger of idealisation of the group which cannot be sustained and which limits the potential growth and is a threat to the group's survival.

The Role of the Group Therapist/Conductor

Foulkes defined group psychotherapy as 'psychotherapy for the group, of the group, including its conductor' [18], emphasising that the therapist is also a group member who learns from, and to an extent is altered by, the group experience. He renamed the group therapist as 'conductor', a term reflecting the orchestra-conductor's fluctuating authority and nuanced facilitatory role. The conductor, in the early stages, is responsible for '*modulating the tempo, linking various instruments together, interpreting the score*' [19]. As the group progresses, the conductor acts more as a facilitator and a convenor rather than a leader, relinquishing his/her authority to the group with exception at times of great anxiety or change in the group where greater containment is needed, for example when members join or leave the group.

Dynamic Administration

The group therapist's primary task, during its early group formation is called dynamic administration. Dynamic administration '*refers to various activities which the conductor performs in order to maintain this setting. The concept includes such apparently mundane tasks such as arranging the furniture in the room and drafting letters to group members which in the face of it might be delegated to a secretary or administrator. The conductor takes on these tasks because they have dynamic significance and have to be woven into the material which forms the analytic process*' [8]. In the early phases of the group the anxiety tends to run high as in other forms of psychotherapy but in a group this is much amplified by the presence of other group members who are effectively strangers. The group may evoke a fear of contagion of others' 'madness or depression', exposure of weakness, vulnerability, helplessness and dependency as well as fear of the responses of others, annihilation of the self and loss of identity in the face of the group. The conductor's authority and leadership style is crucial at this point.

Particularly in the early stages of joining a group, patients may find ways to reduce anxiety by challenging the boundaries of the group, for example forming subgroups or deciding to meet outside the sessions. This undermines the task of the group and may also repeat early life boundary violations. The analyst's firm, curious but non-critical authority is required in these circumstances in order to recover safe boundaries and the capacity for the group to act as a safe and effective container [20].

The Conductor's Interventions

The conductor is responsible for cultivating the group's therapeutic culture. He/she is simultaneously a conductor, convenor and a group member, generating exchange in order to facilitate communication. As the group progresses, and the search is on for the 'language of the group', communication moves from monologue, to dialogue and then, in a mature group, to discourse [21].

Psychoanalytic concepts – transference, countertransference, projection and projective identification are drawn upon and are helpful in understanding the powerful processes within the group. Transference is understood not only as vertical (from patient to therapist or from therapist to the group) but also horizontal (between patients) and from the patient to the group as a whole. Attention is paid to both verbal and non-verbal communication. Interventions can be directed towards anyone person in the group, or towards the group as a whole. Free-floating discussion is the group analytic equivalent to psychoanalytic free association when meaning emerges via metaphors, dreams, feedback, exchange of ideas, feelings and narratives, all 'capable of bringing moments of significance and illumination where change can take place' [21].

The Conductor's Subjectivity

The conductor is both a 'participant and an observer' and 'not a neutral bystander in the group's ever changing processes' [9]. There can therefore be no proper examination of the interactions and pathology in groups without also examining oneself as a group member. The conductor's unconscious is activated from the very start, group events are unknown and unpredictable and the anxiety evoked also affects the conductor. Therefore, in order to qualify as a group analyst, the therapists themselves need a rigorous experience of being a patient in a group.

The way the group functions will in part be related to the conductor's strengths, vulnerabilities and blind spots. For example, if the conductor's anger or frustration for the group is not adequately processed, then the group can get stuck and patients may find themselves unable to express aggression, rage and hatred [22]. The conductor should also be acutely aware of the impact of sociocultural events and social unconscious forces on the individual's and group's development and how this continuously gets re-enacted in the here and now of the group.

Some Important Concepts in Group Analytic Psychotherapy

The Matrix

Foulkes believed that the transformational nature of the group lay in the group's 'Matrix', the hypothetical web of interpersonal and transpersonal communications that takes place in the group. The word 'matrix' originates from the symbolic derivation of the womb, emphasising the group's generative and containing properties. This concept is central in group analytic theory but is also at times seen as a nebulous and confusing concept. It forms an ever-changing, non-linear, interactive process among its members, and the group as a whole is the active agent of transformation and change.

The transpersonal refers to universal themes that are unconsciously shared and go 'through' a person, whereas the interpersonal relates to the interaction between people and to the potential interactive processes that take place in the group.

Location of Disturbance and 'Autistic Mumbling' of the Symptom in the Group

Mental health difficulties can be considered as disturbances of relating, and all forms of illness occur within a network of relationships. Psychological disturbance is understood as being 'located between people'. This allows for a conceptualisation of psychopathology as an expression of a disturbance of communication and relating that goes beyond any one individual and is in fact located in the whole group. This becomes manifest and available for understanding when treatment is offered in a group. This is a very helpful way of thinking about illness and disorder as it reduces scapegoating or excessive focus on any index member as being the disturbed one. Pathology and illness can be enabled and constrained by the individual and the group. For example, the repetition of a symptom (a patient who talks week after week about a physical sensation of pain or a mental symptom such as low mood) might leave people in the group feeling bored and uninterested. This repetition of the same symptom can function to block communication between people in the group and the symptom can be seen as 'autistic mumbling' that attacks the capacity to relate with others as it just mumbles to itself. When this is understood as a process that is unconsciously reinforced by more than one person in the group, then the autistic mumbling can have shared ownership and people can begin to talk about deeper anxieties and fears. This is an example of how a moment of deeper understanding can be a point of potential transformation if seized. The individual learns to communicate distress via other means, neurotic symptoms can reduce and narcissistic preoccupation markedly abates.

Mirroring and Resonance

Past interpersonal struggles are repeated and explored through the group's interactional processes under the conductor's watchful analytic stance. Foulkes and Anthony [23] likened the group to a 'hall of mirrors' where unconscious aspects of oneself can be experienced as located in someone else in the group. This process of mirroring can become very clear in the group, and its recognition can be transformative. In contrast, malignant mirroring [18] is a form of negative mirroring where unwanted and repressed aspects of oneself can become stuck and rigidly located in the other. A typical example of this is when a patient states '*this group is full of depressed and boring people and is bringing me down*' when they are actually referring to their own depression and their desire to locate it outside themselves.

Other transformative experiences in a group include 'resonance' where suddenly and unexpectedly something expressed by one patient can strike a chord and deeply move another in the group. Foulkes refers to resonance as the: shared '*reaction in response to a stimulus*' when members discover a '*share-able common key, common coin*' with which they can communicate [6]. For example, a story brought by a patient of being anxious and angry when they encountered a homeless person in the street may reverberate and resonate deeply with another patient's experience of not belonging. The conductor may then attempt to explore this as a communication from the group as a whole with regard to what type of '*home*' one is looking to find in group therapy.

Social Unconscious

Another important group analytic concept is the 'social unconscious', a '*second nature*' of '*which the individual is unaware*'. Hopper, a psychoanalyst and group analyst, viewed the social unconscious and the individual unconscious as inseparable. He conceptualised the social unconscious as '*the existence and constraints of social, cultural and communicational arrangements of which people might be unaware or partially aware*' and emphasised the penetrating forces of society acting upon the individual which are vital for understanding a person and their groupings, in every form and structure [24].

Setting Up a Group, Indications and Contraindications

Group Composition and Membership: Selection Process

The small analytic group is a heterogeneous, slow-open, stranger group consisting of approximately eight patients and a group conductor/therapist. 'Slow open' means that patients can join and leave after a certain duration while newcomers join and the group continues. 'Stranger' means that patients do not know each other before they first meet for the group and they are encouraged to only meet during the group. Normally these groups convene once a week for 90 minutes, some groups may meet twice weekly. In many of these groups there is no specified ending date and members can remain in the group for as long as required. Lorentzen [25], a group analyst in Norway, has shown positive outcomes in patients who attend short-term groups of less than a year's duration.

Patients in the group usually have various mental health difficulties, come from different sociocultural backgrounds and are generally of mixed gender, ethnicity, employment and marital status, although some single-sex groups are available. Groups with this diversity are called 'heterogeneous'. 'Homogeneous' groups are set up to address one specific primary problem, for example eating disorders or sexual abuse.

As with all forms of psychotherapy, careful consideration should be given as to whether this form of treatment is likely to be helpful to this patient at this point in time. This occurs as part of an initial consultation process with the patient. The group therapist carefully considers what type of group the patient may be best suited to.

Initial Consultation

The consultation process varies in duration but typically consists of two to three sessions. Factors to be considered during the one-to-one meetings with the patient are reasons for seeking psychotherapy, his/her response to previous therapeutic encounters, anxieties and thoughts about joining the group, resentment, ambivalence and resistance observed in relation to psychotherapy but more importantly on entering a group process. Particular emphasis is placed on previous experiences in groups such as families, school, university, peers, friendships, sports teams, colleagues etc. It is important to take note, for example, how the patient ranks in birth order with regard to other siblings in the family and what his/her role had been in relation to this. Was he/she an only child who was never used to sharing or was he/she one of many and felt lost among his/her siblings? How much will this be played out in the group and how might he/she think about this during the initial consultation? Can he/she find his/her voice in a group? Other group treatments offered in the past and response to them will also be considered. Exploration of these issues informs the therapist as to how a patient might form part of a therapy group, where attention and space is shared with other patients. This is different to individual therapy where the patient will have the therapist all to him/herself. Common anxieties about joining a group include that the past may become repeated within the group – which is exactly why group therapy may be indicated.

Vignette

Jasmine had a history of repeated abusive relationships. During the consultation process she was initially opposed to group therapy, saying she was worried that in a group she will simply take on every one else's problems and again feel like a doormat whom others exploit. The group therapist was able to explain how this is exactly why group therapy could be seen as the treatment of choice in providing a live arena in which just this pattern can be seen, understood and changed in the safety of a therapeutic setting.

The therapist's feelings in relation to the experience with the patient in the room (counter-transference) is also important just as it would be if one was assessing for suitability for individual psychotherapy. Can the therapist work with this patient or is there something unbearable felt in the room in relation to this patient that might not be tolerated or be possible to explore during the therapeutic endeavour? Can this be worked through and contained with the therapist maintaining the capacity to think or not?

There are wide inclusion criteria for an analytic heterogeneous group. Patients presenting with anxiety, depression, relationship difficulties, struggling to negotiate developmental and transition points in their lives, and a history of unprocessed trauma, bereavement or loss can be suitable [26]. Patients need to have a degree of insight and motivation to change, some capacity to relate, and curiosity about the sharing process of the group. They should show commitment during the consultation process with punctual and reliable attendance, which is a good prognostic sign for future group attendance. Group therapy can be indicated when relationship factors are key to the presentation with the expectation these difficulties will become manifest and possible to explore within the group.

Vignette

Mark has a pattern of repeated conflicts with authority figures after growing up with a dominating and physically abusive father. This has affected his employment due to conflict with bosses, he has dropped out of individual therapy and does not follow medical or psychiatric advice. In the group, members recognise how he tries to challenge and also undermine the therapist's authority – they are both sympathetic and also challenging and he feels sufficiently supported to talk about how frightened he was of his father, and how this has affected all his subsequent relationships.

Exclusion Criteria

Potential exclusion criteria for group psychotherapy are:

- Extreme paranoia
- Paranoid personality disorder
- Psychotic symptomatology
- Acutely suicidal states of mind
- Acute uncontained crises
- History of extreme violence or uncontrolled past or recent impulsive and explosive behaviour

Supervision

Discussing potential referrals in supervision is vital as the supervision group's 'third eye' can assist in ensuring a safe and balanced group composition, taking also into account countertransference responses not only from the presenting therapist but also from the rest of supervision members; supervision too is helpfully informed when carried out within a group. For example, a therapist may have positive responses towards a patient during the consultation process and no concerns with regard to joining his/her group, while supervision peers may pick up hostility and resentment, suggesting further work is needed in order to gain a fuller picture. This process allows deeper anxieties to come to light during the next session which may have remained 'hidden' during the initial meeting. Addressing such anxieties before potentially joining a group allows a realistic consideration of how one might experience or behave in the group, and the balance between ambivalence and commitment once he/she joins. Therapists normally prefer to see the patient in the room where the group will take place so that a patient can have a more direct experience of the physical setting which could put him/her in touch more acutely of what it might be like to join the group.

Setting Up a Group: Practical Considerations

In the preceding sessions of a new member joining the psychotherapy group, the therapist explores the newcomer's and also the existing patients' thoughts, feelings and anxieties with regard to the imminent new arrival. Importantly, the newcomer is prepared for the likely interpersonal, interdependent experience that will be encountered in the group and the existing group members prepared for the arrival of the new member and their responses to this change in the group. In addition, the following essential questions about practical aspects of group therapy need to be explored:

- Can the potential newcomer attend this particular group consistently and reliably at this particular day/time in view of work or other commitments?
- Can he/she commit to a minimum of a year in the group?
- Will he/she be a complete stranger in this group apart from knowing the therapist? (The aim is for this to be a stranger group so that crossover from actual past relationships is kept to a minimum and the group is a confidential, neutral space for new relationships to emerge where reflection is possible.)

The conductor makes the prospective newcomer aware of the following group principles prior to joining:

- Members should know and call each other by their first names only
- Confidentiality is paramount and what is presented in the group remains in the group unless the therapist decides to break confidentiality in the exceptional circumstances of imminent high risk to self or others. To this effect, no contact is advised between patients outside the group sessions
- Regular and punctual attendance is encouraged as well as notice of absences.
- It is strongly recommended that a patient commits to the group for a minimum of a year
- When deciding to leave the group, the patient is advised to give at least a few months' notice

Any violation of these principles is considered to be a 'boundary incident' and is viewed as a non-verbal communication requiring careful exploration. These principles are addressed during the consultation as part of the preparation process. The conductor watches for conscious and unconscious reactions when these are discussed with the patient.

The existing members are also informed in advance of the newcomer's arrival. Therapists vary as to what information they divulge to the group about the newcomer.

Common anxieties about joining a group include knowing another patient beforehand, taking on others' problems when they have enough problems themselves, not having enough space in the group to explore their own issues, having to put up with an aggressive patient in the group, not having anything in common with others. The therapist can attempt to allay or explore some of those fears during the preparation period. For example, confidentiality is an essential parameter that needs to be introduced very early on in the consultation. The therapist should ensure as far as possible that this is a stranger group but on very rare occasions, someone might know someone else in the group, despite the conductor's careful selection process. Under these circumstances, the patient needs to feel in safe hands with a therapist who will address this straight away in the group so that a decision is made whether it would be appropriate for both patients to co-exist in the group or whether the newcomer may have to leave and a new group to be found for him/her. The common anxiety of encountering someone aggressive and 'out of control' in the group may need to be thought in relation to the patient's own aggressive and unacceptable impulses that may seem to be out of control. Not having anything in common with others might reflect an early experience of not belonging and always feeling different. The decision to leave a group is also importantly addressed within the group to consider all factors, including unconscious processes, which may be informing this decision.

Vignette

Mati had grown up with a younger brother who represented his country at athletics and whom he felt had usurped his position in the family. He presented with marital problems and difficulty loving his young son whom he felt absorbed all his wife's attention. After a year in the group during which he engaged well he abruptly announced he wished to leave. This followed a new younger man joining the group and Mati was greatly helped when advised of the importance of staying and working through feelings of sibling rivalry and anxiety about replacement, anger and displacement in the group.

Conclusion

Group analytic psychotherapy addresses the individual in the group, the group in the individual and the space in between. It places emphasis on the relationship between self and other, the interpenetration of the personal self and the social self and the understanding of both individual and social unconscious creative and destructive processes occurring between people. Attention to both content and process is required at all times with focus on both verbal and non-verbal communication.

The psychotherapy group provides a live setting in which to address one's own difficulties and to gain a deeper understanding of the self and others. In this rich therapeutic arena, one's own unconscious contributions to both difficulties in relating as well as increased knowledge of one's own strengths and resources can be achieved in a life-changing manner.

In contrast to individual psychotherapy, in which the dyadic relationship between therapist and patient provides the focus of intense attention, in the group there continuously exist multiple transference and countertransference responses (both vertical: between patient and therapist and horizontal: between patients) providing ample opportunities to consider how we relate and fail to relate, understand and misunderstand. With time, this process equips the individual with more insight into the self but also with the social and interpersonal tools to have a more fulfilling life increasing resilience, well-being as well as concern and compassion for the self and other.

The group is a journey and not the destination. What is critical is the complexity of the process and the challenges it presents. Complexity in the group is about the convolutions of the dialogue that leads to discourse, the struggle with the presence of boundaries and the absence of direction, with continuous tension between the individual and the group. What emerges is not a solution but new vistas, a new narrative of relationships.

In a small therapeutic group, the reality is that no one alone has the power to decide how change is going to emerge and what shape it will take. Through the co-creation, interdependence and continuous interactive discourse of its members, one can actively make a 'home among strangers' [21].

The best advocate for this approach is the patient. Therefore, I conclude with parts of a poem from a patient about a group (copyright consent given). The poem speaks of the power of transformation and hope that this approach can offer.

Seven years in a group

> When I was young and quite depressed
> Full of loss and pain and grief
> I joined a group of troubled souls
> All searching for relief
>
> As told we tried to share our lives
> We sat together twice a week
> And though our words were quite apart
> My dreams began to leak
>
> I found the group spoke out today
> But used the voices of my past
> I thought that I had run away
> I found my childhood held me fast
>
> I'd always thought I owned myself
> I now found out I was on loan
>
> . . .
>
> My group became my other selves
> They even seemed to share my skin
> I couldn't tell whose mind was whose
> And in my turn I sucked them in
>
> But in a while I found I could
> Without the guilt of being wrong
> Decide which parts I wished to own
> And which to pass along . . ..
> *R Brown, 2011*

References

1. RCPsych Psychotherapies. www.rcpsych.ac.uk/mental-health/treatments-and-wellbeing/psychotherapies?searchTerms=GROUP%20PSYCHOTHERAPY [Accessed 6/11/2020]

2. Yalom ID. *The Theory and Practice of Group Psychotherapy*, 5th ed. New York: Basic Books, 2005.

3. De Mare P. Michael Foulkes and the Northfield experiment. In M Pines, ed., *The Evolution of Group Analysis*. London: Routledge. 1983; pp. 218–31.

4. Pines M. *The Evolution of Group Analysis*. London: Jessica Kingsley Publishers, 2000.

5. Bion WR. *Experiences in Groups*. London: Tavistock Publications Ltd, 1961.

6. Foulkes SH. *Selected Papers: Psychoanalysis and Group Analysis*. London: Karnac Books, 1990.

7. Wotton L. Between the notes. *Group Anal* 2012; 46(10): 48–60.

8. Behr H, Hearst L. *Group-Analytic Psychotherapy: A Meeting of Minds*. London: Whurr Publishers Ltd, 2005.

9. Foulkes SH. *Therapeutic Group Analysis*. London: George Allen & Unwin, 1964.

10. Stacey R. *Complexity and Group Processes: A Radically Social Understanding of Individuals*. Hove: Brunner-Routledge, 2003.

11. Stacey R. Affects and cognition in a social theory of unconscious processes. *Group Anal* 2005; 38(1): 159–76.

12. Zinkin L. Malignant mirroring. *Group Anal* 1983; 16: 113–26.

13. Shermer VL, Pines M. *Ring of Fire. Primitive Affects and Object Relations in Group Psychotherapy*. London: Routledge, 1994.

14. Hinshelwood RD. Attacks on the reflective space: containing primitive emotional states. In VL Schermer, M Pines, eds., *Ring of Fire. Primitive Affects and Object Relations in Group Psychotherapy*. London: Routledge. 1994; pp. 86–106.

15. Nitsun M. *The Anti-group: Destructive Forces in the Group and Their Creative Potential*. London: Routledge, 1996.

16. Brown D. Pairing Bion and Foulkes. In RM Lipgar, M Pines, eds., *Building on Bion*. London: Jessica Kingsley Publishers. 2003; pp. 153–80.

17. Hopper E. *Traumatic Experience in the Unconscious Life of Groups*. London: Jessica Kinsgley Publishers Ltd, 2003.

18. Foulkes SH. *Group Analytic Psychotherapy: Methods and Principles*. London: Gordon and Breech, 1975.

19. Barwick N. Core concepts: what does the conductor do? Part 1. In N Barwick, M. Weegman, eds., *Group Therapy. A Group-Analytic Approach*. London: Routledge. 2018; pp. 51–69.

20. Zinkin L. The group as container and contained. *Group Anal* 1989; 22: 227–34.

21. Schlapobersky J. *From the Couch to the Circle: Group-Analytic Psychotherapy in Practice*. London: Routledge, 2016.

22. Papanastassiou M. The Pygmalion concept in group analysis. The conductor's anti-group and the search for the group as a container. *Group Anal* 2019; 52(1): 36–50.

23. Foulkes SH, Anthony EJ. *Group Psychotherapy: The Psychoanalytic Approach*. Harmondsworth: Penguin, 1965.

24. Hopper E, Weinberg H. *The Social Unconscious in Persons, Groups and Societies*. London: Karnac Books; 2011.

25. Lorentzen S. *Group Analytic Psychotherapy. Working with Affective, Anxiety and Personality Disorders*. Hove: Routledge, 2013.

26. Brown D. Assessment and selection for group. In J Roberts, M Pines, eds., *The Practice of Group Analysis*. London: Routledge. 1991; pp. 55–72.

Mentalizing in Psychiatric Practice

Chapter

12

Anthony W. Bateman

The concept of Mentalizing is a recent theoretical development that has made a major contribution to our understanding of, and capacity to clinically work with, patients with a variety of different disorders. This has been particularly significant in the treatment of borderline personality disorder (BPD). Mentalizing draws upon psycho-analytic, cognitive and relational models of psychological functioning, attachment theory and neuroscience. It is central to psychiatric practice for a number of reasons. First it is a transdiagnostic concept and so is applicable to a range of mental health conditions spanning childhood to old age [1]. Second its position as a well-developed component of the literature on neurobiology and higher-order cognition (HOC) gives it a central place in neuropsychiatry and cognitive psychology [2]. The component of HOC that is called mentalizing has the capacity to rearrange processes within the brain and assure 'business as usual' notwithstanding adverse conditions.

- Mentalizing is thinking about actions in terms of thoughts and feelings
- Reflective mentalizing is using knowledge of these mental states to master life challenges (metacognitive mastery, or the ability to respond to psychological challenges effectively on the basis of psychological knowledge or reflective mentalizing) or designating thoughts as 'just thoughts' that do not need to be acted on or that, by contrast, need to be seriously and maturely considered [3]
- Affective mentalizing and mentalized affectivity [4] is a higher-order process above cognition including cognition regarding emotions

Mentalizing increases resilience to adversity, protecting psychological vulnerable individuals from relapse, and improving therapeutic outcomes [5]. Focussing on mentalizing helps people consider how teams, systems and services interact to facilitate or undermine interventions and the delivery of services; a non-mentalizing team and system has a negative impact on clinical care by creating an environment that impedes the implementation of reliable and responsive pathways to care and the realisation of skilful treatment [6].

What Is Mentalizing?

Mentalizing as a concept arose from a dynamic, interpersonal understanding of mental processes. It describes a particular facet of the human imagination: an awareness of mental states in oneself and in other people, particularly in explaining their actions [7]. It involves perceiving and interpreting the feelings, thoughts, beliefs and wishes that explain what people do. This entails an awareness of someone's circumstances, their prior patterns of behaviour and the experiences to which the individual has been exposed. Similarly, to mentalize ourselves entails an acceptance of our prior experiences, their influence on us and an awareness of our current context.

The idea that mentalizing is an act of imagination implies that any act of mentalizing is by its very nature uncertain; internal states are opaque, changeable, and quite often difficult to pin down, even in one's own mind. This means that any attempt to make sense of mental states is vulnerable to error or inaccuracy. Usually we recognise and rapidly correct errors when our understanding fails to produce a coherent narrative of ourselves and others. But this emphasis on the imagination, and the intrapersonal and interpersonal uncertainty this entails, creates great potential as well as significant vulnerabilities – our reliance on our imagination to explain experience generates our social complexity and cultural creativity, but also leaves us vulnerable to psychological disorder and psychic distress. Persistent failures in mentalizing lead to psychiatric symptoms [8]. We fail to interpret our own internal states accurately, we misperceive what is happening in the external world, we overemphasise or undervalue our selves in the world. In short as our mentalizing decreases we no longer have a robust illusion of personal integrity and continuity and our mental processes fragment.

Although mentalizing functions as a single entity or aptitude, neuroscientists have identified four different components, or *dimensions*, to mentalizing [9], which reflect different social-cognitive processes. They are:

1. Controlled versus automatic mentalizing
2. Mentalizing the self versus mentalizing others
3. Mentalizing with regard to external versus internal features
4. Cognitive versus affective mentalizing

Controlled mentalizing reflects a serial and relatively slow process, which is typically verbal and demands reflection, attention, awareness, intention and effort. The opposite pole of this dimension, automatic mentalizing, involves much faster processing, tends to be reflexive and requires little or no attention, intention, awareness or effort. It is used in daily interaction when assumptions are made about mental states which underpin conversation and perspective; they serve the individual well as long as the assumptions have a level of accuracy.

The self–other mentalizing dimension involves the capacity to mentalize one's own state – the *self* (including one's own physical experiences) and/or the state of *others*. The two are closely connected, and an imbalance signals vulnerability in mentalizing both others and the self. Individuals with mentalizing difficulties are likely to preferentially focus on one end of the spectrum, although they may be impaired at both.

Mentalizing can involve making inferences on the basis of the *external* indicators of a person's mental states (e.g. facial expressions) or figuring out someone's *internal* experience from what one knows about them and the situation they are in. From the perspective of clinical assessment, the internal–external distinction is particularly significant in helping clinicians understand why some patients appear to be seriously impaired in their capacity to 'read the mind' of others, yet they may be hypersensitive to facial expressions or bodily posture, giving the impression of being astute about others' states of mind. The external focus can make a person extremely vulnerable to the observable behaviour of others.

Cognitive mentalizing involves the ability to name, recognise and reason about mental states (in oneself or others), whereas *affective* mentalizing involves the ability to understand the *feeling* of such states (again, in oneself or others), which is necessary for any genuine experience of empathy or sense of self.

What Is Ineffective Mentalizing?

To mentalize effectively requires the individual not only to be able to maintain a balance across these dimensions of social cognition but also to apply them appropriately according to context [8]. In an adult with personality disorder, for example, consistently imbalanced mentalizing on at least one of these four dimensions would be evident. From this perspective, different types of psychopathology can be distinguished on the basis of different combinations of impairments along the four dimensions which are referred to as different mentalizing profiles.

If an imbalance of mentalizing becomes fixed the mental processes become dominated by modes of mentalizing known as:

- Psychic equivalence
- Teleological mode
- Pretend mode [10]

In psychic equivalence thoughts become facts, images are real and internal understanding is the same as external reality leading to delusions, for example. Clinicians describe this initially as 'concreteness of thought' in their patients. There is a suspension of doubt, and the individual increasingly believes that their own perspective is the only one possible.

In teleological mode understanding motives of others is determined by what happens in the physical world – 'he did not text me so it means he did not love me'. The teleological mode appears in patients who are imbalanced towards the external pole of the internal–external mentalizing dimension – they are heavily biased towards understanding how people (and they themselves) behave and what their intentions may be in terms of what they physically do.

In pretend mode there is a decoupling of mental states from external influence so the patient functions in an isolated world uninfluenced by mental states of others; the person is unable to hold more than one version of reality simultaneously. In more extreme cases, this may lead to feelings of derealisation and dissociation.

Psychopathology and Mentalizing

Psychiatric symptoms and syndromes arise in the context of a failure of mentalizing; the mentalizing problems may either be a core component of the disorder and lead to symptoms or rather be the result of the mental changes. This is evidenced by the major psychiatric categories of personality disorder, mood disorder and psychosis, all of which have been shown to be associated with mentalizing problems.

The Mentalizing Model of Borderline Personality Disorder (BPD)

An underlying failure in mentalizing and its relationship to adversity and attachment has been presented as a model for BPD [8, 11].

Mentalizing develops in the context of attachment relationships throughout childhood and adolescence. Secure attachment processes facilitate robust mentalizing while disorganised and insecure attachment processes, especially in the context of developmental trauma and neglect, undermine the acquisition of stable mentalizing. A core feature of BPD is poor mentalizing, with different problems arising at different stages of the disorder, dependent on the mentalizing profile of the individual [12–14].

The mentalizing profile of a patient with BPD tends to show imbalance in all the dimensions of mentalizing:

1. There is often an unstable self-representation and sometimes an over-reliance and acceptance of other representation and a domination of affective processing and automatic mentalizing, and reliance on external mentalizing
2. The attachment system in BPD may be disordered [15], and the problems of the attachment system may create a vulnerability in relation to interpersonal interaction and intimate relationships [16, 17]
3. There is suggestive evidence that mentalizing can protect from the expression of symptoms and it is the failure of that protection (resilience) that makes someone symptomatic [18]
4. Developmentally, the quality of attachment and mentalizing interact in complex causal ways: while a benign attachment context is considered to enhance mentalizing, understanding and overcoming adversity entails the enhancement of mentalizing in the process of overcoming the trauma [19]

Mentalizing in Mood Disorder

In depression the situation is different. The disorder itself impacts on mentalizing and most studies have found that the duration and severity of depression negatively influences mentalizing capacities. Clinical experience and a growing body of research suggest that disturbed mood impairs individuals' ability to mentalize [20, 21]. When depressed individuals attempt to mentalize, mentalizing is likely to be distorted, with excessive self-preoccupation and ineffective mentalizing modes dominating, for example psychic equivalence in which feeling bad means 'I am bad' [22]. Mentalizing is shut down and the individual shows hypomentalizing with poverty of thought, inability to access emotion, and experience of body and mental emptiness. Studies have quite consistently reported impairments in mentalizing, based on a wide variety of tasks, in patients with both unipolar and bipolar disorder [23].

In bipolar disorder mentalizing potentially becomes excessive with over-recruitment of the cognitive processing system leading to hypermentalizing [24]. Beliefs about the self and an understanding of the motives of others are not grounded in reality and become overly complex and intricate. This is a form of pretend mode in which the patient cannot accept difference in self and other representations. Importantly, these changes in mood disorders have been found to predict relapse in major depression and have been demonstrated in euthymic patients, even when basic cognitive dysfunctions associated with depressed mood were controlled for. This finding clearly suggests that mentalizing impairments continue to exist outside depressive episodes and thus may be involved in the onset and recurrence of mood disorders.

Mentalizing in Psychotic States

In psychotic states there is a reliance on low level mentalizing. Mental states lack differentiation and there is a breakdown between self and other, internal and external experience – self and other boundaries become permeable, thoughts become facts (psychic equivalence), mental images have the quality of reality (psychic equivalence), misunderstandings abound (teleological mode). However, phenomenologically, psychosis is defined not solely by symptoms of hallucinations and delusions, but also by a disturbance in mentalizing of self, which can be expressed in a number of different forms of psychotic subjectivity. Normally a sense of self-agency and capacity for self-regulation, established in the context of embodied engagements with caregivers during infancy, gradually fosters control and regulatory capacity over bodily signals, which is essential in establishing a minimal self [25]. The ubiquity and consistency of bodily cues firmly ground the individual's basic sense of continuity as an integrated continuous being. Dysfunctions within the sensory and self-monitoring processes necessarily alert the individual to attend to and manage states of vulnerability threatening the basis of self-integrity. Self-integrity is manifestly disturbed in schizophrenia and other disorders such as autistic spectrum disorders or other neurode-velopmental conditions [26].

Within this framework, a mentalization-based approach provides a legitimate starting point to address the central problem of psychosis – that of alterations in sense of self. Evidence also suggests that attachment and mentalizing may not represent causal factors in the development of psychosis [27] but rather represent key protective factors that can (a) attenuate the clinical course of emerging psychosis in those at increased risk and (b) sustain recovery in affected individuals. In other words, a mentalization-based approach to psych-osis seeks to enhance protective mechanisms in the early part of the disease, and to strengthen the 'non-psychotic' part of the personality [28, 29] in affected individuals, to promote resilience to life challenges.

Loss of the capacity to mentalize plays a key role in the development of mental distress, and robust and stable mentalizing increases resilience to social and personal set backs. A focus on generating mentalizing may therefore be helpful in the treatment of a range of psychiatric disorders either as the main target for intervention or as an adjunct to other treatment.

Mentalizing as a Focus for Psychiatric Intervention

Mentalizing is no different from any other mental activity – it improves with practice! So clinicians need to focus on mentalizing as a target of intervention by making mental states the subject of scrutiny whatever the intervention model they are using. A range of interven-tions stimulate mentalizing process and although these have been organised into a package known as mentalization-based treatment (MBT) [30, 31], all clinicians can engage in stimulating mentalizing process in their daily practice.

Attitude

The attitude of the clinician is crucial. The psychiatrist's task is to stimulate a mentalizing process as an essential aspect of any therapeutic interaction. Thinking about oneself and others develops, in part, through a process of identification in which the clinician's ability to use his mind and to demonstrate a change of mind when presented with alternative views is internalised by the patient, who gradually becomes more curious about his own and others' minds and is consequently better able to reappraise himself and his understanding of others. In addition, the continual reworking of perspectives and understanding of oneself and others in the context of stimulation of the attachment system and within different narrative contexts is key to a change process, as is the focus of the work on current rather than past experience.

Not-Knowing Stance

The 'not-knowing or mentalizing stance' [31] is part of this general therapeutic attitude and is central to ensuring that the psychiatrist maintains his curiosity about his patient's mental states. A common confusion has been that being a not-knowing clinician is equivalent to feigning ignorance. The clinician has a mind and is continually demonstrating that he can use it! He may hold alternative perspectives to the patient and if so this is a perfect moment for further exploration

In the role of clinician, you are naturally pulled into excess passivity or activity. Mentalizing entails striking a balance in which assumptions are actively questioned, probed and explored. It is especially productive to challenge patients' unreasonable assumptions about you and it is recommended that this is done through a series of therapeutic steps:

1. Empathy in relation to the patient's current subjective state
2. Exploration and clarification and, if appropriate, challenge
3. Identifying affect and establishing an affect focus
4. Mentalizing the relationship

Detailed discussion of these therapeutic interventions can be found in [31].

Arousal

Arousal undermines mentalizing. It is important to maintain arousal levels in a session within an optimal range – not too high so that mentalizing is overwhelmed, and not too low so that mentalizing becomes severely restricted. The aim is to help a patient manage arousal and become sensitive to levels of arousal and specific contexts that undermine mentalizing. Any intervention that is delivered with the primary aim of de-escalating excess affect and/or decreasing anxiety and/or increasing arousal can be used.

Contrary Moves

Mentalizing is a flexible, responsive process. In contrast non-mentalizing is fixed and rigid. The clinician focusses on increasing the patient's capacity to use different components of the dimensions of mentalizing in relation to context. For example, in everyday life it might be appropriate to use more cognitive aspects of mentalizing, in an important negotiation perhaps, and yet at another moment in the meeting to be sensitive to the emotional states of oneself and others if the negotiation is to be completed successfully. A patient who is overwhelmed by emotion may not be able to represent his/her states of mind to him/herself or to others and so loses the chance of someone else helping him/her with how he/she feels. Maintaining some cognitive sense of the bewilderment of the other might allow enough expression of the content of the emotion to enable another person to offer appropriate comfort. So the immediate task of the clinician is to help the patient maintain balance between the different poles of each dimension of mentalizing; move the patient towards an internal focus if they are excessively externally focussed or vice versa, heighten the affective component if the cognitive state of mind is to the fore, or vice versa, and so on.

Affect and Significant Events

A focus on affect in the context of significant events, especially in those involving relationships and personal interactions, is often considered to be a process of focussing on the patient's current affective state, identifying the what he/she is feeling, and labelling the emotion. This is only part of the focus on affect that is central to the practice of MBT. While important, this process is not sufficient to characterise the affect focus within a session. The patient must begin to identify the specific aspects of an interaction to which they are sensitive, develop ways of managing the affect they experience, and eventually become aware of them before they overwhelm their capacities to manage. To this end the clinician and patient identify affects as they arise during events and then label them as emotions to be monitored over time in treatment itself. So the process is the identification of these important affects and sensitivities and their recognition as and when they are triggered in a session. It is often the clinician's task to try to identify such affects so that they become available as part of the joint work. Identifying the affect is an important step in MBT because it links general exploratory work of affect to relational sensitivity. So it is within the patient–clinician interaction that detailed work is done to understand how relational processes interfere with mentalizing.

Mentalizing the Relationship

It has been suggested that the patient–clinician relationship in terms of transference is not used in MBT [32]. Perhaps it is the vigilant attitude to the use of the interpersonal relationship to promote mentalizing that has led to this view. Practitioners are cautioned firstly about the commonly stated aim of transference interpretation, namely to provide insight, and secondly about genetic aspects such as linking current experience to the past because of their potential iatrogenic effects. But equally 'mentalizing the relationship' is a key component of mentalizing intervention and so we have set out a series of steps to be followed to minimise the risk of harm.

The issue is the mentalizing capacity of the patient and its relationship to arousal. Complex interventions such as those related to detail of patient–clinician interaction or the genesis from the past of current states require a thoughtful and reflective patient if they are to be effective. A non-mentalizing patient who holds rigid mental perspectives and who has limited access to the richness of past experience is unlikely to be able to hold other perspectives in mind while he/she compares them to his/her own, particularly if they are complex and subtle. He is likely to feel overwhelmed; far from stimulating a mentalizing process the intervention compounds non-mentalizing by increasing anxiety. The patient panics, feeling incapable of considering the clinician's fully mentalized and coherent intervention. Structuring of mental processes occurs and the patient becomes more rigid and insistent about his own point of view.

1. The first step is the full validation of the experience the patient is having about the relationship with the clinician. The clinician seeks to see the perspective of the patient without implying the experience is a distortion. The danger of the genetic approach to working with transference is that it might implicitly invalidate the patient's experience

2. The second step is to identify and explore some of the detail of the patient experience – when did they first notice it, what are their thoughts about it. As the events which generated the feelings in the relationship are identified and the behaviours that the thoughts or feelings are tied to are made explicit, sometimes in painful detail, the contribution of the clinician to these feelings and thoughts will become apparent

3. The third step is for the clinician to accept his contribution towards the patient's experience. The patient's experience of his interaction with the clinician is likely to be

based on a partially accurate perception of the interaction, even if they are based on a small component of it. It is often the case that the clinician has been drawn into the relationship and acted in some way that is consistent with the patient's perception of him/her. It may be easy to attribute this to the patient, but this would be completely unhelpful

4. The fourth step is collaboration in arriving at an alternative perspective. Mentalizing alternative perspectives about the patient–clinician relationship must be arrived at in the same spirit of collaboration as any other form of mentalizing. The metaphor used for training is that the clinician must imagine sitting side by side with the patient rather than opposite him. They sit side by side looking at the patient's thoughts and feelings, where possible both adopting an inquisitive stance about them. The fifth step is for the clinician to present an alternative perspective, and the final step is to monitor carefully the patient's reaction as well as one's own

Some of this process can be considered as mentalizing the 'counterrelationship' which is broadly the clinician presenting his own perspective. It is best to think of it as 'being ordinary' in the sense of considering what would you say or do if your friend told you this or behaved in this way towards you. This is not a licence for you to behave in any way you please or to say whatever you like – any more than you would do in a respectful relationship with a friend. Rather, it is advocating openly working on your state of mind in therapy in a way that moves the joint purpose of the relationship forward, keeping your and your patient's mentalizing on-line. To do this you often will have to speak from your own perspective rather than from your understanding of your patient's experience.

Evidence for Effectiveness of Mentalizing as a Target of Treatment

Originally developed for the treatment of BPD, MBT, in keeping with mentalizing as a transdiagnostic concept, has been tested in a range of disorders and subjected to a number of randomised controlled trials.

An initial study of MBT for BPD [33] compared its effectiveness in the context of a day hospital programme with routine general psychiatric care for patients with BPD. Treatment took place within a routine clinical service and was implemented by mental health professionals without full psychotherapy training who were offered expert supervision. Results showed that patients in the day hospital programme showed a statistically significant decrease on all measures in contrast to the control group, which showed limited change or deterioration over the same period. Improvement in depressive symptoms, decrease in suicidal and self-mutilatory acts, reduced inpatient days, and better social and interpersonal function began after 6 months and continued to the end of treatment at 18 months. Follow-up at eight years [34] showed patients treated in MBT remained better than those receiving treatment as usual but their general social function continued to be somewhat impaired. Nevertheless, significantly more were in employment or full-time education than in the comparison group and only 14 per cent still met diagnostic criteria for BPD compared to 87 per cent of the patients in the comparison group who were available for interview.

A partial replication study of this original day hospital trial has been completed by an independent group in the Netherlands showing that good results are achievable within mental health services away from the instigators of the treatment [35–37]. Further evidence for this is presented by Petersen et al. [38] who treated a cohort of 22 patients with personality disorders with once-weekly mentalization-oriented group therapy for up to three years following a stabilisation phase in a day treatment programme. There was no dropout from treatment. Significant improvements were observed on symptoms, interpersonal function, social adjustment, and vocational status, and there was significant reduction in use of services.

An outpatient version of MBT was developed and was the focus of a further randomised controlled trial [39]. This randomised controlled trial tested the effectiveness of an 18-month MBT in an outpatient context (MBT-OP) against a structured clinical management (SCM-OP) approach for treatment of BPD [40]. Patients randomised to MBT-OP showed a steeper decline of both self-reported and clinically significant problems, including suicide attempts and hospitalisation. It appears from this study that although structured treatments improve outcomes for individuals with BPD, a focus on specific psychological processes brings additional benefits to structured clinical support. MBT is relatively undemanding in terms of training so it may be useful for implementation into general mental health services.

Further research on mentalizing and MBT has provided evidence that mentalizing failures can be a useful target for treatment in adolescents with behavioural and affective problems. In one study in an inpatient setting, a reduction in hypermentalizing (but not other forms of mentalizing) from admission to discharge appeared to be associated with a reduction in adolescent borderline symptoms from admission to discharge [13]. The presence of hypermentalizing can also distinguish between adolescents with borderline personality pathology, adolescents with other psychiatric disorders and healthy control adolescents on the basis of self-report [41]. Finally, mentalizing of the self (as operationalised through measures of experiential avoidance) was found to predict an increase in borderline symptomatology over the course of a one-year follow-up period in 881 adolescents recruited from the community [42]. That hypermentalizing can be reduced through a mentalization-based milieu approach to treatment [24] accords well with the results of a recent study in Denmark that showed a reduction in borderline symptoms in adolescents with borderline symptoms taking part in mentalization-based group therapy [43].

The effectiveness of a MBT approach in adolescents was derived from a randomised clinical trial conducted by [44]. In this study, 80 adolescents (85 per cent female) consecutively presenting to mental health services with self-harm and co-morbid depression were randomly allocated to either MBT-A or treatment as usual (TAU). Adolescents were assessed for self-harm, risk-taking and mood at baseline and at 3-monthly intervals until 12 months. Their attachment style, mentalizing capacity and BPD were also assessed at baseline and at the end of the 12-month treatment. Results indicated that MBT-A was more effective than TAU in reducing self-harm and depression. This superiority was explained by improved mentalizing and reduced attachment avoidance and reflected improvement in emergent BPD symptoms and traits.

Treatment for adolescents commonly includes family work and there is considerable development of mentalizing with families as a treatment intervention [45, 46]. More recently a families-based mentalizing intervention has been described for those families supporting a close person with BPD. In a delayed-treatment randomised controlled trial of a mentalization-based intervention for families or significant others living with or supporting a person with BPD 56 family members/significant others were randomised either to immediate Families and Carers Training Support (MBT-FACTS), a supportive and skills-based programme consisting of five 1.5- to 2-hour evening meetings, delivered by trained family members, or to delayed intervention [47]. The primary outcome was adverse incidents reported by the family member in relation to the person with BPD. Family members randomised to immediate intervention showed a significant reduction in reported adverse incidents between themselves and the identified patient in the second phase of treatment compared with those randomised to delayed intervention. Secondary outcome measures showed family functioning and well-being improved more in the immediate-treatment group; changes were maintained at follow-up. There were no differences in depression, total anxiety and total burden; both groups showed improvement on all these measures. Findings show that the MBT-FACTS programme delivered by families to families supporting a person with BPD reduces reported adverse incidents within the family. Further studies are needed to show whether this reduction improves outcomes for the individual with BPD.

Finally studies suggest that MBT may be useful in a range of disorders with data being reported on the use of MBT in treatment of people with antisocial personality disorder (ASPD) [48, 49], substance use disorder (SUD) [50] and eating disorders [51]. Individuals with BPD who were co-morbid with ASPD are more likely to show improvements in symptoms related to aggression when given standard outpatient MBT than those offered a structured protocol of similar intensity but excluding MBT components. This study suggests MBT may be a potential treatment for ASPD particularly in terms of its relatively high level of acceptability and promising treatment effects.

Mentalizing Milieu, Teams and Systems

Developing a secure, cohesive team is essential for effective treatment of patients with complex problems and for generating creative teamwork and a well-functioning unit that delivers skilful intervention. In essence, a team has to define one of their tasks as generating integrated interventions tailored to each patient. Any patient needs to experience a team which has an integrated and coherent understanding of them. Experiencing radically different perspectives of themselves from different members of the team will lead to anxiety and fragmentation. Teams need to work assiduously on a shared representation of each patient so that interventions are synergistic and facilitate more robust self-representation. The development and maintenance of a mentalizing clinician in the context of a team is a primary aim of Adaptive/Adolescent Mentalization-Based Integrative Treatment (AMBIT) [52].

The aim of the AMBIT model is to address the key features and challenges of working within complex systems using mentalizing as the integrating principle [53]. The model captures four key arenas:

- **Work with clients:** managing risk and non-engagement in a population that is often not conventionally help-seeking
- **Work with the team:** managing workers' experiences of anxiety, frustration and isolation, and the risk of them experiencing professional shame and burning out
- **Work with networks:** addressing inevitable disintegrations across multi-agency and multi-professional networks, and the frustrations that these evoke
- **Learning at work:** sustaining an openness to change from familiar (if frequently ineffective or exhausting) patterns of working towards the (assumed) riskiness of evaluating outcomes and trying new approaches.

Keeping a healthy morale when treating patients with severe personality disorders and other complex psychiatric problems can be challenging for several reasons. First, patients are emotionally challenging, at times becoming hostile to staff members and undermining their therapeutic confidence. Second, change in personality disorder is slow, which can lead to pessimism among members of the team. Third, splits in the team, whether arising from problems among the patients or within the team itself (which at this point may have divergent experiences and mental representations of the patient), commonly manifest themselves as disagreements about treatment that may become polarised, making it hard for individuals not to blame one another for management or treatment difficulties. Fourth, intermittent crises can lead to an onerous workload and constant anxiety about risk. Finally, in the event of a patient's suicide this has a profound effect on not only the individual clinician who was caring for the patient but also the whole team.

Sustaining and maintaining a secure, organised team with a healthy, enthusiastic morale can be achieved through working within a coherent treatment model. Mentalizing as a unifying and organising principle works well for this purpose because clinicians with divergent views about psychopathology relate to the generic nature of mentalizing as a mental process. A mentalizing milieu is created in which the focus is on clinician mental states along with those of the patient. The primary aim of interventions, whatever theoretical model being used, is to facilitate more robust mentalizing in the patient team supervision and group peer interaction reflects this.

References

1. Bateman A, Fonagy P. *Handbook of Mentalizing in Mental Health Practice*. Washington DC: American Psychiatric Publishing, 2012.

2. Rudrauf D. Structure-function relationships behind the phenomenon of cognitive resilience in neurology: insights for neuroscience and medicine. *Adv Neurosci* 2014; 2014: 1–28.

3. Sharp C, Fonagy P, Goodyer I. *Social Cognition and Developmental Psychopathology*. Oxford: Oxford University Press, 2008.

4. Jurist EJ. Mentalized affectivity. *Psychoanal Psychol* 2005; 22: 426–44.

5. Fonagy P, Allison E, Campbell C. In A Bateman, P Fonagy, eds., *Mentalizing, Resilience, and Epistemic Trust. Handbook of Mentalizing in Mental Health Practice*, 2nd ed. Washington DC: American Psychiatric Association Publishing. 2019; pp. 63–77.

6. Bales D, Verheul R, Hutsebaut J. Barriers and facilitators to the implementation of mentalization-based treatment (MBT) for borderline personality disorder. *Personal Ment Health* 2017; 11: 118–31.

7. Fonagy P, Gergely G, Jurist EL, Target M. *Affect Regulation, Mentalization and the Development if the Self*. New York: Other Press, 2002.

8. Fonagy P, Luyten P. A developmental, mentalization-based approach to the understanding and treatment of borderline personality disorder. *Dev Psychopathol* 2009; 21: 1355–81.

9. Lieberman MD. Social cognitive neuroscience: a review of core processes. *Annu Rev Psychol* 2007; 58: 259–89.

10. Fonagy P, Bateman A. The development of borderline personality disorder: a mentalizing model. *J Pers Disord* 2008; 22: 4–21.

11. Fonagy P, Campbell C, Bateman A. Update on Diagnostic Issues for Borderline Personality Disorder. *Psychiatric Times* July 2016; 33(7).

12. Luyten P, Fonagy P, Lowyck B, Vermote R. Assessment of mentalization. In A Bateman, P Fonagy, eds., *Handbook of Mentalizing in Mental Health Practice*.

Washington DC: American Psychiatric Association Publishing. 2012; pp. 43–66.

13. Sharp C, Ha C, Carbone C et al. Hypermentalizing in adolescent inpatients: treatment effects and association with borderline traits. *J Pers Disord* 2013; 27: 3–18.

14. Ensink K, Normandin L, Target M et al. Mentalization in children and mothers in the context of trauma: an initial study of the validity of the Child Reflective Functioning Scale. *Br J Dev Psychol* 2015; 33: 203–17.

15. Choi-Kain LW, Fitzmaurice GF, Zanarini MC, Laverdiere O, Gunderson JG. The relationship between self-reported attachment styles, interpersonal dysfunction, and borderline personality disorder. *J Nerv Ment Dis* 2009; 197: 816–21.

16. Gunderson J, Lyons-Ruth K. BPD's interpersonal hypersensitivity phenotype: a gene–environment–developmental model. *J Pers Disord* 2008; 22: 22–41.

17. Deckers JW, Lobbestael J, van Wingen GA et al. The influence of stress on social cognition in patients with borderline personality disorder. *Psychoneuroendocrinology* 2015; 52: 119–29.

18. Berthelot N, Ensink K, Bernazzani O et al. Intergenerational transmission of attachment in abused and neglected mothers: the role of trauma-specific reflective functioning. *Infant Ment Health J* 2015; 36: 200–12.

19. Luyten P, Fonagy P. Mentalizing and trauma. In A Bateman, P Fonagy, eds., *Handbook of Mentalizing in Mental Health Practice*, 2nd ed. Washington DC: American Psychiatric Association Publishing. 2019.

20. Weightman MJ, Air TM, Baune BTFP. A review of the role of social cognition in major depressive disorder. *Front Psychiatry* 2014; 5: 179–83.

21. Luyten P, Fonagy P. The stress–reward–mentalizing model of depression: an integrative developmental cascade approach to child and adolescent

depressive disorder based on the research domain criteria (RDoC) approach. *Clin Psychol Rev* 2018; 64: 87–98.

22. Lemma A, Target M, Fonagy P. *Brief Dynamic Interpersonal Therapy: A Clinician's Guide*. Oxford: Oxford University Press, 2011.

23. Billeke P, Boardman S, Doraiswamy PM. Social cognition in major depressive disorder: a new paradigm? *Transl Neurosci* 2013; 4: 437–47.

24. Sharp C, Vanwoorden SJ Hypermentalizing in borderline personality disorder: a model and data. *J Infant Child Adolesc Psychother* 2015; 14: 33–45.

25. Fotopoulou A, Tsakiris M. Mentalizing homeostasis: the social origins of interoceptive inference. *Neuropsychoanalysis* 2017; 19: 3–28.

26. Hobson P. Concerning knowledge of mental states. *Br J Med Psychol* 1990; 63: 199–214.

27. Debbané M, Benmiloud J, Salaminios G et al. Mentalization-based treatment in clinical high-risk for psychosis: a rationale and clinical illustration. *J Contemp Psychother* 2016; 46: 217–25.

28. Bion WR. Differentiation of the psychotic from the non-psychotic personalities. *Int J Psychoanal* 1957; 38: 266–75.

29. Debbané M, Salaminios G, Luyten P et al. Attachment, neurobiology, and mentalizing along the psychosis continuum. *Front Hum Neurosci* 2016; 10: 406.

30. Bateman A, Fonagy P. *Mentalization Based Treatment: A Practical Guide*. Oxford: Oxford University Press, 2006.

31. Bateman A, Fonagy P. *Mentalization Based Treatment for Personality Disorders: A Practical Guide*. Oxford: Oxford University Press, 2016.

32. Gabbard G. When is transference work useful in dynamic psychotherapy. *Am J Psychiatry* 2006; 163(10): 1667–9.

33. Bateman A, Fonagy P. The effectiveness of partial hospitalization in the treatment of borderline personality disorder –

a randomised controlled trial. *Am J Psychiatry* 1999; 156: 1563–9.

34. Bateman A, Fonagy P. 8-year follow-up of patients treated for borderline personality disorder: mentalization-based treatment versus treatment as usual. *Am J Psychiatry* 2008; 165: 631–38.

35. Bales D, van Beek N, Smits M et al. Treatment outcome of 18-month, day hospital mentalization-based treatment (MBT) in patients with severe borderline personality disorder in the Netherlands. *J Pers Disord* 2012; 26: 815–20.

36. Bales DL, Timman R, Andrea H et al. Effectiveness of day hospital mentalization-based treatment for patients with severe borderline personality disorder: a matched control study. *Clin Psychol Psychother* 2015; 22: 409–17.

37. Bales D, Timman R, Luyten P, Busschbach J, Verheul R. Implementation of evidence-based treatments for borderline personality disorder: the impact of organizational changes on treatment outcome of mentalization-based treatment. *Personal Ment Health* 2017; 11(4): 266–77.

38. Petersen B, Toft J, Christensen L et al. A 2-year follow-up of mentalization orientated group therapy following day hospital treatment for patients with personality disorders. *Personal Ment Health* 2010; 4: 294–301.

39. Bateman A, Fonagy P. Randomized controlled trial of out-patient mentalization based treatment versus structured clinical management for borderline personality disorder. *Am J Psychiatry* 2009; 1666: 1355–64.

40. Bateman A. Treating borderline personality disorder in clinical practice. *Am J Psychiatry* 2012; 169: 1–4.

41. Somma A, Ferrara M, Terrinoni A et al. Hypermentalizing as a marker of borderline personality disorder in Italian adolescents: a cross-cultural replication of Sharp and colleagues' (2011) findings. *Borderline Personal Disord Emot Dysregulation* 2019; 6: 5. doi:10.1186/s40479-019-0104-5.

42. Sharp C, Kalpakci A, Mellick W. First evidence of a prospective relation between avoidance of internal states and borderline personality disorder features in adolescents. *Eur Child Adolesc Psychiatry* 2015; 24: 283–90.

43. Bo S, Sharp C, Beck E et al. First empirical evaluation of outcomes for mentalization-based group therapy for adolescents with BPD. *Personal Disord* 2017; 8: 396–401.

44. Rossouw T, Fonagy P. Mentalization-based treatment for self-harm in adolescents: a randomized controlled trial. *J Am Acad Child Adolesc Psychiatry* 2012; 51: 1304–13.

45. Asen E, Fonagy P. Mentalization-based therapeutic interventions for families. *J Fam Ther* 2012; 34: 347–70.

46. Midgley N, Alayza A, Lawrence H, Bellew R. Adopting minds: a mentalization based therapy for families in a post-adoption support service: preliminary evaluation and service user experience. *Adopt Foster* 2018; 42: 22–37.

47. Bateman A, Fonagy P. A randomized controlled trial of a mentalization-based intervention (MBT-FACTS) for families of people with borderline personality disorder. *Personal Disord* 2019; 10(1): 70–9.

48. Bateman A, Fonagy P, Bolton R. Antisocial personality disorder: a mentalizing framework. *Focus (Am Psychiatr Publ)* 2013; XI(2): 178–86.

49. Bateman A, O'Connell J, Lorenzini N, Gardner T, Fonagy P. A randomised controlled trial of mentalization-based treatment versus structured clinical management for patients with comorbid borderline personality disorder and antisocial personality disorder. *BMC Psychiatry* 2016; 304: 304–11.

50. Philips B, Wennberg P, Konradsson P, Franck J. Mentalization-based treatment for concurrent borderline personality disorder and substance use disorder: a randomise controlled feasibility study. *Eur Addict Res* 2018; 24: 1–8.

51. Robinson P, Hellier J, Barrett B et al. The NOURISHED randomised controlled trial comparing mentalization-based treatment

for eating disorders (MBT-ED) with specialist supportive clinical management (SSCM-ED) for patients with eating disorders and symptoms of borderline personality disorder. *Trials* 2016; **17**: 549–63.

52. Fuggle P, Bevington D, Cracknell L et al. The Adolescent Mentalization-based Integrative Treatment (AMBIT) approach to outcome evaluation and manualization: adopting a learning organization approach. *Clin Child Psychol Psychiatry* 2015; 20(3): 419–35.

53. Asen E, Campbell C, Fonagy P. Social systems: beyond the microcosm of the individual and family. In A Bateman, P Fonagy, eds., *Handbook of Mentalizing in Mental Health Practice*. Washington DC: American Psychiatric Association Publishing. 2019; pp. 229–43.

Part II Applied Psychotherapeutic Thinking

Psychological Approaches to Affective Disorders

Sue Stuart-Smith

Introduction

The term affective disorders encompasses a range of conditions that affect mood and emotional functioning. It includes unipolar and bipolar disorder as well as anxiety states. This chapter covers the psychodynamic processes involved in depression and anxiety. Key factors that play a role in predisposing, precipitating and perpetuating these conditions are outlined. Along with psychoanalytic theory, the chapter draws on attachment theory and affective neuroscience.

Although psychiatric diagnostic systems classify them separately, there is considerable overlap between anxiety and depression as evidenced in the high levels of concurrent symptoms that are generally seen. For example up to 60 per cent of patients of patients with generalised anxiety disorder have been found to meet the criteria for major depressive disorder and about 50 per cent of patients with panic disorder experience an episode of major depression [1, 2].

The Subjective Experience of Depression

Depression is characterised by the loss of both motivation and pleasure in life. An underlying flatness of mood is accompanied by persistent feelings of worthlessness which are sustained by negative, ruminatory thoughts. The depressed person suffers from mental pain and finds themselves shut out from aspects of experience they have previously experienced as good, pleasurable or beautiful. This aspect of the condition is vividly portrayed in the following lines from Shakespeare's *Hamlet* [3].

> *I have of late—but wherefore*
> *I know not—lost all my mirth, forgone all custom of*
> *exercises; and indeed it goes so heavily with my*
> *disposition that this goodly frame, the earth, seems to*
> *me a sterile promontory, this most excellent canopy,*
> *the air, look you, this brave o'erhanging firmament,*
> *this majestical roof fretted with golden fire, why,*
> *it appears no other thing to me than a foul and pestilent*
> *congregation of vapours.*

When the mind is overtaken by negative affects like this, the sufferer is unable to benefit from relationships or other experiences that might be consoling or replenishing and this state of disconnection in itself helps perpetuate the condition. Sleep and appetite which are also life sustaining are almost invariably disrupted too. In Hamlet's case, this profound alteration of mental state follows his father's unexpected death. The context in which it occurs makes it hard for him to mourn his loss and he contemplates both revenge and suicide. As will become clear, an inability to mourn plays a pivotal role in the underlying psychology of depression.

Mourning and Melancholia

The earliest psychoanalytic theories about the origins of depression, or melancholia as it was then called, identified a reaction to loss as a central feature of the condition. Karl Abraham, one of Sigmund Freud's colleagues, was the first psychoanalyst to write about the association between loss and depression. In 1911, he suggested that early life losses and/or a lack of affection in childhood might predispose to depression in later life [4]. Then in 1917, Freud published a paper entitled Mourning and Melancholia[5]. This work is considered seminal, not only because of its contribution to the understanding of depression, but also because it describes how Freud came to recognise the extent to which the mind is actively engaged in internal relationships and it therefore marks the beginning of 'object relations' as a development in psychoanalytic theory. This development involved a shift away from a focus on the instincts and drive theory towards a recognition that early life relationships are represented within the psyche and thereby unconsciously influence psychic functioning. Object relations theory, which emerged in the mid-twentieth century, built on this recognition through the work of Ronald Fairbairn, Melanie Klein and Donald Winnicott [6].

In Mourning and Melancholia, Freud observes that both states involve a loss of interest in the outside world and a high level of internal preoccupation that leaves little energy for other purposes. He refers to mourning as psychological work. Memories of the lost loved one are repeatedly returned to and a range of painful feelings are experienced at different stages, including sadness, anger and guilt. This emotional work gradually leads to an acceptance of the reality of the loss and allows for a recovery of interest and enjoyment in the outside world so that the ego becomes free to form new attachments. Melancholia too can be triggered by bereavement or rejection but in contrast to the ever-present awareness of loss in mourning, the melancholic may withdraw the loss from consciousness, making it less apparent as a cause.

In mourning, Freud writes, it is the world that is rendered 'poor and empty' whereas in melancholia, it is the ego itself that is experienced as impoverished or worthless. The low self-worth that typifies melancholia involves a highly active process of self-denigration and self-criticism. Freud observes that it is as if part of the ego has turned on itself in judgement and that in order to do this, it takes itself as an object. He also notes that the melancholic's self-criticisms are invariably disproportionate and are typically found on closer inspection to resemble complaints against the lost loved one. In this way, he concludes, the self-reproaches of the melancholic may be understood as displaced attacks on the lost love object.

Freud was curious as to how this might come about and he hypothesises that the lost object has been taken in to the ego through a process of unconscious identification. A narcissistic identification like this means there is no separation, so the pain of loss can be mitigated and denied. Furthermore, in directing recriminations towards the self, feelings of guilt towards the lost person are also reduced. Freud writes:

Thus the shadow of the object fell upon the ego, and the latter could henceforth be judged by a special agency, as though it were an object, the forsaken object.

Later on, he named this judgemental agency the superego in order to differentiate it from the ego [7].

Freud outlines how the unconscious processes involved in melancholia are an attempt to deal with internal conflict arising from opposing feelings of love and hate and the accompanying guilt over angry or aggressive impulses. Ambivalence is an element of every love relationship but in depression, the hostile feelings are unconscious, they have been repressed and are redirected towards the ego. The nature of the attacks varies but it often takes on a punitive or sadomasochistic quality. Generally, it can be said that the power of the superego is linked to the severity of the depression and in its most destructive form can lead to self-harm and suicide. Freud points out that the ego can only kill itself if it treats itself as an object and in doing so, splits off aggressive and murderous impulses that are then directed towards the self. A pull towards suicide in the context of loss can also represent a way of seeking continued proximity to the lost object and be an attempt to resolve unbearable pain and fears of disintegration triggered by grief.

Freud identifies a narcissistic aspect to depression because of the extent to which it involves the sufferer turning away from object relating and withdrawing into the self. The negative internal relationship between the ego and superego forms a vicious circle that means that an adjustment to loss is unable to proceed; hence Freud came to regard melancholia as a pathological form of mourning.

A Case of Frozen Grief

Mr R had been suffering from depression for over 12 months when he was referred for psychotherapy. He had originally been treated at home by the crisis team because of persistent suicidal ideation. Antidepressant medication had helped him to some extent but he remained withdrawn from his wife and children and had been unable to return to work.

When he attended for the psychotherapy assessment the therapist was struck by the detached and matter-of-fact account he gave of his father's death two years previously. His father had been rushed to hospital following a sudden collapse and the last few days of his life had been spent in an intensive care unit. The therapist tried to make a link between this traumatic event and his depression but Mr R was reluctant to consider the possibility, insisting that he had coped with it. However, he then told the therapist that his memory of his father was fixed on those last few days when he was lying in bed unconscious, attached to tubes. He was troubled by this and wished he could recover happier memories of his father.

During the second assessment consultation Mr R became tearful when the therapist commented that with the loss of his good memories of his father, it was as if he had not only lost his father physically but had lost him in his inner world as well. This was the first time since his father's death that he had shed tears and he then described how as the eldest son he had taken on the role of supporting his mother in her grief. It became clear that Mr R had been unable to mourn himself and that he was living in a state of frozen grief. It also emerged that he had felt unable to live up to his father's high expectations and doubted his own capacities as a result. As a consequence, along with love and respect for his father, he harboured strong feelings of resentment.

Mr R embarked on a course of weekly therapy in which he was gradually able to acknowledge and express painful feelings. At the same time, he became aware of his own ageing and mortality. These sessions were often exhausting for him and he became anxious that the therapy was making him worse. He started to miss sessions and might well have broken off treatment but was helped to continue with the encouragement of his psychiatrist.

About four months into the therapy he arrived for a session in a more animated state than usual and immediately spoke of a period of his childhood when he and his father used to go fishing together. These trips had been enjoyable for both of them and the recovery of these memories was a relief to him. Following on from this it became possible to explore in more detail the negative aspects of their relationship linked to his father's tendency to put him down. This had intensified after he started secondary school and for a long period, he barely spoke to his father. It seemed to the therapist that he had been shutting his father out of his mind in a similarly angry way following his death. With the therapist's help, Mr R began to understand that he had internalised his father's undermining of him in the form of the relentless self-denigration he suffered from.

As therapy progressed, Mr R came to recognise that while his father could be rigid and domineering, he also had anxious and insecure traits. In turn, Mr R became less harsh on himself and his mood and energy gradually lifted.

The case of Mr R illustrates the link between depression and a difficulty in dealing with ambivalent feelings, particularly aggression. The nature of the relationship with his father had offered little opportunity for his angry feelings to be safely expressed and detoxified. The work of mourning his loss and integrating his hostile feelings took place in the therapy.

The Neurobiology of Attachment

It used to be thought, and sometimes still is, that a 'reactive' type of depression which arises in response to life events like Mr R's can be differentiated from a more biological or 'endogenous' form of depression. But human psychology and neurobiology are inextricably linked. The systems that relate to bonding and attachment are particularly important in understanding the origins of affective disorders. The neuroscientist, Jaak Panksepp who pioneered the field of affective neuroscience has hypothesised that depression emerged in the course of evolution as an adaption that promotes survival through conserving the energy of infant mammals when separation distress becomes unduly prolonged [8].

The field of affective neuroscience is focussed on the basic emotional operating systems in the brain which we share in common with other mammals and which have the power to override higher cerebral processes. These are implicated in many of the psychiatric disorders and in depression and anxiety, it is the panic/grief system that is most powerfully implicated. Experiences of loss, separation and rejection all set in motion a cascade of neurobiological changes that involve, among others, the oxytocin, opioid and dopamine systems. Disruptions to these are associated with many of the symptoms seen in affective disorders and may help explain why these disorders are so common [9].

The significance of disrupted attachment is confirmed in research that shows that the experience of a major loss in childhood is associated with an increased risk of depression later in life [10]. Early childhood loss is also associated with bipolar disorder [11] and panic disorder [12].

The long-term vulnerability that arises through adverse childhood experiences arises, at least in part, as a result of neuroendocrine changes involving the hypothalamic–pituitary–adrenal axis. These alter the stress response of the developing brain in a way that predisposes to depression and anxiety in later life. Other effects that have been demonstrated include changes in the hippocampus, amygdala and orbitofrontal cortex [13]. In contrast, the experience of good relationships that lead to secure attachment patterns can confer some protection, which is why John Bowlby regarded attachment as the 'bedrock' of human psychology [14].

Childhood experiences of attachment give rise to internal working models of relationships [15]. Interactions with caregivers, in particular the quality of maternal attunement and mirroring, influence the development of neural networks involved in affect regulation. This direct effect on brain structure and functioning has been demonstrated using neuroendocrine markers and fMRI studies [16]. This evidence confirms psychoanalytic theories about the importance of early emotional containment and explains why when containment is lacking there is an impaired ability to recognise and regulate feelings.

A Case Involving Early Life Loss

Mrs H was in her early thirties when she started psychotherapy. Four years previously she discovered that her husband was having an affair with his former girlfriend. She had only been married to him for a few years and was profoundly shocked by the revelation and began to suffer from anxiety and depression. After he left her, her functioning deteriorated rapidly and she was admitted to hospital for a brief period having been found in a distressed and confused state standing by the edge of a motorway bridge near her home.

Once the divorce was finalised, she thought she would be able to move on with her life but this did not happen. Her anxiety levels increased and she became convinced that her friends were fed up with her for being so stuck. These thoughts were feeding her low self-esteem and causing her to isolate herself. She started to experience panic attacks and increasingly found it hard to leave the house. She could not understand why she was unable to move on with her life, particularly as she no longer wished to be reunited with her husband.

The psychotherapy assessment revealed that her early life experience was an important contributing factor in her difficulties. She was the eldest of two children and when she was about three years old, her mother developed post-natal depression following the birth of her brother. It was severe enough for her mother to be hospitalised for a time. It seemed that during this period she received little attention from either her father or the aunt who helped the family out. If she did get attention she was made to feel she was being a nuisance and that her baby brother took precedence. As a result she felt intensely lonely and recalled crying herself to sleep.

Life at home improved when her mother returned but she experienced marked separation distress when she started school. It seemed that yet again she was being a nuisance and her feelings could not be tolerated. The therapist made a link between her recent experience of rejection by her husband and her emotionally traumatic separation from her mother as a child. Mrs H was then able to recognise that she was isolating herself now much as she had felt isolated then and that the anxieties she was experiencing now were in part associated with this much earlier period of her life.

This case illustrates how an experience of loss can reawaken unconscious emotional memories related to an earlier life loss. Mrs H's early life disruption and the emotional deprivation she suffered from gave rise to an insecure pattern of attachment. A parent suffering from a mental illness as her mother did may find it hard to be emotionally available to a child. The child in turn can become overly preoccupied by the parent's state of mind and end up like Mrs H lacking an awareness of her own emotional processes. When she started attending therapy, her anxiety was causing her to avoid social contact. With the therapist's help she was able to see that this was helping to perpetuate her condition. She also responded to the emotional containment in the therapy. The process of being helped to make sense of her feelings was a new experience for her.

The Contribution of Melanie Klein

Melanie Klein's theories build on Freud's earlier work. She describes how a person's response to loss in adult life is influenced by earlier life losses that are then reactivated. These include the very first kinds of loss that are experienced in infancy involving the breast, or breast substitute through weaning, as well as the repeated comings and goings of the baby's mother or main carer [17].

Developmentally, such experiences precipitate a phase that Klein identified as a prototype of mourning which she termed 'the depressive position' and she believed that the developmental resolution of the depressive position helps equip an individual to cope with losses later on in life. In other words, it lays down a template for mourning. That is not to say that it is a one-off achievement, anxieties associated with the depressive position need to be reworked throughout life, particularly when there is a need to adapt to change.

Whereas paranoid-schizoid anxieties revolve around survival of the self, depressive position anxieties focus on the survival of the object that is depended on. Overcoming these anxieties involves acceptance of ambivalent feelings and gives rise to an integration of good and bad aspects of the object.

Klein describes how, in order to overcome experiences of loss and associated anxieties, there needs to be a good internal object that is robust and can function as a source of strength and consolation. She makes the point that a secure and caring object in the inner world actually helps someone to find, or rather re-find, these qualities when they are needed in the external world. Conversely, when a good object is lacking, a pattern may become set up that leads to further isolation and loss in subsequent relationships.

Klein recognised that developmentally, there is a healthy aspect to depressive anxieties and feelings of guilt, because as long as they are not too severe, they help to stimulate the wish to repair and restore. She writes: '*Side by side with the destructive impulses in the unconscious mind both of the child and of the adult, there exists a profound urge to make sacrifices, in order to help and to put right loved people who in phantasy have been harmed or destroyed.*' [18]. In contrast, when the superego remains in a primitive state, as it is in the paranoid-schizoid position, and operates in a self-destructive way, repair feels impossible and feelings of shame and guilt may be so great that they need to be heavily defended against.

The Psychoanalytic Understanding of Psychotic Depression

Richard Lucas emphasised the need to recognise the psychotic element that is hidden in major depressive disorder [19]. The internal world is dominated by a relationship in which a vulnerable ego is in thrall to an omnipotent superego. There is a loss of insight and little capacity to reflect or consider alternative attitudes to the self. The disproportionate sense of guilt, self-denigration and self-blame means that it is extremely difficult to reason with a patient in this state. Lucas described how the clinician needs to *'tune in to the psychotic wavelength'* and thereby come to better understand the nature of the disturbance in the inner world. In his view this internal situation is likely to contribute to the typical biological symptom of diurnal mood variation. Patients may feel worse on waking because in their sleep and their dreams, their unforgiving internal world has assumed dominance. Daytime brings scope for reality testing and as the day progresses patients start to feel better because their experience of external reality is much less harsh than their internal reality.

Different Types of Anxiety and Their Origins

Anxiety has an adaptive function. It enhances survival by alerting the subject to danger and much like depressive feelings and mourning, a certain measure of anxiety is associated with health.

Freud thought that anxiety functions as a 'signal' of something that represents danger in the unconscious mind. In response to this the ego mobilises defences in order to prevent the dangerous thoughts or impulses from emerging into consciousness. Just as an episode of depression may not be associated by the patient with a rejection or loss, so patients who are suffering from anxiety may have no idea why they are anxious. The role of the therapist in this situation is to try to understand the unconscious processes that may be driving the anxiety and to help the patient recognise the defences that are involved in perpetuating the situation.

In psychoanalytic theory there is a developmental hierarchy of anxiety [20]. Psychotic anxieties related to fears of fragmentation and disintegration are considered the most basic and primitive form of anxiety. Next are the persecutory and paranoid anxieties associated with the paranoid-schizoid position.

Separation anxiety relates to the fear of losing the object and arises in the depressive position. For Klein, much of its power derives from a child's aggressive impulses towards the object who leaves them and the fear that the object will be damaged or disappear as a result. Bowlby focussed on it as a direct consequence of the real experience of parental loss and emotional neglect [21]. In practice, the two are often overlaid and a combined effect is seen. Separation anxiety can lead to various kinds of safety and reassurance-seeking behaviours and may express itself as agorophobia or excessively dependent traits.

Castration anxiety is the dominant oedipal anxiety. This relates to fears of punishment for forbidden desires for the opposite sex parent and the wish to take the place of the same sex parent. In later life, this can manifest itself as anxiety about being successful and a wish to avoid envy or jealousy because of unconscious fears of retaliation. This can lead to the seemingly paradoxical situation in which someone becomes depressed or anxious following an achievement or happy life event.

Superego anxiety plays a major role in affective disorders, particularly in depression. Developmentally, the superego is formed as a result of internalised relationships with parents and other authority figures but it is not entirely based on real relationships and is partly shaped by the fantasies that surround a child's destructive and hateful feelings. In terms of pathology, it is the quality of the superego that matters. A healthy superego is a source of both motivation and morality. An overactive and harsh superego is likely to be associated with perfectionistic traits and associated feelings of never being good enough. Children who experience neglect or abuse often internalise a sense of the self as bad because it is the only way to make sense of the way they are being treated. The victim–abuser dynamic they are exposed to is likely to be replicated internally between the superego and the ego. A punitive superego such as this is powerfully depressogenic.

A Case Involving Unconscious Guilt

Miss A was in her early thirties when her mother was diagnosed with cancer and started a lengthy course of chemotherapy. She had suffered from previous episodes of depression in her twenties and had been taking antidepressants for many years but her mother's illness triggered a serious set back. She found herself struggling to cope with everyday life and increasingly retreated to her bed.

She was the youngest of three children with two older brothers. In the middle phase of her childhood, her father's work took him abroad and her mother struggled to manage the children on her own. She was expected to do many of the household chores and her mother would punish her in a physically abusive way if she did not. As a result she grew frightened of her mother and harboured a deep resentment about the extent to which her brothers were favoured.

When Miss A started attending therapy, her mother was still receiving treatment and had suffered a number of complications. From the beginning, the therapist was struck by the nastiness of Miss A's self-recriminations. She spoke of feeling bad inside and her negative ruminations had a savage quality to them. After a time, the therapist was able to link these to her powerful feelings of grievance about the abuse she had experienced as a child.

Being able to explore her feelings of hatred and resentment without judgement or blame helped Miss A feel understood. Gradually, it became possible to look at her own prickly and difficult behaviour towards her mother now. Recognising her part in maintaining the difficult relationship between them helped her respond to her mother in a different way and as her feeling of responsibility for her mother's illness reduced, she began to experience some feelings of compassion for her.

It seemed that, in Miss A's unconscious, her mother's illness had provided a frightening confirmation of the destructive power of her hatred and had amplified her feelings of guilt. In this way, depressed patients may feel omnipotently responsible for damage to their objects and feel that neither symbolic or real repair is possible. In Miss A's case, an inner process of reparation was set in motion as a result of the therapy and it was then mirrored externally in the improved relationship to her mother that began to emerge.

The Role of Manic Defences and the Psychoanalytic Understanding of Bipolar Disorder

Klein's work on manic depressive states describes how powerful manic defences such as omnipotence, idealisation, contempt and denial can be called into play in order to deal with the painful affects associated with loss and feelings of deficiency. A fundamental aspect of the manic position is a triumph over objects and any feelings of dependence on them. Rather than working towards reparation, various forms of instant or magical restoration may be used so that the experience of loss and/or guilt is quickly negated. Klein thus distinguished between manic reparation which is based on omnipotent control and healthy reparation which is based on concern and care for the object.

Manic states of mind can be understood as a solution to an unbearable internal burden of guilt or shame arising from a relentlessly undermining superego. In mania, the ego temporarily achieves freedom from the superego by detaching from it. Lucas described how the manic phase can be regarded as '*The uncoiling of a clockwork spring that has been progressively tightened during the depressive phase*' [19, p. 201].

For patients with bipolar disorder, the mainstay of treatment is undoubtedly pharmacotherapy but a psychodynamic approach can help them develop an understanding of the psychological precipitants of such episodes. Even if the patient is unable to benefit from this kind of insight, clinicians and relatives involved in their care can gain from understanding potential emotional triggers.

A Breakdown of Manic Defences

Mr P was in his fifties when he was referred for psychotherapy from the outpatient department because he was not responding to medication. He had a previous history of depression and this episode was triggered when he was made redundant following a company takeover.

Throughout most of his adult life, his self-esteem had been vested in his success at his job, his attractiveness to women and his love of driving fast cars. His wife had remained loyal to him, although throughout their marriage he had neglected her while conducting a series of extra-marital affairs.

In the therapy, he had a tendency to be condescending towards the therapist and would move rapidly away from discussing anything that might evoke painful feelings. It emerged that when he was in his teens, his mother had suddenly announced she was leaving the family home to live with another man. He became estranged from her and had little contact with her after this time. His younger brother expressed considerable distress throughout this period while he felt he was superior in not showing such weakness. He consciously blanked the experience of abandonment out and saw himself as self-sufficient.

Mr P had strong narcissistic traits and, in the sessions, it was difficult for him to experience any vulnerability. There were a few occasions when he was able to do this but he would invariably miss the following session, saying that something more important had come up. He found it hard to take in and acknowledge the therapist's contributions and had a habit of repeating her interpretations subsequently as if they were his own ideas. This gave rise to strong counter-transference feelings of anger and irritation.

Mr P's strategy of seeking excitement through cars and women had functioned as a manic defence over a long period of time and had served to protect him from feelings of inadequacy and rage. The loss of his job led to a collapse of these defences and as a result he became depressed. The case illustrates the difficult countertransference feelings that may need to be managed when split-off feelings are projected into the therapist. In dismissing the value of the therapist's ideas, he was making her redundant, much as his employer and his mother had done to him. It turned out that he had a similar way of relating to his psychiatrist too.

The Process of Therapy

As in any therapy, the therapist's first task in treating an affective disorder is to try to understand the nature of the patient's mental pain and establish a sense of meaningful contact. This requires sensitivity and patience on the part of the therapist as patients may be cut off from their feelings or overwhelmed by anxiety. The very nature of depression means that the patient may find it hard to believe in the possibility of change and as a result, it is often the therapist who has to carry the belief that change might be possible.

Once a safe enough setting has been established, the patient may begin to express deep-rooted feelings. It is important for the therapist to be able to bear these painful feelings without resorting to reassurance or solution seeking. In this way the therapeutic space can function as a safe container. Feelings can be explored and understood so that they become to be more manageable.

Some of the work that takes place in therapy involves helping the patient develop a capacity for mentalisation [22]. This is an important part of any therapy in which there has been early life deprivation leading to impaired self-reflection and recognition of feelings. Mentalising allows feelings to be thought about rather than acted on. As this capacity develops, the patient will benefit from an ability to 'step back' from powerful anxieties and other feelings and be less likely to be overwhelmed or act out on them.

The harsher the superego, the more likely it is that the therapist interpretations will be experienced as criticisms. This pattern will need to be acknowledged and worked through. Over time, the therapist's non-judgemental stance is crucial in allowing for some modification of the superego. It provides a different view of the self from the patient's internal critique and means that a more understanding and compassionate way of relating to the self can be internalised. The existence of powerful defences against feelings of loss, guilt and hostility means that a negative therapeutic reaction at some point during the therapy is not uncommon in patients with affective disorders.

Both psychoanalysis and attachment theory emphasise the centrality of relationships in human psychology and the developmental need to mourn loss and separation [23]. This is why the ending of therapy is such a crucial phase of treatment. Themes of separation and loss inevitably come to the fore and it therefore presents an important opportunity for the patient to anticipate and work through an experience of loss. It is not uncommon for there to be a degree of relapse at this point, so it is important that the ending is planned to allow time for this work to take place.

Sometimes patients or clinicians feel it is necessary to make a choice between psychotherapy or medication. It may be thought that medication will limit a patient's emotional responsiveness to therapy, whereas in practice it is often the other way round and drug treatment can help reduce levels of anxiety and depression that would otherwise impede a patient's ability to engage in a therapeutic relationship. The combination of brief psychodynamic psychotherapy and medication has been found to give an improved outcome and enhance quality of life in major depressive disorder [24]. In panic disorder, a combination of brief psychodynamic psychotherapy and medication has been found to reduce relapse rates more effectively than medication alone [25].

Patients suffering from recurrent depression or treatment-resistant depression will need a longer-term course of psychodynamic psychotherapy and there is evidence to support this. The Tavistock Adult Depression study found significant improvements in patients undergoing an 18-month course of psychotherapy [26]. These findings were most apparent two years after therapy ended. This delayed therapeutic benefit supports the idea that the effects of psychodynamic therapy emerge over a longer time course than other kinds of therapy.

Conclusions

There is an overlap in the aetiology and symptomatology of depressive and anxiety disorders which can be traced developmentally to disrupted attachment relationships and early experiences of loss. These in turn make it harder to negotiate subsequent experiences of separation, loss and rejection. Emotional deprivation and a lack of positive affirmation in childhood are liable to be internalised in the form of an overly harsh superego which plays a central role in the negative ruminations and depressive thinking that gives rise to feelings of despair and a sense of low self-worth. When they first present, patients often do not link their symptoms of depression or anxiety to recent or past life events. This means that taking a detailed life history is essential in order to identify the predisposing and precipitating factors that may be at work and through gaining this understanding, the psychiatrist can explore options for psychological treatment in a more meaningful way.

References

1. Gorman JM, Coplan JD. Comorbidity of depression and panic disorder. *J Clin Psychiatry* 1996; 57(Suppl 10): 34–41.

2. Brown TA, Campbell LA, Lehman CL, Grisham JR, Mancill RB. Current and lifetime comorbidity of the DSM-IV anxiety and mood disorders in a large clinical sample. *J Abnorm Psychol* 2001; 110(4): 585–99.

3. Cantor PA. *Shakespeare: Hamlet*. Cambridge: Cambridge University Press, 2004.

4. Abraham K. Psychoanalytic investigation and treatment of manic-depressive insanity and allied conditions. *Psychoanal Rev* 1913; 1: 231.

5. Freud S. Mourning and melancholia. *J Nerv Ment Dis* 1922; 56(5): 543–5.

6. Greenberg JR, Mitchell SA. *Object Relations in Psychoanalytic Theory*. Cambridge, MA: Harvard University Press, 1983.

7. Freud S. The ego and the id. In J Strachey, ed., *The Standard Edition of the Complete Psychological Works of Sigmund Freud, Volume XIX (1923-1925): The Ego and the Id and Other Works*. London: Hogarth Press. 1961; pp. 1–66. (Original work published 1923)

8. Panksepp J, Watt D. Why does depression hurt? Ancestral primary-process separation-distress (PANIC/GRIEF) and diminished brain reward (SEEKING) processes in the genesis of depressive affect. *Psychiatry* 2011; 74(1): 5–13.

9. Panksepp J. *Affective Neuroscience: The Foundations of Human and Animal Emotions*. Oxford: Oxford University Press, 2004.

10. Shapiro MB. The social origins of depression: By G. W. Brown and T. Harris: its methodological philosophy. *Behav Res Ther* 1979; 17(6): 597–603.

11. Li J, Precht DH, Mortensen PB, Olsen J. Mortality in parents after death of a child in Denmark: a nationwide follow-up study. *Lancet* 2003; 361(9355): 363–7.

12. Kendler KS, Neale MC, Kessler RC, Heath AC, Eaves LJ. Childhood parental loss and adult psychopathology in women: a twin study perspective. *Arch Gen Psychiatry* 1992; 49(2): 109–16.

13. Nemeroff CB. Paradise lost: the neurobiological and clinical consequences of child abuse and neglect. *Neuron* 2016; 89 (5): 892–909.

14. Bowlby J. *Separation, Anxiety and Anger: Attachment and Loss*. London: Hogarth Press, 1973.

15. Bowlby J. *Attachment and Loss*. New York: Basic Books, 1969.

16. Schore AN. *Affect Regulation and the Origin of the Self: The Neurobiology of*

Emotional Development. New York: Routledge, 2015.

17. Klein M. *The Writings of Melanie Klein. Love, Guilt and Reparation and Other Works*. London: Hogarth Press. 1975; p. 341.

18. Klein M. Mourning and its relation to manic-depressive states. *Int J Psychoanal* 1940; 21: 125–53.

19. Lucas R. The psychotic wavelength. *Psychoanal Psychother* 2008; 22(1): 54–63.

20. Gabbard GO. *Psychodynamic Psychiatry in Clinical Practice*, 5th ed. Arlington: American Psychiatric Publishing, Inc., 2014.

21. Bowlby J. Developmental psychiatry comes of age. *Am J Psychiatry* 1988; 145(1): 1–10.

22. Bateman AW, Fonagy PE. *Handbook of Mentalizing in Mental Health Practice*. Arlington: American Psychiatric Publishing, Inc., 2012.

23. Holmes J, Slade A. *Attachment in Therapeutic Practice*. London: SAGE, 2017.

24. De Jonghe FE, Kool S, Van Aalst G, Dekker J, Peen J. Combining psychotherapy and antidepressants in the treatment of depression. *J Affect Disord* 2001; 64(2–3): 217–29.

25. Wiborg IM, Dahl AA. Does brief dynamic psychotherapy reduce the relapse rate of panic disorder? *Arch Gen Psychiatry* 1996; 53(8): 689–94.

26. Fonagy P, Rost F, Carlyle JA et al. Pragmatic randomized controlled trial of long-term psychoanalytic psychotherapy for treatment-resistant depression: the Tavistock Adult Depression Study (TADS). *World Psychiatry* 2015; 14(3): 312–21.

<table>
<tr><td>Chapter</td></tr>
<tr><td>**14**</td></tr>
</table>

Psychological Approaches to Psychosis

Jo O'Reilly

We can't cure a patient of their delusional world unless we understand the conditions in which they became necessary.

Sigmund Freud

This chapter will describe the psychological processes thought to underlie psychosis and how these approaches can assist our understanding and management of psychotic disorders. There is no single model for complex conditions and the main theoretical underpinnings and treatment approaches derived from psychodynamic, systemic and cognitive behavioural frames of reference will be outlined. Clinical examples will illustrate the application of these ideas in clinical care.

Psychodynamic Approaches to Psychosis

The madman is a waking dreamer.

Kant [1]

A psychodynamic approach to psychosis builds upon the following ideas:

1. Psychotic symptoms represent a return to psychological processes which are normal in infancy and childhood
2. The content of psychotic symptoms has meaning and expresses material from unconscious areas of the mind
3. Psychotic symptoms tend to be created by primary process mental activities, rather like dreams, so the meaning may be disguised
4. The personal biography of the patient provides material which may be key to understanding the presentation
5. Psychological mechanisms in psychotic functioning include projection of internal experiences into the outside world, a rupture in the contact with reality, denial, rationalisation and loss of the ability to symbolise leading to concrete thinking
6. Delusions and hallucinations may be an attempt to rebuild contact with external reality and to find meaning after a breakdown has occurred
7. There is a psychotic and non-psychotic part of the mind in us all, with potential to revert to more psychotic ways of mental functioning under conditions of psychic strain
8. Psychotic symptoms are common and are brought to the attention of services when they overwhelm the ability to function and behave within usual parameters

The origins and development of these concepts will be outlined in this chapter, which will also consider what can be learnt about the mind from the investigation of psychotic functioning. Clinical examples will be described to illustrate how a psychodynamic approach helps to understand patients presenting with psychosis and can assist in their management.

Freud and Psychosis

The ideas of the insane have more in common with ordinary human concerns than might seem the case at first. Seemingly normal behaviour may in fact be much more bizarre when examined closely.

Sigmund Freud [2]

One of the earliest psychoanalytic explorations of psychosis was based upon Freud's study of the memoirs of Daniel Paul Schreber, a judge who had a florid psychotic breakdown [3]. Schreber recorded his experiences meticulously in his memoirs and Freud applied himself to studying his account of his complex delusional system and hallucinatory experiences. Freud's ideas formed the foundations of early psychoanalytic explorations of psychosis.

Freud considered Schreber's symptoms to be understandable, meaningful and linked to early childhood conflicts and anxieties, particularly in terms of his relationship with his father. Thus, his symptoms contained a 'fragment of historical truth' (see Chapter 2). He recognised powerful processes of projection in his delusional symptoms, and therefore how a more extreme version of normal psychological functioning was operating despite the highly bizarre nature of the beliefs and experiences. He saw Schreber's experience of his own mind fragmenting as projected outside himself and transformed into the belief that it was the world itself that was collapsing. Freud was able to shed light on the meaning of the psychotic symptoms by realising they followed similar processes to dreams, and as conveying vital information, both about the underlying issues behind the development of the psychosis for Schreber, and also how the deeper strata of the mind operates.

Freud saw the 'central catastrophe' in psychosis as being the fragmentation of the mind and loss of contact with reality in response to becoming overwhelmed with anxiety. He described how loss of meaningful connection with the world precedes the development of delusions and hallucinations – an anxiety state which forewarns of psychosis and which we may refer to nowadays as delusional mood. Freud recognised how Schreber's state of mind became calmer as his delusions intensified and attributed this phenomenon to the restoration of certainty and meaning provided by the psychotic symptoms. This provides an understanding of how the distress and agitation of some patients seems to decrease as their delusional world becomes more crystallised in their minds; as if the delusions provide an alternative reality which although distressing may be preferable to the reality which led to the original breakdown.

Thus, Freud set the scene for an approach to psychosis that seeks meaning in the symptoms. He saw psychosis as a response to an external reality which has become unbearable for a fragile mind to apprehend, and recognised delusion formation as an attempt to re-find meaning in a more tolerable form. Freud described the development of delusions as *'like a patch where originally a rent had appeared in the ego's relation to the external world'* [4]. In addition to the noise and tumult of the psychotic symptoms Freud also noted the presence of a sane aspect of the patient, acting like '*a detached observer*' during psychotic illness.

Freud was writing over 100 years ago; psychological understanding has developed considerably since then and some of his conclusions have been challenged and modified. However, as the case below illustrates, his early and groundbreaking ideas continue to provide helpful insights into psychotic patients' predicaments.

> *Verity was an inpatient with a relapse of a psychotic illness, diagnosed as schizoaffective disorder. Her children had been taken into foster care as she was unable to adequately look after them. As her mental state stabilised she became increasingly preoccupied with her family and an access visit was arranged. On the day of the visit she became very agitated, distressed and persecuted making demands on the staff about the terms upon which she was prepared to see the children, none of which were possible to meet. She then said she had pain due to all the cracked eggs in her ovaries and was too unwell to go ahead with the visit. She settled quietly in her bed showing no sign of any physical discomfort.*

Verity's belief that her eggs were 'cracked', a term also used to describe madness, could be seen as an expression of her anxiety that her children had been damaged by her illness. The symptom presents this in disguised form as it is too painful for her to consciously know. This is akin to how our dreams may represent deep fears, wishes and urges from the unconscious areas of the mind – rather like the Trojan horse they can enter the citadel of conscious thought only disguised as something else. As Verity's delusional beliefs developed, meaning that the visit was cancelled, she became less distressed. In this way the psychotic symptom has provided a solution to the problem and also allowed it to be expressed, using displacement, into a more acceptable physical pain. She did not seek medical attention for the abdominal pain she describes, suggesting that she also knows this to not be an expression of a physical health problem and in this way remains in contact with reality; rather like knowing a dream is a dream.

In considering what the symptoms may mean staff can be encouraged to really listen to their patient's experiences and to understand better the underlying difficulties. Management can then be offered which is more in keeping with these issues, as in this case when her key nurse talked to her quietly about how her children were doing, which Verity listened to intently. The psychosis becomes material to be heard and thought about rather than a symptom to be treated.

Freud's ideas contributed the following main themes to the understanding of psychosis:

1. **Delusions are seen as psychologically determined phenomena, based upon powerful projection into the external world of disturbing mental contents**
2. **The central catastrophe in psychosis is the initial loss of meaningful contact with reality and fragmentation of the mind under conditions of excessive stress**
3. **Delusions and hallucinations are secondary symptoms to the original breakdown and are attempts to reconstruct a new reality with meaning and structure after the old reality has been given up**
4. **In remodeling reality, psychological processes similar to the primary process activity of dreams are revealed, such as wish fulfilment, lack of notion of time, hallucinatory realisation of repressed desires, displacement and condensation**
5. **Psychotic symptoms, like dreams, convey important material towards understanding the patient and their underlying difficulties**

Psychosis and Early Development

Humankind cannot bear too much reality.

T S Eliot [5]

If a primary feature of psychotic processes is a rupture in the relationship with reality, and the recreation of an alternative, the processes by which we learn about and come to terms with the world around us can provide important information about what happens when this falls apart in psychosis. Psychoanalytic ideas about early development and how a relationship with reality is forged and stabilised in the mind can provide a basis for understanding how this can unravel in later life.

We are not born with an understanding of ourselves, the external world and the boundary and relationship between the two. These have to be learnt and the earliest days of life outside the mother's body present immediate challenges for the developing mind. The infant has to find a way to withstand, differentiate, organise and understand the bombardment of all his experiences, his internal sensations and urges and encounters with the external world and people in it, now he is outside the mother's body. He also needs to manage and to make sense of the mother's absences while in a state of helplessness and dependency upon her care to survive. The challenges and psychological processes of normal infancy and childhood shed light on some aspects of psychotic processes in later life if the relationship with reality breaks down in psychosis. Psychotic symptoms from a psychodynamic perspective are seen as the intrusion into adult life of developmentally early modes of mental functioning.

Paranoid-Schizoid Functioning and Unconscious Phantasy

In her recognition of the intensity of infantile emotional life, and her description of the paranoid-schizoid position, Melanie Klein observed how the processes of early emotional life have much in common with psychotic functioning [6]. She saw the activities and structures of the mind as being primarily relationship seeking, or object related. During infancy and childhood, the self is constantly engaged in imaginary processes of either doing something to another or being done to. These themes are often expressed in childhood play. The splitting processes of paranoid-schizoid functioning allow for an initial binary differentiation between good and bad. States of distress are attributed to the actions of harmful others, persecutory objects, whose intent is to cause the distress. These archaic malign objects contain all projected aspects of the infant's aggression or rage and the self is imagined to hold only goodness. This is the world of primitive object relationships, of projected states of mind into others, of an imagined pain-free state constantly under threat from a malign other. Klein believed that unconscious phantasies such as these form the basic structures of the unconscious mind. She observed how the infant interprets his bodily sensations, appetites and instincts including aggression and libido in terms of relationships. There is an initial truth in this as all his experiences depend upon the response of another – hunger is because he has not been fed for example, and a pain in the stomach is given meaning as an intrusion by another who is intent on harm.

These early phantasies linger and continue to provide meaning in the depths of the mind, an unconscious populated by primitive object relations, the world of binary concrete splitting, acting upon and being done to, and a self who is undifferentiated from primitive good and bad figures. These primitive object relations continue to give meaning to our experiences in subliminal ways – comments such as 'you will be the death of me', or 'you're breaking my heart' revealing how our ongoing meaning-making processes are built upon these primitive interpretations of a good self being acted upon by another's harmful intent.

In psychosis, these early primitive object relations are brought to the foreground of consciousness and intrapsychic pain is transformed into a problem between the self and a persecutory other. The external world becomes dominated by projected elements of one's own mind, in a similar way to the child's conception of the world.

> Giles, an isolated and troubled young man, had long-standing conflicts with his neighbours, in part due to his keeping antisocial hours and playing loud music. He developed a psychotic belief that his neighbours were harming him by leaking poison into his flat, which he renamed Nirvana, and he showed a complete disregard for any role on his part in the difficulties.

This illustrates the return to more primitive forms of object relating, with the idea of an entirely good self under threat by the harmful intents of another – hallmarks of paranoid-schizoid functioning. Giles' own intrapsychic difficulties had been transformed into an interpersonal issue with the illusion his own self was Nirvana-like and beyond reproach. The splitting in the mind between good self in relation to a bad object has re-emerged and his symptoms resonate with early unconscious phantasies. In Giles' mind the neighbours became the problem and his own troubled internal states have become a problem in the outside world.

Symbolisation and Psychosis

We need to be able to symbolise in order for there to be space between ourselves and our experiences, otherwise we are simply in them. The ability to form mental representations of our experiences is the basis of mentalization and thought. The infant needs to be able to develop mental representations of his mother in order to separate from a merged state with her and to develop a sense of himself and the other with boundaries between them. In early life, psychic experience is felt to be the entire reality, a world of 'psychic equivalence', concrete and absolute states [7]. Symbolisation allows for our experiences to have an as-if quality which distinguishes thoughts and feelings from concrete reality, allowing for example words to describe feeling bad rather than the world having become entirely bad.

The ability to symbolise is learnt through repeated experiences of nurture and attunement, in which the child's experiences are gathered, named and understood. The screams of persecution from paranoid-schizoid states become modified into a calling out from a baby who is able to hold the mother in his mind and to wait. This is accompanied by an increasing sense of the workings of his own mind, of his own volition, agency and wishes. The infant's sense of himself becomes less confused with the other as he develops the ability to use symbols and metaphors and to tolerate uncertainty and ambiguity. Hannah Segal [8] described how the concrete thinking which characterises psychosis is due to the loss of the ability to symbolise, meaning psychic reality is indistinguishable from external reality – she called this **symbolic equation**, a return to the concrete experiences of early life. The certainty which accompanies many psychotic states, and the loss of any 'as-if' mode of thinking, indicates the ability to symbolise has become compromised. Concrete functioning also affects the nature of the transference relationships meaning that a psychotic transference may develop and this can profoundly distort the nature of relationships. Seemingly random acts of aggression on inpatient units for example can illustrate how the other has become concretely equated with a bad feeling or thought.

> *Paul had a relapse of paranoid schizophrenia when his mother started a relationship with a new partner. After a period of agitation and tearfulness he developed the delusional belief that he was the son of a prophet. He became calmer as the delusion gathered form, stopped his medication and assaulted his distressed mother after accusing her of trying to brainwash him when she tried to persuade him otherwise. Any anxiety or feelings of loss had been projected into his mother whom he then had to vigorously defend himself against – reality and ordinary concern had become a threat to his delusional reality.*
>
> *As Paul's psychosis developed he believed concerned family members were trying to control his thoughts by telepathy. To his mind this was a concrete fact and he boarded up the windows and door of his flat to keep the brainwaves out. He smashed the potted plants his mother had given him as he believed them to be spying on him on his mother's behalf and refused all contact with his key worker, deeming him the 'Anti-Christ'. When treated with medication he still had some paranoid thoughts about his family and their intentions towards him but was able to see these as anxieties and suspicions; in a more psychotic state there was no thoughts representing an as-if position; he knew they were harmful and he had to concretely keep them out.*

This case illustrates both Paul's return to primitive object relations in which his own projected concern and distress was experienced as an attack from his mother, and also how, through concrete processes, the pots had become equated with her and had to be destroyed. His external environment had become populated by the fears and concerns of his own internal states, with the loss of the reality of his good connection with his mother and any notion of painful feelings of exclusion and rejection. His previously good relationship with his key worker had also been transformed through a concrete and psychotic transference, the key worker becoming identified with all that was bad.

Hallucinatory Wish Fulfilment

In early life, if distress levels are too high, or the containing function of another is insufficient, the baby may turn to alternative sources of comfort and versions of reality that he creates in his own mind – referred to as **hallucinatory gratification.** For example, a distressed and hungry baby who refuses the nipple may gain some temporary respite from sucking at his own finger. This is accompanied by the psychic experience of omnipotence, a turning away from another and an experience of being able to meet all his needs himself.

Under conditions of intense mental strain in adult life, the mind may again turn to its own devices and create an alternative universe as a solution to a frustrating, depriving or terrifying external world. This alternative reality may refute just the situation which has led to it; for example, the omnipotence of paranoid beliefs within which the patient is of central and undeniable importance, as opposed to a reality of social exclusion and isolation. These solutions may seem bizarre as they are provided by primary process, gratification-seeking mental activity, with their origins in the hallucinatory wish fulfilment activities of infancy.

Thus, through her description of paranoid-schizoid function, Klein came to understand psychosis as a state in which less developed forms of psychic functioning come to the fore. Extreme projection of the turbulent and disturbing contents of the mind are expelled into the outside world and experienced as reality, meaning that the patient is surrounded by tantalisation, threats and persecutors. The attribution of parts of one's own mind to another leads to the loss of separation and boundaries between self and other, with fear of intrusion and control from outside. Extreme splitting into absolute states of good and bad means that relationships become distorted and bizarre, and a delusional world in which the patient is often omnipotent and of central importance may be created, guided by the principles of hallucinatory wish fulfilment. Vulnerability, loss, dependence, painful exclusions and rejections are made non-real as the psychotic mind replaces these ordinary concerns and turns towards the creations of their own mind, with delusional and less painful alternatives.

Kleinian Contributions to Understanding Psychosis

Melanie Klein and her colleagues contributed the following ideas towards understanding psychosis:

1. Emotional life in infancy is characterised by extreme projection, concrete thinking, splitting and confusion of internal and external states, processes also seen in psychosis
2. Psychotic processes originate from paranoid-schizoid functioning. Paranoid mechanisms, and psychotic object relationships and phantasies are likely to be returned to throughout life when triggered by excessive anxiety
3. Unconscious phantasy underlies every mental process, activity and symptom
4. The ability to symbolise is crucial in psychological development and concrete thinking is a hallmark of a failure of symbolisation
5. The development of an alternative reality, guided by hallucinatory wish fulfilment, is seen in early life and also in psychosis

Klein's ideas developed the psychoanalytic model that psychotic processes are present in the psychological biographies of us all and were followed by a flowering of interest in both the psychoanalytic treatment of psychotic patients and developing the theoretical understanding of psychosis.

Oedipal Triangulation: The Tent Peg Which Secures the Mind

Psychoanalytic thinking has continued to develop ideas about psychosis based upon how the infant builds up and structures his knowledge of the world. Jacques Lacan [9], a French psychiatrist and psychoanalyst, described how the closeness of the early relationship with the mother is also a source of anxiety. Through the provision of milk she can decide the infant's fate and in a state of dependency and helplessness he has to work out where she goes in her absence, how to understand 'the space behind the mother' [10]. The ability to tolerate the presence of another in the mother's life, the representation of the paternal, provides a painful but containing answer to this primary dilemma. The triangulation this provides structures the mind and frees the child to establish his own identity and boundaries. The world is no longer made up of random events or limitless possibilities. Rather like the inner sheet and the fly sheet of a tent, the oedipal tent peg as it were provides the necessary space between the dyadic and secures the structure through triangulation, preventing the tent linings from being overly detached or stuck together.

Lacan also wrote about the triggers which can release psychotic symptoms, describing these as often occurring at some important maturational step and changes in the individual's situation, such as leaving home, marriage or loss [11]. At these times any vulnerability in symbolic triangulation may become exposed, revealing the underlying struggle to maintain separation from the primary object and to establish boundaries around one's own thoughts and agency. A restless search to find meaning and connections between oneself and others in the outside world may then ensue. Lacan links this to the intense interest in the secret connections between things commonly seen in psychotic states as the quest for early answers to the 'facts of life' [12] has not been adequately secured and accepted.

Benjamin developed florid symptoms of psychosis in his first term at university, when he left home for the first time. His father had left when he was young and his mother had become very depressed. It seemed he had functioned rather as the man of the house while growing up. At university he became perplexed and seemed to have lost his sense of himself and what he was there for. He became endlessly preoccupied with an estates agent's sign which had his surname and the name of another person on it. He interpreted this as a signal of a secret relationship involving his father. He spoke of being 'deleted' and paced the streets in a state of perpetual and unresolved activity. He was allocated a key nurse who commented he seemed unable to care for himself without the mental health team, while also relating to her with hostility, as if she was a threat.

It seemed Benjamin had prematurely developed an identity as a man in the absence of his father and the close proximity of his mother had allowed this structure to support him psychically until he moved away. This separation seems to have exposed his underlying psychological fragility, confusion about his place in the world and what had happened between his parents; the transition to independence had exposed the lack of symbolic support to manage this. His relationship with the mental health team seemed to convey both his intense dependency and fear of becoming overwhelmed by the close proximity of another, suggesting early difficulties in establishing his own ego boundaries and distance from his objects.

Psychotic and Non-Psychotic Parts of the Personality

In some corner of their minds there was also a normal person hidden like a detached spectator, watching the hubbub of illness go by.
Sigmund Freud [13]

The idea of there being both a psychotic and non-psychotic part of the mind, first described by Freud as the 'sane spectator', has been further developed particularly by Wilfred Bion [14], and more recently, Richard Lucas [15]. Bion considered psychotic processes to be universal, and that the likelihood of a psychotic breakdown depended upon the balance between the effective influences of the psychotic and non-psychotic processes. The psychotic part attacks awareness of internal and external reality and has an active muscular quality, using powerful projective processes to evacuate troublesome awareness and emotions out of the mind and into the external world. In addition, in psychotic states a violent form of splitting occurs in which the non-psychotic parts of the mind are fragmented and expelled. This external reality then becomes populated with what Bion called **bizarre objects** in which the individual comes to be surrounded not only by expelled feelings but also by the parts of himself which are able to recognise reality, to hold insight and to observe oneself. Paul's smashed plant pots could be seen as an example of bizarre objects containing projected parts of his own mind.

Hallucinations, Bizarre Objects and Thought Disorder

Bion's ideas provide a psychological model to understand the nature of hallucinatory processes, as the entire perceptual apparatus of the mind is expelled into the outside world [16]. The ability to think about oneself, to observe oneself and to question oneself are ejected from the mind and are experienced as persecutions of being under surveillance, talked about and accused from external sources. These ideas continue to be in keeping with psychological models in which hallucinatory processes represent an externalisation of internal experiences and an inability to differentiate them.

Bion also described the psychotic part of the personality as launching attacks on linking between thoughts and ideas, creating thought disorder and non-sense. Lacan added further ideas about thought disorder, describing how the problem for the psychotic is that there are too many possible meanings at every potential juncture of thought as oedipal structuring has not provided a sufficient anchoring and limiting role.

These processes leave the patient very dependent on others to understand them and to look after them. The almost wholesale projection of self-knowledge and self-awareness into others can mean the mental health team holds and needs to function in keeping with key aspects of the patient's own mind. A common example may be the complete absence of awareness of a patient's past and more recent history while they become intensely preoccupied with their delusional world; it is the team who need to know the past vulnerabilities, recent challenges and hold concern for the future.

> Charity was admitted to a psychiatric ward convinced that the television commentators were talking about her, and that the weatherman was providing a running commentary on the 'storms and sunshines' which predicted her future. She believed she was being monitored by devices in tinned food and had padded her food cupboard with blankets to prevent this. She was utterly preoccupied with these beliefs, feeling under total surveillance, banished her TV to the cellar of her home and was malnourished. She had seemingly no awareness of her other circumstances or relationships and was utterly dependent on ward staff to know about her life history, previous illnesses, family relationships and physical needs. She agreed however to hospital admission and was compliant with her medication and treatment on the ward.

In Charity's case it seemed the psychotic part of her personality had projected all awareness of her mental state and its deterioration into the television, and awareness of her feelings of hunger and need for nourishment into the food tins, which had become bizarre objects monitoring her and trying to control her from the outside.

For Bion and Freud there is always some contact with reality even in the most disturbed mental states. Hence the patient who is convinced they need brain surgery to remove a microchip implanted in their brain but happily remains under the care of a psychiatric team rather than a neurosurgeon, or Charity's compliance with an involuntary admission and psychotropic medication. The non-psychotic part of Charity's mind, although under powerful pressure from the psychotic, seemed to know she needed the care of the mental health team.

Loss, Mourning and Psychosis

Loss has a central place in psychological development and the challenges of negotiating this may predispose to mental disorder (see Chapter 2)

Manic defences are universal and used frequently. They act to protect the individual from excessive anxiety or persecution related to loss. Although usually linked with bipolar affective disorder, manic processes are powerfully operative in other forms of psychosis. Under the sway of the manic defence, reality is denied; omnipotence reigns, there is no vulnerability or dependence and the impact of loss is negated.

> Troy grew up in a household with three older sisters and his mother; the father left the family when he was two, effectively abandoning them. Troy became a talented footballer and seemed to hold a special position both as the man of the household and at school, where he was revered for his sporting prowess. He was however released from his contract with an academy for a premier league football team and he became manic shortly after. On admission to the psychiatric ward he believed he was a sporting superstar, able to impregnate women with a touch of his finger. It seemed his experience of rejection and helplessness in relation to loss was denied, and he had created an alternative reality in which he was omnipotent and grandiose. Troy struggled as he responded to the medication and as his mania started to recede he became non-compliant with treatment, seeming to prefer the delusional world he had created to the painful realities of loss and shame.

This case also illustrates how psychotic symptoms, even bizarre and distressing, may serve an important function for a mind which does not feel equipped to manage reality. This preference for delusional alternative may underly treatment resistance and non-compliance commonly seen in working with psychotic patients.

A psychodynamic approach therefore links the mental processes of infancy with the psychological processes of psychosis in later life. Hallmarks of psychotic functioning such as concrete thinking and absolute certainty, primitive representations of good and bad, experiencing external reality as containing looming threats which seek to intrude and control, feelings of being acted upon, hallucinatory experiences and delusion formation can be helpfully considered from this perspective, enabling the patient's dilemmas to seem more understandable and less estranged from ordinary human concerns than their symptoms may suggest. A model which accepts the psychosis as a meaningful communication and psychotic material as functioning rather like dreams and operating under primary processes can be helpful in equipping staff and supporting their curiosity in understanding what is being expressed.

Psychodynamic Approaches to Working with Psychosis

In general individual or group psychodynamic psychotherapy is not recommended as a treatment approach for most cases, although psychodynamically trained therapists do continue to work with psychotic patients after careful assessment of the likely risks and benefits. Treatment resistance can be a considerable obstacle for psychotherapy and whether the intervention is likely to lead to meaningful change needs to be carefully considered.

However, a psychoanalytic approach does provide a framework for understanding the patient's experience and considering the underlying issues, taking into account the life story of the patient, developmental challenges and triggering events. NICE guidelines in the UK recommend the use of psychoanalytic principles to help health care professionals to understand the experiences of people with psychosis and their interpersonal relationships [17].

The delivery of care through multidisciplinary teams represents a concerted effort to engage patients in therapeutic relationships with mental health staff towards supporting recovery; however, this task is often confounded by the persistence of the psychosis and the difficulties in engaging in therapeutic relationships which can thwart recovery. A psychodynamic approach can also help to shed light on the relational aspects of the patient's difficulties as these are expressed to the team.

The bizarre, florid and bewildering presentations of psychotic patients – or the quiet oddness and the underpinning beliefs accompanying them of many who do not usually present to services – contain rich material for those seeking to explore and to fathom the workings of the mind.

Systemic Approaches to Psychosis

Chapter 9 describes how a systemic approach to mental disorder considers how relationships and patterns of communication in families contribute to the genesis and maintenance of psychological disturbance. A systemic approach to psychosis sees the identified patient as expressing a fundamental problem which needs to be addressed within the family system.

Features of a systemic approach to psychosis include

1. Recognition of the fundamental importance of addressing family and other close relationships in psychosis
2. Focus upon the role of high levels of expressed emotions and contradictory communications (double bind hypothesis) in the genesis and relapse of psychotic illness
3. A convincing and robust evidence base
4. Inclusion within NICE guidelines
5. Paucity of suitable services

Family interventions have the best evidence base of all psychological therapies for psychosis. Systemic approaches to working with psychosis are built upon the premise that growing up in an environment where the child consistently receives mixed messages about how to feel and behave can lay the foundations for psychotic disturbance [17]. Research in the 1970s showed that high expressed emotion significantly predicts relapse in schizophrenia [18] and further studies showed that the use of family therapy could significantly reduce this [19]. The development of these ideas and their application is outlined further in Chapter 9.

For a time in the UK services offering family interventions for psychosis were developed but this has not been maintained in most of mainstream psychiatric practice. The NICE guidelines 2014 recommend a family intervention for at least 10 sessions and up to 1 year. [20, recommendation 1.3.7.2]. It is surprising given the evidence base, how scanty provision is within the NHS for family interventions. In a more recent development, the Open Dialogue Approach explicitly recognises the importance of psychological development and relationships in psychiatric breakdown as described in Chapter 26 and has the potential to bring both psychoanalytic and systemic thinking to the forefront of clinical practice.

Cognitive Behavioural Approaches to Psychosis

Key aspects of a cognitive behavioural approach to psychosis include:

1. Psychological distress plays a role in the development of psychosis, including trauma and difficulties with self-esteem
2. Psychotic processes are part of a continuum with more normal states of mind, and delusions may not be so different from everyday beliefs

3. The beliefs and experiences have meaning
4. There is also present a part of the patient who can be helped to observe and to consider the delusional beliefs and perceptions
5. The delusional beliefs may serve a protective function against underlying feelings and thoughts which are troubling

Although a cognitive behavioural therapy (CBT) approach considers cognitive processes at a rational level and does not concern explicitly itself with unconscious processes, there is some common ground with psychodynamic ideas. A CBT approach to psychosis assumes the presence of a non-psychotic part of the mind able to establish a therapeutic alliance and to think about the content of the psychotic symptoms from a different, non-psychotic perspective.

Kingdon and Turkington [21] proposed a general framework for working with psychotic patients which they termed the **normalising strategy**, pointing out similarities between hallucinations and paranoid symptoms and experiences common in ordinary functioning. CBT has led to treatment approaches based on assessment of delusional beliefs and establishing a therapeutic alliance which enables exploration and seeking evidence behind a delusional belief [22]. Normalising strategies provide an approach for weighing up and questioning delusional beliefs, using techniques such as peripheral questioning and socratic questioning to enable the belief to be clarified and the evidence for and against it assessed. This engages the mind at the level of logical argument. A further CBT technique for working with psychosis includes recognition that the delusion may be serving a protective function and is linked with strong states of affect, referred to as a **hot cognition**. A different approach would then be taken using **inference chaining** which seeks to get behind the delusion – particularly with grandiose beliefs – which may be defensive against self-doubts and low self-esteem.

CBT for psychosis is not a single psychological model, and there are a varied combination of techniques depending on the stage of the illness and symptoms. There has been a major interest in extending the original CBT model, from additional perspectives such as Mindfulness, Acceptance and Commitment Therapy, Metacognitive Therapy, Narrative Therapy [23] and Compassion-Focussed therapy. Common to all models is the central role of considering the meaning of the intrusive symptoms, and the behavioural and emotional response of the individual in dealing with the symptoms.

A key aspect of the approach is the development of a formulation as Table 14.1 illustrates. Examples of therapeutic aims include reducing distress, improving coping skills, developing alternate explanations for distressing experiences, changing attentional process through training, changing meaning, changing core beliefs and changing behaviour through exposure and behavioural experiments. CBT for psychosis has been well researched and shows symptom relief across a range of measures [24].

Table 14.1 shows an example of a formulation used with the patient by a CBT therapist to identify the predisposing, precipitating and maintaining factors for their psychotic symptoms as a basis for treatment.

Schema-focussed therapy addresses the core underlying beliefs in psychosis, for example 'I am inferior', and looks at the evidence for these beliefs, including in lived and imagined scenarios. In contrast to a normalisation approach this accepts that the delusion has meaning, rather than is a misbelief which can be corrected through rational thought. This can provide the basis for the generation of alternative explanations and reduction of the need for the beliefs.

Table 14.1 CBT formulation for psychosis – a clinical example

Predisposing factors		
Life experiences	Core beliefs: self and others	Rules for living
Family history of psychosis	*I am in danger*	*If I let my guard down, I will*
Bullying in school	*I don't fit in*	*be attacked*
Sexual abuse in teenage	*I am different*	*Hide true self!*
Altered perceptions when	*I am bad*	*Don't get close to others*
using drugs	*People are going to be cruel, malevolent*	*Never trust anyone!*

Precipitating factor: external and internal intrusive events

External activating event, e.g.	Alienating experiences, e.g.	Unusual sensory perceptions, e.g.
Rejection, humiliation, other	Surroundings seem strange	Hearing own name spoken aloud
threat to self-esteem or safety	Time passes slowly or faster	Sounds, whispering, voices inside or outside head
Co-workers laughing when I made a mistake	Feeling of unreality	Strange visual perceptions, visions
	People appear or sound strange	Somatic sensations without attributable cause
	Difficulty in concentrating	
	Difficulty in thinking	

Maintaining factors: secondary appraisal and reactivation of core beliefs

They have started again	*Am being watched*	**World is dangerous, strange**
They will attack me	*I have to protect myself*	
They will humiliate me	*I can't cope with this*	
People know what I think	*I am losing my mind*	
	I will lose control	

Maintaining factors: threat-focussed attention and cognitive biases

- Hyperarousal
- Perceptual bias: e.g. selective attention to threat
- Memory biases
- Source monitoring bias (attribute self-generated thoughts to others)
- Hindsight bias
- Self-serving bias – blaming others for failure
- Covariation bias – overestimation of causality and underestimation of chance
- Reasoning bias – mind reading, personalisation, jump to conclusions
- Negative expectation bias (pessimism)
- Belief inflexibility bias – I know I am right, as I can feel it (emotional reasoning)
- Confirmation bias (bias against disconfirmatory evidence)

Maintaining factors: reinforcement through consequences

Emotional consequences	Behavioural consequences	Social consequences
Fear	Avoid people	Withdrawal
Anger	Safety behaviours	Loneliness
Despair	Be on the guard	Reduced interests
	Scan environment for danger	Stigma
	Rumination	
	Drug abuse	

NICE guidelines recommend that adult patients with schizophrenia are offered CBT over 16 planned sessions on a one to one basis with the aims of:

- Establishing links between thoughts, feelings or actions and their current or past symptoms and or functioning
- Re-evaluation of perceptions, beliefs or reasoning and how this relates to their target symptoms

The CBT should include at least one of the following:

- Monitoring thoughts, feelings or behaviours with respect to the symptoms
- Promoting alternative ways of coping with the target symptom
- Reducing distress, improving functioning [20, recommendation 1.3.7.1]

Conclusion

It is possible to know just about everything about schizophrenia as a disease without being able to understand one single schizophrenic [25]

Psychological perspectives offer an approach to psychosis based upon meaning, understanding and curiosity about the patient's personal biography and relationships. Symptoms, however bizarre, are viewed as providing key insights into the patient's inner world and attention is paid to the content and form of the delusional beliefs and hallucinations. Patient care is informed by an approach which seeks to understand both acute breakdown and the psychological factors which may contribute to chronicity and treatment resistance. There are different models which may diverge in terms of their aims and application but hold in common an overarching approach with a specific focus upon the symptoms and their meaning for the individual as a basis for clinical care.

Acknowledgements

I am very grateful to Dr P J Saju for his help with the CBT section of this chapter.

References

1. Kant I. *Verush über die Krankheiten des Kopfes*. Konigsberg, 1764.

2. Freud S. Psychoanalytic notes on an autobiographical account of a case of paranoia. In J Strachey, ed., *The Standard Edition of the Complete Psychological Works of Sigmund Freud, Volume XII (1911–1913): Case History of Schreber, Papers on Technique and Other Works*. London: Hogarth Press. 1958; pp. 9–82. (Original work published 1911)

3. Schreber DB. Memoirs of My Nervous Illness. New York: New York Review Books, 2000.

4. Freud S. Neurosis and Psychosis. In J Strachey, ed., *The Standard Edition of the Complete Psychological Works of Sigmund Freud, Volume XIX (1923–1925): The Ego and the Id and Other Works*. London: Hogarth Press. 1961; pp. 149–53. (Original work published 1924)

5. Eliot TS. Burnt Norton. In *Four Quartets*. Vol. 1. 1936.

6. Klein M. Notes on some schizoid mechanisms. In *The Writings of Melanie Klein*. Vol. 3. *Envy and Gratitude and Other Works*. London: Hogarth Press. 1946; pp. 1–24.

7. Target T, Fonagy M. Playing with reality: II. The development of psychic reality from a theoretical perspective. *Int J Psychoanal* 1996; 77: 459–79.

8. Segal H. Notes on symbol formation. In *The Work of Hannah Segal: A Kleinian Approach to Clinical Practice.* New York: Jason Aronson. 1957; pp. 49–65.

9. Miller J-A (ed.). *The Seminars of Jacques Lacan. Book III. The Psychoses, 1955–1956.* London and New York: Taylor and Francis. [Reprinted New York: W. W. Norton & Company, 1997]

10. Lacan J. *La relation d'objet. Les formations d'inconscient 1957–8.* Ed JA Miller Paris: Seuil, 1998.

11. Lacan J. *De La Psychose Paranoiaque Dans ses Rapports Avec la Personalitie.* Paris: Seuil, 1932.

12. Money-Kyrle R. *The Collected Papers of Roger Money-Kyrle.* Ed. D Meltzer. Strathtay: Clunie Press, 1981.

13. Freud, S. An outline of psychoanalysis. The psychical apparatus and the external world. In J Strachey, ed., *The Standard Edition, of the Complete Psychological Works of Sigmund Freud, Volume XXIII (1937–1939): Moses and Monotheism, An Outline of Psycho-Analysis and Other Works.* London: Hogarth Press. 1964; p. 202. (Original work published in 1940)

14. Bion WR. Differentiation of the psychotic from the non-psychotic personalities. In *Second Thoughts.* New York: Jason Aronson. 1957; pp. 43–64.

15. Lucas R. *The Psychotic Wavelength: A Psychoanalytic Perspective for Psychiatry.* Hove: Routledge, 2009.

16. Bion WR. On hallucination. In *Second Thoughts.* New York: Jason Aronson. 1957; pp. 65–85.

17. Bateson G, Jackson DD, Haley J, Weakland J. Towards a theory of schizophrenia. *Behav Sci* 1956; 1(4): 251–4.

18. Brown GW, Birley JL, Wing JK. Influence of family life on the course of schizophrenic disorders: a replication. *Br J Psychiatry* 1972; 121: 241–58.

19. Pilling S. Bebbington P, Kuipers E et al. Psychological treatments in schizophrenia: I. Meta-analysis of family intervention and cognitive behaviour therapy. *Psychol Med* 2002; 32(5): 763–82.

20. NICE. Psychosis and schizophrenia in adults: prevention and management. NICE Guideline CG178. 2014.

21. Kingdon D, Turkington D. *Cognitive Behavioral Therapy of Schizophrenia.* Hove: Lawrence Erlbaum Associates, 1994.

22. Turkington D, Siddle R. Cognitive therapy for the treatment of delusions. *Adv Psychiatr Treat* 1998; 4: 235–42.

23. Rhodes J, Jakes S. *Narrative CBT for Psychosis.* Hove: Routledge, 2009.

24. Dobson K, Dozois J. *Handbook of Cognitive-Behavioural Therapies,* 4th ed. New York: Guilford Press, 2019.

25. Laing RD. *The Divided Self.* London: Penguin Books. 1964; p. 33.

Personality Disorder

15

Tennyson Lee

A Clinical Scenario

Ms N, a 27-year-old woman has been urgently referred to the community psychiatric service by her General Practitioner. The psychiatrist Dr R feels anxious about the encounter as the receptionist says Ms N has been 'abusive and challenging'. Ms N informs Dr R she saw her boyfriend Tom talking to his ex-girlfriend and has since had urges to take an overdose.

Ms N brightens up in the meeting. On mental state examination she is not clinically depressed. She says she has no further thoughts of harming herself. Dr R spends an hour with Ms N and despite his initial misgivings has found the meeting interesting and pleasant. He informs her he will discharge her as things seem stable and will arrange a follow-up appointment. In a second the atmosphere switches. Ms N becomes furious and says she wants to be admitted. Taken aback, Dr R starts explaining his recommendation. Ms N abruptly stands up, saying 'You don't have a clue do you? I've got more pills at home why don't I just go and take them all'.

How can we understand this encounter? What defence mechanisms is Ms N using? What is the short- and longer-term management? What are the options for therapy? What is the prognosis? This chapter will address some of these issues.

Objectives of Chapter

1. To describe the epidemiology of personality disorder (PD) – its distribution and determinants
2. To describe key aspects of assessment and treatment of PD to inform evidence-based clinical practice

Introduction

Personality in all its variety and presentations has captured our interests for a long time – Hippocrates, born 460 BC, was already grappling with the concept through the four humors, black bile, yellow bile, blood and phlegm. An imbalance was thought to influence personality as melancholic, choleric, saguine and phlegmatic. The history of the study of personality is laudable for its attempts at (1) systematising (including through categorisation, resulting in the present ICD and DSM classification systems) (2) interest in psychopathy and (3) attempts at linking personality to biology (with initial forays like phrenology now replaced by significant developments in neuroscience) [1].

Personality consists of the dynamic organisation of enduring patterns of cognition, emotion, behaviour and motivation, and ways of relating to others that characterise an individual [2]. PD may be thought of as occurring when these patterns lead to significant difficulties for the individual or those around them.

The concept of PD has been criticised on several dimensions:

Scientifically: personality is a dimensional entity to which a categorical approach denies reality. There is a lack of an empirical base for existent PD categories.

Clinically: there is considerable overlap between different specific PDs. The classification is polythetic, as not all diagnostic criteria are necessary for making a diagnosis. As only five out of nine criteria need to be met for a diagnosis of borderline PD (BPD) [3], 151 different combinations are possible. Two individuals can have a diagnosis of BPD and only share one out of nine criteria, suggesting considerable differences within this diagnostic group.

Socially: the diagnosis is stigmatising. Psychiatrists have more critical and negative attitudes towards PD than other mental disorders [4, 5].

Problematic as the diagnosis may be, PD is an important condition given its prevalence and impact on the individual with the disorder, their families, services and wider society.

A note on use of the term PD in this chapter. When used PD refers to personality disorders in general. It should be noted however that the evidence base for treatment of PD is based on BPD, and sections of the chapter referring to treatment are referring to treatment of BPD.

Epidemiology of PD

The epidemiology of PD is under-researched and fraught with methodological problems. Table 15.1 summarises key figures [6]. The wide range of prevalence estimates across studies is likely to be due to differences in samples and measurement instruments.

Community: the prevalence of at least one PD is estimated at 12 per cent [7], and of each specific PD varies between 0.1 per cent (schizoid) and 2.5 per cent (histrionic) [8]. Males and females have a similar rate of diagnosis of at least one PD, although there are gender differences in the diagnosis of specific PDs (e.g. antisocial PD (ASPD) is more common in males). PD is higher in the young, those with low educational achievement, unemployed and divorced [9].

Primary care: patients with PD tend to present with medical symptoms in primary care [10]. Yet when formally studied, PD prevalence is 10 to 30 per cent, with one in four of those attending primary care having a diagnosis of PD [11]. This suggests under-detection in routine practice.

Secondary care: between 40 per cent and 92 per cent of psychiatric outpatients [12] and about 50 per cent of psychiatric inpatients [13] meet criteria for a PD.

There is considerable co-morbidity. Over half of people with PD also meet criteria for at least one other major psychiatric disorder, for example mood disorders and anxiety disorders [9]. All PD clusters are significantly associated with increased rates of anxiety, mood, externalising (i.e. conduct disorder, attention-deficit hyperactivity disorder) and substance use disorders [9]. Nearly half of those meeting criteria for any PD also met criteria for a second PD diagnosis and 14 per cent met four or more individual PD diagnoses [14].

Table 15.1 Median prevalence (per cent) PD in community-based studies using DSM-IV [6]

Paranoid	Schizoid	Schizotypal	Histrionic	Antisocial	Borderline	Narcissistic	Avoidant	Dependent	Obsessive
1.1	0.9	0.6	1.8	1.2	1.1	0.4	1.5	0.8	3.2

Self-Harm

Compared with individuals without PD, those with PD are significantly more likely to engage in intentional self-harm in all its forms, namely suicidal deaths, suicidal attempts and non-suicidal self-injury [15]. PD is very high among patients presenting to treatment following intentional self-harm (23–55%) and suicidal deaths (13–56%) [15]. The odds of dying by suicide is 15–38 times higher for people with PD than for those in the general population [15]. This wide range is due to being based on different samples (primary care and hospitalised patients). PD has been found to be present in nearly 30 per cent of suicide attempts [15] and 10 per cent of BPD patients do eventually kill themselves [16].

Across the Life Cycle

Children and youth: there is a firm basis for establishing early diagnosis and treatment of BPD in adolescents. This basis includes: (1) BPD is as valid and reliable diagnosis in adolescence as it is in adults based on phenomenology, stability, risk factors, separation of course and outcome from other disorders and efficacy of treatment for BPD [17]. (2) It has an estimated prevalence of 1–3 per cent in the community, 11–22 per cent in outpatients and 33–49 per cent in inpatients [17].

Old age: PD is a condition that seems to improve with age, the prevalence of PD among older people in the community is estimated to be about 10 per cent [18].

Culture

Culture is relevant in both the expression and assessment of PD. Regarding *expression*, ICD-11's description of PD acknowledges the role of culture by specifying '*The patterns of behaviour characterizing the disturbance cannot be explained primarily by social or cultural factors*' [19]. Regarding *assessment* the ICD and DSM systems make cultural assumptions as they are framed by Western norms of personality functioning, putting self before relational aspects. Differences in expression, and assessment, of PD may be a factor in epidemiological findings regarding PD as in the two following studies. A systematic review of ethnic variations in prevalence and treatment of PD found significantly lower prevalence and range of treatment offered in non-white versus white subjects [20]. A study of inpatients found that compared with white subjects, PD was significantly less prevalent in non-white ethnic groups [21].

Aetiology

PD is a developmental disorder, and development occurs within a social context. Thus rather than focussing on isolated aetiological mechanisms it is more appropriate to incorporate multiple levels of analysis at individual (e.g. genetics, temperament and adversity), family and socioeconomic levels [22]. Specific genetic mechanisms have not been identified and are unlikely to be found, as PD is influenced by multiple genes each having a small effect. Epigenetics indicates the need for a more transactional model whereby the potential for genetic expression is shaped through environmental influences [23]. Disruptions in early attachment, in combination with biological vulnerability, contribute to problems with sense of self and other disturbances of identity characteristic of PD. The dynamic nature of personality as understood by psychodynamic theory thus becomes linked to our biology.

Assessment in PD

Accurate assessment and diagnosis of PD is problematic, given the wide range of non-discriminant symptoms *and* extensive co-morbidity. It is therefore essential to retain what the key purpose of the assessment is, namely to identify:

1. *What is the problem?* The problem is usefully seen as having two components – *caseness* (what is the diagnosis – at both psychiatric and psychological (i.e. the formulation) levels) and *impact* (which may be seen as a measure of severity and therefore determining what level of treatment is required)
2. *What is the treatment* based on (1) the problem as described above and (2) on the ability of the patient to make use of what is offered? Is one thinking of management at primary, psychiatric and/or psychological level?

Thus, when assessing PD it is useful to keep the concepts of *caseness* (the psychiatric diagnosis), *impact* (of the individual's difficulties on himself and others) and *frame* (how ready is the patient to benefit from psychotherapy in terms of e.g. stability of living conditions, level of chaos in their lives, psychoactive drug dependence) in mind. *Caseness* and *impact* help in determining what is the problem, and *impact* and *frame* help determine what is the appropriate treatment.

ICD-11 and DSM-5

ICD-11

A version of ICD-11 was released on 18 June 2018 and it is planned that Member States will start reporting using ICD-11 on 1 January 2022.

The ICD-11 classification of PD [24] is groundbreaking and was developed in response to problems identified with PD diagnosis as described above. It does away with the specific PD diagnoses, instead adopting a dimensional approach to personality and focussing on personality traits. The steps are:

1. identify if a PD is present (problems in functioning of aspects of self and/or with others which are 'pervasive', 'enduring' and have significant impact)
2. assess level of severity (mild, moderate or severe)
3. assess which is the predominant trait domain (negative affectivity, disinhibition, detachment, dissociality and anankastia). Given the importance many clinicians place on BPD, the ICD-11 task group have accepted that this diagnosis will be retained

DSM-5

While the original specific classifications have been retained as they were in DSM-IV, there is an alternative model for PD which translates well with ICD-11 in its emphasis on self and other, levels of personality functioning, and trait domains identified [25].

These developments in ICD-11 and DSM-5 are an important step. They are 'clinically near' as they focus on personality functioning through the prism of *self* or interpersonal (i.e. '*other*') dysfunction. This is consistent with psychoanalytic theories of personality, in particular contemporary object relations theory with its emphasis of the individual's internal representation of himself and of others [26]. Secondly, the dimensional nature of personality and PD is accepted through the focus on severity. This not only makes clinical sense but is also backed by research, for example, generalised severity is the most important single predictor of current and prospective dysfunction [27]. The above-mentioned importance for the busy clinician of establishing *caseness* and *impact* is borne out by the ICD-11 and DSM-5 guidelines.

Screening for PD

The standardised Assessment of Personality – Abbreviated Scale (SAPAS) [28] is a useful screening tool. It has eight items as below.

In general, do you have difficulty making and keeping friends?

Would you normally describe yourself as a loner?

In general, do you trust other people?

Do you normally lose your temper easily?

Are you normally an impulsive sort of person?

Are you normally a worrier?

In general, do you depend on others a lot?

In general, are you a perfectionist?

A score of three items correctly identified the presence of DSM-IV PD in 90 per cent of participants. It is recommended as feasible for routine use in clinical settings where a high prevalence of PD is expected and is thus suitable for psychiatric, not primary care, settings.

A more sophisticated screening tool, used widely in the PD services, is the Structured Clinical Interview for DSM (SCID), which is a semi-structured interview that takes around 90 minutes to complete.

The Function of Assessment at Different Levels of Care

The different function of assessment at different levels of care is a useful guide for clinicians.

At primary care and general psychiatry level: the function is PD detection and the decision whether to manage or refer on. If management is to occur at either of these levels, more specific formulation and diagnosis is required.

At psychotherapy service or PD service level: the function here is confirmation whether PD is present and the decision whether to offer therapy. If therapy is to be offered, is the level of psychological intervention supportive (shoring up defences) or to enable psychic change (challenging defences)? As personality can be seen as the organisation of defence mechanisms, achieved by dint of hard work by the individual to get him/her through life (or not), he/she resists giving up these mechanisms – whether consciously or unconsciously. If the syntonic component of his/her defences is too great, he/she may not be up for psychic change (even if he/she claims to be).

The *treatment contract* is a critical component of treating patients with more severe PD. It sets the treatment frame (essential for this patient group whose chaotic presentation directs all therapeutic activity to symptom fighting rather than tackling the underlying issues) and defines the responsibility of the patient (e.g. regular attendance, undertaking to address self-harming behaviour) and service (e.g. providing a safe and stable environment).

While different evidence-based treatments place different emphases on the treatment contract, how the patient responds to the expectations of the treatment contract is in itself a useful part of the assessment.

Treatment

Psychological and Psychiatric Management

There is an evidence base for the treatment of PD but it is small and exists for BPD [29] (see Table 15.2). No single therapy stands out as more effective [30]. Recent meta-analysis of specialist therapy for BPD suggests outcome changes are modest and unstable [16].

An evidence-based treatment not appearing in Table 15.2 is Systems Training for Emotional Predictability and Problem Solving (STEPPS). This is a manualised cognitive-behavioural skills based 20-week programme with a systems component to include the patient's 'system', for example her family members, friends and key professionals [32]. If one considers the essence of personality is one's relationship to oneself and others, a systems approach seems a key ingredient to therapy.

Well-defined, manualised general psychiatric treatments include structured clinical management (SCM) [33] and general psychiatric management (GPM) [34]. These compare well to the more specialised treatments. Given the high prevalence of BPD in non-specialist services and that general clinicians may not have the interest, or resources, for specialist training, these manualised treatments allow optimisation of general psychiatric care.

The psychological understanding of BPD which places difficulties with attachment and identity as core underpins the treatment models recommended and evidenced base for services managing PD. Table 15.3 serves as a useful preliminary checklist for clinicians to assess their state of readiness to provide an effective service to patients with BPD.

Medications

There is no robust evidence for the use of medications to treat PD. The NICE guidelines recommend avoiding the use of medications for BPD or individual symptoms. Despite this, it is estimated that 92 per cent of BPD patients had received psychotropic medication, mainly antidepressant or antipsychotic [35].

Medications treatment for PD is essentially a trial of one. A practical approach to prescribing includes monitoring the transference and countertransference (for reasons why the psychiatrist may be prescribing – for example, is it due to the extreme demand of the patient who projects an urgency in the psychiatrist to do something even if it lacks evidence for its utility), to educate the patient regarding which symptoms are being targeted and potential side effects, to set the duration for the trial of therapy, to negotiate before starting that the medication will be stopped if there is no improvement, to prescribe defensively (e.g. give prescriptions weekly) and to monitor carefully [36].

Specific PDs

This chapter mainly covers BPD, antisocial (or dissocial) and narcissistic PD (NPD), the former two as the PD diagnoses most frequently made, and the latter for its relative neglect within services.

Table 15.2 Evidence-based treatments for borderline personality disorder[a]

	Transference-focussed psychotherapy (TFP)	Mentalisation-based treatment (MBT)	Cognitive analytic treatment (CAT)	Schema-focussed therapy (SFT)	Dialectical behavioural therapy (DBT)
Theoretical background	• Psychoanalytic • Object relations • Drive theory	• Psychoanalytic • Development theory • Attachment theory Cognitive	Psychoanalytic Cognitive	Cognitive behavioural therapy (CBT)	Cognitive behavioural therapy Dialectical theory
Key concepts	Identity diffusion Aggression Object relations Primitive defence mechanisms	Mentalising[b] Loss of mentalising (psychic equivalence, teleological, and pretend modes) when arousal too low or too high (frequently in context of attachment difficulties)	Self states Reciprocal roles and procedures	Schemas Schema modes Coping strategies	Emotion dysregulation Invalidating environment
Mechanisms of change	Increased integration of concept of self Increased awareness of the unconscious	Increased mentalisation	Change in reciprocal procedures	Change in maladaptive schemas	Learning new behaviour Synthesising opposing ideas
Patient–therapist relationship	Therapist neutrality Exploration of relationship	Collaborative Therapist not assume an expert stance Exploration of relationship	Non-collusive	Collaborative Reparenting	Dialectical relationship – acceptance and change
Treatment goals	Integration of identity Improved relationship to self and others	Increase ability to mentalise within an attached relationship	Recognise and revise unhelpful patterns	Identify and modify schema	Emotion regulation Distress tolerance Interpersonal effectiveness

Table 15.2 (cont.)

	Transference-focussed psychotherapy (TFP)	Mentalisation-based treatment (MBT)	Cognitive analytic treatment (CAT)	Schema-focussed therapy (SFT)	Dialectical behavioural therapy (DBT)
		Improved relationship to self and others			Control over behaviour
Techniques	Interpretation Transference Countertransference Technical neutrality	Enhancing mentalising (including about the transference) Keeping patient's mentalising difficulties in mind	Description (writing letter to patient) Identifying roles patient adopts and expects	Identifying schemas Guided discovery	Problem solving Validation Skills training Affect control Mindfulness
Framework	Individual 2 × week 1 year Outpatient	Group and individual 2–5 × week 18 months Outpatient/day hospital	Individual 1 × week 6 months[c] Outpatient	Individual 1–2 × week 1 year Outpatient	Group and individual 2 × week 1 year Inpatient/outpatient

[a] The columns from left to right are in the order from most psychoanalytic to least psychoanalytic in approach.
[b] Mentalising is both an implicit and explicit process by which we make sense of others and ourselves, in terms of intentional mental states.
[c] CAT is the shortest duration of the treatments in the table.
Adapted from Lee, 2016 [31].

Table 15.3 Recommendations for services managing PD from the evidence base treatments

Dimension	Indicator
Within the clinical encounter	
Clinician	Equipped to work with patients with PD? (clinician's personality, training, sense of organisational support)
Clinician–Patient	Focus on therapy relationship
	Clear treatment model: manualised, structured,
	Hierarchy of intervention (e.g. prioritising patient safety, then breaks to the treatment frame need to be attended to before deeper psychological treatment can occur)
	Activity on part of both patient and therapist expected
	Primary clinician who works with the patient
	Treatment objectives defined
	Roles of patient and therapist defined, including limits of roles
	Guidelines on crisis management agreed upon
	Emphasis on collaboration
	Attention to structure and frame – e.g. use of treatment contract
	Coherence in theory and practice
	Long term (12–18 months)
	Importance of supervision and consultation stressed
Beyond the clinical encounter, i.e. the wider system	
Family	Involvement
Wider services	Organisational willingness and support
	Integration and good communication with other services
	Easy access to emergency services, medical review, inpatient admission when required with clear plan for re-establishment into community
	Well integrated with services encouraging voluntary and/or return to work schemes

Emotionally Unstable Personality Disorder Borderline Type (ICD-10) – Alternatively Borderline Personality Disorder (in DSM-5)

Epidemiology: BPD has a point prevalence of 1 per cent in the community (comparable to that of schizophrenia) although it is under-recognised by primary care clinicians. It has rates of 12 per cent in outpatient psychiatric clinics and 22 per cent in inpatient psychiatric clinics [37].

Course and prognosis: while BPD was believed to be a lifelong disorder, it has a good prognosis, for example 75 per cent of BPD patients regained close to normal function by the age 35–40, and 90 per cent had recovered by age 50 [38]. A 10-year follow-up of BPD patients found 50 per cent recovered (Global Assessment of Functioning 61 or higher), 86 per cent remission (not meeting DSM-III-R caseness) [39]. However, although impulsive symptoms (e.g. overdosing or cutting) remit earlier, affective symptoms change less, and these patients are less likely to find employment, stable partners or bear children [40].

Clinical: it is useful for the busy clinician to think along the dimensions of thought, affect, behaviour and interpersonal relations when considering a diagnosis of PD. The diagnosis can be made in ICD-10 Diagnostic Criteria for Research or DSM-5 if five or more of the following are present:

Cognition: identity instability, transient, stress-related paranoia or severe dissociation* (*appears in DSM-5 only)

Affect: affective instability, feeling of emptiness, inappropriate or intense anger

Behaviour: impulsivity in a destructive way, recurrent self-harm

Interpersonal: fear of abandonment, unstable and intense personal relations

A critique of the diagnostic criteria above is that it contributes little to a psychological understanding of the patient. Kernberg's concept of Borderline Personality *Organisation* (which is not synonymous with BPD but incorporates this diagnosis, among others (including narcissistic, antisocial and histrionic PD) comes in use here. Kernberg views Borderline Personality *Organisation* as comprising (1) *ego weakness* (the ego being unable to manage the demands of the id, superego and reality), (2) *primary process thinking* (the kind of fantastical thinking we have when we dream), (3) use of *primitive defence mechanisms* (e.g. splitting, projective identification, idealisation, denial, omnipotence, devaluation) and (4) *pathological internal objects* which are typically of a persecutory or idealising nature [41].

Transference and countertransference: countertransference may be considered as the total emotional reaction of the therapist to the patient. It comprises the contribution of the therapist (i.e. therapist's transference) and the patient (via projective identification). The patient's contribution is a source of information regarding his internal world (i.e. his internal objects). Characteristics of the countertransference to individuals with BPD are that they are often rapidly developing, intense, unstable, confusing and exert the pressure to 'do something'.

The strength of feeling aroused in the clinician in working with patients with PD is intense enough to invoke the concept of 'countertransference hate'. Clinicians often balk at this term, preferring to think they are at most merely irritated. This position denies the level of aggression of this condition (which may be more overt through threats or acts of deliberate self-harm but is frequently covert and therefore missed). If not processed, countertransference hate may manifest in a range of affects including anxiety, irritation, avoidance, denial and passivity. Components of countertransference hate include *malice* (when the therapist may tend to be sadistic or cruel) and *aversion*. Aversion is the most dangerous to the patient as it may tempt the therapist to abandon the patient. Recognition and processing of the countertransference is thus vital to allow the clinician to accept, tolerate and contain these intense feelings [42]. Thus a sudden decision to discharge a patient with BPD needs to be checked for whether this is acting out on the countertransference.

Co-morbidity with BPD is high:

Other psychiatric disorders: there is considerable co-morbidity with the following conditions (prevalence of co-morbidity in brackets): mood disorders (32–83%), anxiety disorders (74%), post-traumatic stress disorder (PTSD; 47%) substance misuse (65%) and eating disorders (14–53%)[43].

Other PDs: There is significant diagnostic co-occurrence with other PDs, for example antisocial, avoidant [44].

A general PD factor has been found to underlie all PD diagnoses [45]. Factor analysis of the DSM PD criteria indicated that they load onto a general factor that includes all the BPD criteria. Thus BPD may be better understood as being at the core of personality pathology, rather then being a specific PD category [45].

Other physical disorders: physical disorders (including digestive and circulatory systems) are more common in patients with BPD than without the disorder [46].

Differential diagnosis of BPD:

While there is co-morbidity between BPD and the conditions below, it is clearly important to distinguish between these conditions when possible.

Affective disorders: in BPD the mood state is for a far shorter period than in affective disorders. Thus compared with *depression*, BPD has far more frequent mood instability (usually lasting hours, not days) which is also more highly responsive to interpersonal life events. Similarly, in comparison with *bipolar affective disorder* (BAD) the high periods in BPD last hours rather than days (note this is still markedly shorter than 'rapid cycling BAD' where the high periods still last days rather than hours). BPD should also be clearly distinguished from type II BAD (defined as having mood swings from depression to hypomania rather than to full mania). The diagnosis of hypomania has requirements defined by duration, severity, time scale and persistence not met by patients with BPD.

Schizophrenia: although the experience of hearing voices in BPD is more accurately viewed as dissociation, the experience is so extreme that individuals often describe what sounds like a psychotic experience. In BPD the auditory hallucinations are of a shorter duration – hours, at most days – compared with schizophrenia.

Attention-deficit hyperactivity disorder (ADHD): hyperactivity and inattentiveness are more marked in ADHD whereas identity disturbance, efforts to avoid abandonment, chronic feelings of emptiness and transient paranoid thoughts characterise BPD.

PTSD: while clinicians may be tempted to diagnose PTSD in patients with BPD it should be kept in mind that there is no clear association between traumatic events in childhood to any specific mental disorder, and that the effects of trauma in BPD do not usually resemble what is seen in PTSD [40].

Autistic spectrum disorders (ASD): the key diagnostic criteria for ASD are social and communication difficulties, strong narrow interests and/or unusually repetitive and stereotyped behaviour. The latter two are useful as discriminant criteria. While there are social and communication difficulties in both conditions, the finding of more emotional dysregulation and dissocial behaviour, and less inhibition in BPD versus ASD [47] are useful indicators for a diagnosis of BPD if these underlie the social difficulties.

To Return to Miss N and Her Treatment . . .

The hierarchy of intervention would be to try to (1) manage the immediate situation by increasing an ability to think, (2) attend to the risk and psychiatric issues and (3) when stability has been reached to consider whether to refer for psychotherapy treatment.

1. Managing the immediate situation entails the ability to tolerate the confusion, and attempting to understand the patient. One can use one's countertransference to understand what is happening, that is, the strong sense of fear and hopelessness the psychiatrist feels as the patient makes to leave the room may indicate the patient's own intolerable feelings being projected into him/her – an example of projective identification

2. Assessment of immediate risk regarding patient safety and short-term decisions regarding psychiatric management – ongoing psychiatric outpatient follow-up or requiring more acute care

3. Referral for psychotherapy – when, why and how? Given the lack of research on these questions, an approach to structure this decision-making is useful. The transtheoretical model of stages of change provides a structure for this [48]. The most relevant stages in PD are:

Precontemplation: the stage in which there is no intention to change behaviour in the foreseeable future. Most patients in this stage are unaware or underaware of their problems. Families, friends, neighbours or employees, however, are often well aware that the precontemplators suffer from the problems. This is the stage at which many patients with PD are, and the stage which psychiatrists struggle with the most regarding unsuccessful referrals for psychotherapy. Given that these patients are far from the therapy frame one can understand that a referral made at this stage is more as a response to the pressure to do something (either originating in the psychiatrist, or being projected into him/her by the patient) than for a clinical indication. Instead of referral, interventions which are more likely to be useful include trying to help the patient to feel understood (e.g. by sharing a psychologically informed formulation), sharing information (e.g. psychoeducation on what PD is), practical interventions (e.g. addressing accommodation problems, severe substance use) and social interventions (e.g. peer support groups) [49].

Contemplation: is the stage in which patients are aware that a problem exists and are seriously thinking about overcoming it but have not yet made a commitment to take action. Contemplators struggle with their attachment to their dysfunctional behaviour and the amount of effort, energy and loss it will cost to overcome it.

Narcissistic Personality Disorder

Epidemiology: the overall low prevalence rates of NPD in both non-clinical and clinical samples may be related to the narrow concept captured in the DSM-5 diagnosis (see below), clinician lack of recognition of NPD and, even when recognised, reluctance to make the diagnosis.

Clinical: the DSM-5 requires a minimum of five of the following diagnostic criteria: grandiose sense of self-importance, preoccupied with fantasies of unlimited success or ideal love, belief in special status, requiring excessive admiration, a sense of entitlement, interpersonally exploitative, lack of empathy, often envious, and being arrogant.

Psychological understanding: the DSM-5 diagnostic criteria are limited as they provide only a partial capture of the problem of narcissism. It describes individuals who are thick-skinned and oblivious but omits the thin-skinned [50] and hypervigilant [51]. While the thin-skinned or hypervigilant individuals are phenotypically different as in being inhibited and shy, the core problem of an inner sense of low self-esteem which is sensitive to how they think others perceive them is the same in both presentations of NPD.

Treatment: there is no clear empirical base for the treatment of NPD. A recent Cochrane review proposal was withdrawn due to the lack of evidence base for treatment of NPD [52].

Antisocial Personality Disorder

Epidemiology rates in forensic settings range from 50 to 80 per cent [53].

Clinical: the ICD-10 requires three of the following criteria: callous unconcern for others' feelings, gross irresponsibility and disregard for social norms; incapacity to maintain enduring relationships; very low tolerance to frustration and a low threshold for discharge of aggression; incapacity to experience guilt or to profit from adverse experience; and marked proneness to blame others or to rationalise behaviour.

Treatment: there is limited evidence for the effectiveness of CBT in different settings, with best evidence for therapy delivered in group format for people with ASPD and substance misuse problems [54]. A subsample of patients from a randomised controlled trial found benefits from MBT for ASPD-associated behaviours in patients with co-morbid BPD and ASPD, including the reduction of anger, hostility, paranoia, interpersonal problems, and social adjustment and concluded that MBT appears to be a potential treatment of consideration for ASPD [55].

Summary

There are many areas requiring further development in the field of PD, including identifying the most active ingredients of successful treatment. Recent developments in assessment and treatment indicate realistic grounds for cautious optimism in addressing PD. The prevalence and impact of PD on the individual, family and society underline the importance of ongoing work in this field.

Acknowledgements

I acknowledge the members of Deancross Personality Disorder service, whose cogent clinical work form the foundation for structuring the material in this chapter.

References

* indicates highly recommended reading

1. Solms ML. The neurobiological underpinnings of psychoanalytic theory and therapy. *Front Behav Sci* 2018; 12: 294.

2. Kerberg OF. What is personality? *J Pers Disord* 2016; 30(2): 145–56.

3. American Psychiatric Association. *Diagnostic and Statistical Manual of Mental Disorders*, 5th ed. Washington DC: American Psychiatric Association, 2013.

4. Lewis G, Appleby L. Personality disorder: the patients psychiatrists dislike. *Br J Psychiatry* 1988; 153: 44–9.

5. Chartonos D, Kyratous M, Dracass S, Lee T, Bhui K. Personality disorder: still the patients psychiatrists dislike? *BJPsych Bull* 2017; 41(1): 12–17.

6. Morgan TA, Zimmerman M. Epidemiology of personality disorders In WJ Livesley, R Larstone, eds., *Handbook of Personality Disorders, Theory, Research, and Treatment*, 2nd ed. New York: Guilford Press. 2018; pp. 173–96.

7. Volkert J, Gablonski TC, Rabung S. Prevalence of personality disorders in the general adult population in Western countries: systematic review and meta-analysis. *Br J Psychiatry* 2018; 213(6): 709–15.

8. Eaton NR, Greene AL. Personality disorders: community prevalence and socio-demographic correlates *Curr Opin Psychol* 2018; 21: 28–32.

9. Huang Y, Kotov R, de Girolamo G et al. DSM-IV personality disorders in the WHO World Mental Health Survey *Br J Psychiatry* 2009; 195: 46–53.

10. Emerson J, Pankratz L, Joos S, Smith S. Personality disorders in problematic medical patients. *Psychosomatics* 1994; 35 (5): 469–73.

11. Moran P, Jenkins R, Tylee A, Blitzard R, Mann A. The prevalence of personality disorder among UK primary care attenders *Acta Psychiatr Scand* 2000; 102: 52–7.

12. Beckwith H, Moran PF, Reilly JG. Personality disorder prevalence in psychiatric outpatients: a systematic literature review. *Personal Ment Health* 2014; 8(2): 91–101.

13. Girolamo GD, Reich JH. *Epidemiology of Mental Disorders and Psychosocial Problems: Personality Disorders*. Geneva: World Health Organization, 1993.

14. Coid J, Yang M, Tyrer P, Roberts A, Ulrich S. Prevalence and correlates of personality disorder in Great Britain. *Br J Psychiatry* 2006; 188(5): 423–31.

15. Turner BJ, Jin HM, Anestis MD et al. Personality pathology and intentional self-harm: cross-cutting insights from categorical and dimensional models. *Curr Opin Psychol* 2018; 21: 55–9.

16. Cristea IA, Gentili C, Cotet CD et al. Efficacy of psychotherapies for borderline personality disorder: a systematic review and meta-analysis. *JAMA Psychiatry* 2017; 74(4): 319–28.

17. Chanen AM, Sharp C. Prevention and early intervention for borderline personality disorder: a novel public health priority. *World Psychiatry* 2017; 16(2): 215–16.

18. Abrams RC, Horowitz SV. Personality disorders after age 50: a meta-analysis. *J Pers Disord* 1996; 10: 271–81.

19. WHO. ICD-11 Clinical Descriptions and Diagnostic Guidelines for Mental and Behavioural Disorders. 2018. https://gcp .network/en/private/icd-11-guidelines /disorders.

20. McGilloway A, Hall R, Lee T, Bhui K. A systematic review of personality disorder, race and ethnicity: prevalence, aetiology and treatment. *BMC Psychiatry* 2010; 10: 33. doi:10.1186/1471-244X-10-33.

21. Hossain A, Malkov M, Lee T, Bhui K. Ethnic variation of personality disorder of 6 years of hospital admissions in East London Mental Health Services. *BJPsych Bull* 2018; 42: 157–61.

*22. Livesley WJ. Integrated modular treatment. In WJ Livesley, R Larstone, eds., *Handbook of Personality Disorders, Theory, Research, and Treatment*, 2nd ed. New York: Guilford Press. 2018; pp. 645–75.

23. Larstone RM, Craig SG, Moretti MM. An attachment perspective on callous and unemotional characteristics. In WJ Livesley, R Larstone, eds., *Handbook of Personality Disorders, Theory, Research, and Treatment*, 2nd ed. New York: Guilford Press. 2018; pp. 324–36.

24. Reed GM, First MB, Kogan CS. Innovations and changes in the ICD-11 classification of mental, behavioural and neurodevelopmental disorders. *World Psychiatry* 2019; 18: 3–19.

25. Bach B, First MB. Application of the ICD-11 classification of personality disorders. *BMC Psychiatry* 2018; 18: 351.

26. Kerberg OF. *Severe Personality Disorders: Psychotherapeutic Strategies*. New Haven: Yale University Press, 1984.

27. Hopwood C, Malone JC, Ansell EB et al. Personality assessment in DSM-5: empirical support for rating severity, style, and traits. *J Pers Disord* 2011; 25(3): 305–20.

28. Moran P, Leese M, Lee T et al. The Standardised Assessment of Personality – Abbreviated Scale (SAPAS): preliminary validation of a brief screen for personality disorder. *Br J Psychiatry* 2003; 183: 228–32.

29. Stoffers JM, Völlm BA, Rücker G et al. Psychological therapies for people with borderline personality disorder. *Cochrane Database Syst Rev* 2012; (8): CD005652.

30. Leishsenring F. Borderline personality disorder *Lancet* 2011; 377: 74–84.

31. Lee T. *Stormy Lives A Journey Through Borderline Personality Disorder*. London: Muswell Hill Press, 2016.

32. Blum N, Black DW, St John D. Systems training for emotional predictability and problem solving In WJ Livesley, R Larstone, eds., *Handbook of Personality Disorders, Theory, Research, and Treatment*, 2nd ed. New York: Guilford Press. 2018; pp. 586–99.

*33. Bateman AW, Krawitz R. *Borderline Personality Disorder. An Evidence-Based Guide for Generalist Mental Health Professionals*. Oxford: Oxford University Press, 2013.

*34. Gunderson JG, Links PS. *Handbook of Good Psychiatric Management for Borderline Personality Disorder*. Arlington: American Psychiatric Publishing, Inc., 2014.

35. Paton C, Crawford MJ, Bhatti SF et al. The use of psychotropic medication in patients with emotionally unstable personality disorder under the care of UK Mental Health Services. *J Clin Psychiatry* 2015; 76 (4): 512–18.

36. Tyrer P, Bateman A. Drug treatment for personality disorders *Adv Psychiatr Treat* 2004; 10:389–98.

37. Ellison WD, Rosenstein LK, Morgan TA, Zimmerman M. Community and clinical epidemiology of borderline personality disorder. *Psychiatr Clin North Am* 2018; 41: 561–73.

38. Paris J, Zweig-Frank H. A 27-year follow-up of borderline patients. *Compr Psychiatry* 2001; 42: 482–7.

39. Zanarini MC, Frankenburg FR, Reich DB, Garrett F. Time to attainment of recovery from borderline personality disorder and stability of recovery: a 10-year prospective follow-up study *Am J Psychiatry* 2012; 167: 663–7.

40. Paris J. Diagnosis of borderline personality disorder. *Psychiatr Clin North Am* 2018; 41(4): 575–82.

41. Kernberg OF. Borderline personality organization. *J Am Psychoanal Assn* 1967; 15: 641–85.

*42. Maltsberger JT, Buie DH. Countertransference hate in the treatment of suicidal patients. *Arch Gen Psychiatry* 1974; 30(5): 625–33.

43. Shah R Zanarini MC. Comorbidity of borderline personality disorder: current status and future directions. *Psychiatr Clin North Am* 2018; 41(4): 583–93.

44. Grilo CM, Sanislow CA, McGlashan TH. Co-occurrence of DSM-IV personality disorders with borderline personality disorder. *J Nerv Ment Dis* 2002; 190(8): 552–4.

45. Sharp C, Wright AG, Fowler JC et al. The structure of personality pathology: both general ('g') and specific ('s') factors? *J Abnorm Psychol* 2015; 124(2): 387–98.

46. Shen C, Hu L, Hu Y. Comorbidity study of borderline personality disorder: applying association rule mining to the Taiwan national health insurance research database. *BMC Med Inform Decis* 2017; 17: 8.

47. Strunz S, Westphal L, Ritter K et al. Personality pathology of adults with autism spectrum disorder without

accompanying intellectual impairment in comparison to adults with personality disorders. *J Autism Dev Disord* 2015; 45: 4026–38.

48. Norcross JC, Krebs PM, Prochaska JO. Stages of change. *J Clin Psychol* 2011; 67: 143–54.

49. Roughley M, Maguire A, Wood G, Lee T. Referral of patients with emotionally unstable personality disorder for psychological therapy: why, when and how? *BJPsych Bull* 2020. http://dx.doi.org/10.1192/bjb.2020.48.

50. Rosenfeld H. Afterthought: changing theories and changing techniques in psychoanalysis. In H. Rosenfeld, ed., *Impasse and Interpretation*. London: Tavistock. 1987; pp. 265–79.

51. Gabbard GO. Two subtypes of narcissistic personality disorder. *Bull Menninger Clin* 1989; 53: 527–32.

52. Stoffers JM, Ferriter M, Völlm BA et al. Psychological interventions for people with narcissisticpersonality disorder. Cochrane Library 2014. www.cochrane.org/CD009690/psychological-interventions-people-narcissistic-personality-disorder [Accessed 27/02/2019]

53. Hare RD. *The Hare Psychopathy Checklist-Revised*, 2nd ed. Toronto: Multi-Health Systems, 2003.

54. Gibbon S, Duggan C, Stoffers J et al. Psychological interventions for antisocial personality disorder. *Cochrane Database Syst Rev* 2010; 16: CD007668.

55. Bateman A, O'Connell J, Lorenzini N, Gardner T, Fonagy P. A randomised controlled trial of mentalization-based treatment versus structured clinical management for patients with comorbid borderline personality disorder and antisocial personality disorder. *BMC Psychiatry* 2016; 16: 304. doi: 10.1186/s12888-016-1000-9.

Complex Post-traumatic Stress Disorder

16

Joanne Stubley

Introduction

In this chapter, the focus will be on the newly emerging diagnosis of Complex Post-traumatic Stress Disorder (C-PTSD). Following a brief overview of the history of the concept and some diagnostic issues that arise, a description will be given of common symptoms and presentations in C-PTSD. A case history will be used to illustrate these points. The chapter ends with a brief outline of some of the principles of treatment.

History of the Concept

Dr Judith Herman, an American psychiatrist and trauma specialist, first used the term Complex Trauma in 1992 to describe a constellation of symptoms that occurred following chronic, repetitive or prolonged trauma. She highlighted that the central feature of the experience was of captivity, being unable to escape from unbearable experiences of helplessness, terror and dread that overwhelmed existing defences. She drew on her clinical experience in working with adult survivors of child sexual abuse, Vietnam veterans and those individuals who had experienced domestic violence to suggest that for many the end result was characterised by a particular presentation of difficulties [1].

Alongside the symptoms of PTSD, which include re-experiencing phenomena, hyper-arousal symptoms and avoidance, Herman suggested that complex trauma might also lead to:

- affect dysregulation
- revictimisation
- dissociation
- somatisation
- identity disturbance

Herman further highlighted that within this group there is development of characteristic personality changes and a vulnerability to repeated harm towards self or others.

It has taken over 25 years for psychiatric classificatory manuals to incorporate a diagnosis of Complex Trauma or Complex PTSD. ICD-11 (the eleventh edition of *The International Classificatory System of Diseases*) will include a diagnosis of Complex PTSD for the first time (C-PTSD) when it comes into effect from 2022. C-PTSD is defined as a disorder that arises after:

> *exposure to a stressor typically of an extreme or prolonged nature and from which escape is difficult or impossible*

ICD-11 describes PTSD as having three core elements:

1. re-experiencing the traumatic event(s) in the present
2. avoidance of these intrusions
3. an excessive sense of current threat

When this definition of PTSD is combined with the following criteria for disturbances in self-organisation, a diagnosis of C-PTSD may be made:

1. disturbances in affects – may include difficulties in emotional regulation (hyperactivation and deactivation), and behavioural disturbances such as self-destructive acts, reckless or violent behaviour
2. disturbances in self-concept – may include feelings of guilt, shame and failure alongside belief in oneself as diminished, defeated or worthless
3. disturbances in relational functioning – difficulty in feeling close to others, avoiding contact with others and lack of interest in personal engagement

Preliminary studies using this ICD-11 definition and incorporating the use of the International Trauma Questionnaire (ITQ) suggest that C-PTSD is common in clinical and population samples and in clinical samples is more commonly observed than PTSD. In a US sample, lifetime prevalence for C-PTSD was found to be 3.3 per cent, with women twice as likely to meet the criteria than men. Prevalence estimates in a US veteran sample were 13 per cent [2]. Cumulative childhood interpersonal violence was a stronger predictor for C-PTSD than PTSD and C-PTSD was associated with a greater co-morbid symptom burden and substantially lower psychological well-being [3].

The inclusion of C-PTSD within ICD-11 has facilitated the development of rating scales such as the ITQ and the publication of studies such as those cited above. It allows for rigorous examination of the descriptor symptom clusters and in time will facilitate a greater understanding of the disorder as a whole. This leaves the evidence base for effectiveness of therapeutic interventions for C-PTSD in its infancy.

Diagnostic Issues

The role trauma plays in mental disorders has been considered and debated throughout the history of psychiatry, psychology and psychotherapy. It has played into the classic nature versus nurture debate and has had a central role in the consideration of the question of biological versus psychological approaches to psychiatry. Splitting may be manifest in the way these debates get played out, as if a side must be chosen and there is no middle ground. It has become increasingly clear that the need to choose a side is no longer relevant to current theory. The virtual explosion in theoretical understanding of the impact of trauma in the last few decades informs us of the complex interplay of genetic predisposition through transgenerational transmission of trauma, early relational trauma's impact on the developing brain and the epigenetic changes it may induce, revictimisation and the kindling effect increasing the risk of adult traumas and problematic outcomes in those who have been traumatised early in life and the complex interplay of traumatic experiences on the body and its biological functioning.

As the impact of trauma, particularly early relational trauma, is becoming clearer, it is also challenging the traditional psychiatric classificatory systems. The use of a diagnosis based on symptomatology, even within a multiaxial framework, fails to capture the complexity of trauma-related disorders. A psychotherapeutic formulation that outlines the biopsychosocial elements to the presentation, I would argue, allows for the best evidence-based practice in relation to the trauma-related disorders. In gaining an understanding of the neurobiological, trauma and attachment theory research, current trauma-informed care requires a psychotherapeutic formulation that addresses the multiple ways in which trauma may have impacted upon that individual and how best to offer interventions in response to this.

It is important to recognise that the trauma-related conditions of Emotionally Unstable Personality Disorder (EUPD) and Dissociative Disorders have considerable overlap. In all of these, there is a strong link to early relational trauma and considerable overlap in clinical presentation is evident between them. All have high rates of co-morbidity including depression, anxiety, substance abuse and eating disorders. Indeed, if an individual presents with a myriad of symptoms that cut across multiple domains, it is indicative of a trauma history.

While it is clear that C-PTSD has considerable overlap with other diagnoses particularly EUPD, there is emerging evidence that C-PTSD has a lower risk of both self-harm and fear of abandonment, and a more stable sense of self than EUPD [4].

While mostly focussed on developmental trauma, it is also important to recognise that C-PTSD may also originate in adult experiences of repeated, prolonged or chronic trauma, which may include the experiences of asylum seekers and refugees, veterans, survivors of torture and survivors of domestic violence.

Clinical Vignette of C-PTSD

Karen was a 45-year-old single mother who lived with her nine-year-old daughter. The GP referral suggested a gradual onset of low mood with increasing hopelessness and despair, accompanied by feelings of guilt and shame. Karen had stopped going out and had been placed on long-term sickness leave from her receptionist role which she had held down for many years. She had no previous contact with mental health services but was an active member of Alcoholics Anonymous (AA), having been abstinent for 15 years. The GP had made this referral as he believed it may have been linked to Karen's daughter disclosing significant child sexual abuse by a family friend in the last six months. Her daughter was being seen by mental health services for children and Karen had engaged in parenting sessions.

In the course of the consultation, Karen disclosed that she had been sexually and physically abused by her father, now deceased. She had been an only child and her mother suffered from a chronic physical condition, leaving Karen as her carer from an early age. Her father was volatile, drank heavily and began sexually abusing Karen from the age of seven. She never disclosed the abuse, which continued after her mother's death, when Karen was 13 years old. At 16 she ran away from home, had a series of abusive relationships, drank to harmful levels and for a period of time lived on the streets. After her third termination of pregnancy 15 years ago, she left her partner and moved into a shelter. She joined AA and began to have a more settled life. During a brief affair with a married man, she became pregnant with her daughter. She entered stable employment as a receptionist and established a good support network of friends.

Since her daughter's disclosure, Karen reported the emergence of nightmares and flashbacks related to her own abuse. She was repeatedly reliving in vivid detail aspects of the sexual abuse, emerging in her dreams and in intrusive images in her mind. She felt constantly on edge and easily triggered by anything related to sexual violence on the television or in the papers. She had virtually stopped sleeping and instead would lie on a mattress outside her daughter's room in the corridor. She had broken off links with most of her friends and had stopped working. She felt increasingly overwhelmed, full of shame and guilt and self-disgust. At these times she also struggled to go to AA meetings and avoided her sponsor. Karen also reported moments when she would shut down, gazing at the television at times for hours on end without remembering anything she had watched. She also reported episodes of losing time, strange dislocated periods where she might find herself suddenly standing on a train station platform or in a shopping centre with no recollection of how she had got there.

The Body in Trauma

When a potentially threatening event occurs, the experience is registered in the brain, particularly the limbic system where the amygdala resides. The amygdala registers the possibility of danger and sets in motion the stress response system to the event to facilitate the fight/flight response through the Sympathetic Nervous System and the release of adrenaline. Activation of the hypothalamus leads to triggering of the HPA (Hypothalamic–Pituitary–Adrenal) axis, central to the stress response, which ultimately leads to the release of cortisol.

The fight/flight response facilitates immediate action. It causes a shutting down of body functions that are not necessary requirements (such as the immune and digestive systems) and gives extra help to those functions most needed. If the danger passes, all of this will usually settle over 20–30 minutes.

However, if the situation is such that fighting or fleeing will not suffice or are deemed to be impossible, the third response is to freeze. This is mediated by the Parasympathetic Nervous System through the Dorsal Vagus Nerve. This is the most primitive reaction in evolutionary terms to danger and involves complete shutdown of our systems, immobilisation and dissociation.

Stephen Porges, a psychiatrist and neuroscientist [5], describes a third element of this system called the Ventral Vagus. This is the most evolutionarily advanced component of the system and links the brainstem, heart, stomach, other internal organs and facial muscles. It is involved in complex processes of attachment, bonding, empathy and social communication. It is opposite in its effects to the sympathetic fight/flight system and shuts down when we are threatened.

If the Stress Response System as outlined above is repeatedly, chronically triggered by trauma such as child abuse, this may have a profound effect on the developing brain. Findings from a number of studies consistently demonstrate higher activation of the amygdala, that part of the limbic system that is the centre for strong emotions such as fear and rage. This higher activation is akin to setting the dial on high for response to any possible threat causing a full-scale Stress Response, with the propensity to chronic activation of the sympathetic nervous system [6].

The hippocampus is responsible for forming memories and in retrieving them also provides context and comparison. Childhood trauma is often associated with smaller hippocampi in adulthood [7]. This can reduce the capacity to measure the degree of threat if one is less able to contextualise against other memories, to learn from experience. So, each danger signal is potentially felt to be extreme and requires the full stress response. Adding to this situation is the recognition that many traumatised children show reduced activation in the ventromedial prefrontal cortex, which is a vital area for emotional regulation, self-reflection and empathy [8].

Research now clearly demonstrates the potential long-term impact of trauma on the body. Felliti showed through his Adverse Childhood Experiences (ACEs) studies the link with childhood trauma and a greater risk of respiratory, cardiovascular disease and diabetes mellitus in adults [9].

Childhood trauma and stress has been linked with shorter telomeres – the caps on the ends of chromosomes – and this is a clear biomarker for ill health and early death [10]. Links have also been established with lower immune responses [11] and higher levels of inflammation.

A Psychoanalytic Model of Trauma

From a psychoanalytic perspective, trauma is thought to pierce the protective shield around the mind so that it is flooded with an excess of external stimulation from the traumatic event. Internally there is a reactivation of anxieties from early life that further overwhelm the individual. This links with Melanie Klein's description of the early infantile state of mind to understand the nature of the anxieties the traumatised patient faces and the defences at their disposal [12]. Thus, the trauma results in a reactivation of powerful, infantile anxieties from the paranoid–schizoid position of early life. The patient is overwhelmed by terror and dread; anxieties of disintegration, persecution and death predominate. There is no sense of protection or trust in the goodness of the world.

Garland, a psychoanalyst and founder of the Tavistock Trauma Unit, also speaks of how trauma results in the loss of the capacity to differentiate between signal anxiety – anxiety experienced when danger threatens – and automatic anxiety – anxiety experienced in an actual situation of danger [13]:

> Thus, traumatized individuals will likely face each new situation, particularly potentially stressful ones, with a greatly heightened sense of threat. The full Stress Response System may then be activated with fight/ flight or freeze inevitably following. Anxieties of dread, horror and persecution may fill the mind, with all trust in the goodness of the world lost. The higher executive functions become overwhelmed meaning that rational, organized thought and measured observation becomes impossible.

The Window of Tolerance

Many trauma therapists employ a notion of the 'window of affect tolerance', first described by Daniel Siegel, a psychiatrist and researcher, in 1999 to describe the shifts between hyperarousal (fight/flight – sympathetic nervous system) and hypoarousal (freeze – para-sympathetic dorsal Vagus) [14]. Siegel suggested there is an optimal zone between these two states where a person can be calm and focussed, able to use their higher cortical, executive functions. This is the window of tolerance.

For traumatised individuals, the window of tolerance is narrow, and they easily shift into either hyper or hypoarousal states. In these states, the capacity to attend, to concentrate and to reflect is impaired and action is far more likely. To manage these states, individuals may employ a variety of means to limit or attenuate the movement out of the window of tolerance.

The hyperarousal (fight/flight) state may lead to attempts to self-medicate through illicit or prescribed drugs or alcohol. The choice of drug is usually predicated on a wish to sedate, to turn off the readiness for threat. Attempts to manage the hyperarousal may also lead to self-harm or eating disturbances. One may postulate that Karen's use of alcohol was perhaps linked to her attempts to sedate her hyperarousal states as an adolescent.

The hypoarousal state, often accompanied by dissociation, may lead to various attempts to enliven one's mental state which may include self-harm, engaging in risk-taking behaviours including promiscuity or using activating substances such as amphetamines or cocaine.

Both responses – to hyper and hypoarousal states – can be seen to increase the potential risk of revictimisation, which I will return to under that section.

Trauma and Memory

Van der Kolk, a psychiatrist and trauma specialist, entitled his book on trauma *The Body Keeps the Score* [15] in response to a recognition of the following:

> The traumatic event does not get processed in symbolic/linguistic forms as most memories are. Because it tends to be organized on a sensori-motor or iconic level - as horrific images, visceral sensations or flight/fight reactions. Storage on a sensori-motor level and not in words is supposed to explain why this type of material does not undergo the usual transforming process.

Partial loss of the hippocampus function prevents a recognition of the context – time and place – making the memories forever seem to be happening in the present. Potentiation of the amygdala gives them an affective strength – they are felt more powerfully in the body, often within the realm of powerful emotions such as fear, rage and panic, with the accompanying Autonomic Nervous System responses of fight/flight or freeze.

Karen's presentation of nightmares and flashbacks would be understood in relation to this, the re-experiencing phenomena are held within the body in this way, so that she lives out the abuse as though it was happening in the present, feeling all of the bodily sensations, images and fight/flight reactions.

Trauma and Attachment

Complex trauma primarily originates in relational trauma – early, severe and chronic traumatic mistreatment by caregivers and/or others.

Main and Solomon described a group of children who had been maltreated and abused by their caregivers [16]. These children showed a pattern of attachment in the Strange Situation Test which was defined as Disorganised. They examined the kinds of interactions evident between mothers and infants in this group and observed caregivers being experienced as either frightened (often of their child's distress) or frightening (intrusive, looming). When these parents were tested using the Adult Attachment interview their narratives were often described as 'unresolved'. Their narratives were generally inconsistent and/or incoherent with many having considerable trauma in their own childhoods. Disorganised infants may often go on to become rigid and controlling children as a way, perhaps, of managing an unbearably frightening and overwhelming world. Disorganised attachment sequelae include deficiencies in reflective capacity [17], increased aggressiveness with peers [18] and general difficulties with affect dysregulation [19]. As adults they are at increased risk of developing serious mental health conditions, particularly trauma based [20].

Attachment research demonstrates a strong correlation between the Disorganised pattern of attachment and childhood trauma. As Liotti describes it [21]:

> *Being exposed to frequent interactions with a helplessly frightened, hostile and frightening, or confused caregiver, infants are caught in a relational trap, created by the dynamics of two inborn motivational systems, the attachment system and the defence (fight-flight) system. The attachment and the defence systems normally operate in harmony (i.e., flight from the source of fear to find refuge in the proximity to the attachment figure). They, however, clash in such a type of infant-caregiver interaction where the caregiver is at the same time the source and the solution of the infant's fear.*

The child is thus caught in a repetitive loop of approach–avoidance conflict which may become a positive feedback loop, intensifying the distress. Neither approach nor avoidance works as a means of self-organisation or as a way to alleviate fear. There is a collapse of the coping strategy and young children in these circumstances are not able to find a way to regulate affect.

Lyons-Ruth describes how these disorganised babies and young children find an organising strategy to cope with their disorganised attachment style by becoming either compulsive caretakers of their parents or aggressively bossy and hostile [18]. It is a way, she postulates, of side-stepping the attachment system through the use of increasingly polarised and false-self relations with the caregiver.

Dissociation

Elizabeth F. Howell, a relational psychoanalyst and traumatologist, describes dissociation as [20]:

> *the searation of realms of experience that would normally be connected.*

Dissociation is a ubiquitous psychic process that may be transient or enduring. It can be used defensively, adaptively or as a form of protection. Examples of dissociation may include trance and mystical states, sleep walking, night terrors, hypnosis, meditation, hypnogogic and hypnopompic phenomena, daydreams, dreams and altered states due to drugs. Dissociation as a defence against overwhelming, unbearable terror and helplessness is part of the hypoarousal, freeze response discussed earlier.

Thus, trauma elicits dissociation which is a discontinuity of experience and memory. Allen describes two components of dissociation [22]. First of all, there is a detachment from the overwhelming experience and secondly a compartmentalisation of the experience so that it is both known and not known. He emphasises that it is initially an adaptive response to fear and psychic pain.

Thus, dissociation results in a piece of traumatic experience being cordoned off and established as a separate psychic state. This experience and its associated affects are associatively unavailable to the rest of the personality but may be experienced as:

- Intrusive images connected to the trauma but otherwise unrecognisable
- Violent or symbolic acting out
- Inexplicable somatic sensations
- Recurrent nightmares
- Anxiety reactions

- Medically unexplained symptoms
- Hallucinations

In severe dissociated states people can behave in organised ways but have no recollection of what they have done or how they have come to be where they are. Karen's shutting down, staring at the television and losing time could be seen as dissociation, a way of disconnecting when feeling overwhelmed. Her losing time and finding herself in situations with no recollection of the journey would also be evidence of dissociation.

In order to understand in more detail what the process is that leads to the development of these kinds of symptoms following traumatic events, it can be helpful to return to the freeze response. Trauma may lead to a fight/flight sympathetic hyperarousal response pattern of PTSD. This has been described by Van der Kolk as 'primary dissociation' [15] and is the most common pattern of PTSD. The other response – the freeze – is a depersonalised, numb reaction in which anxiety does not occur and the person becomes 'detached', observing events as if from a distance from the self and often feeling separated from the body. This is secondary dissociation. This psychological distancing has initially a protective function in preventing hyperarousal, allowing an attention to task without becoming overwhelmed by terror. However, if relied on chronically, this process results in a person living much of their life in a depersonalised state.

There is often an intellectual understanding of what may be occurring but in the absence of an emotional response. Chronic childhood trauma may lead to an association between alexithymia (no words for emotions) and secondary dissociative states. Repeated entry into secondary dissociative states may produce progressively more marked departures from external reality and consciousness for self.

Thus, early abuse increases the likelihood of disorganised attachment through the impaired capacity for affect regulation and the use of pathological dissociation as a defence, which then inhibits further attachment communications and interactive regulation.

Trauma and Words

Childhood trauma is linked to reduced activity in language centres such as Broca's area [15], affecting the capacity to put emotional states (what is being experienced in the body) into words.

Victims of trauma and abuse have also been shown to have a smaller corpus callosum. These fibres connect the right and left hemispheres, allowing communication between the emotional experience and processing, empathy and bonding of the right and the logical, rational, language centre of the left hemisphere. As Music describes [23]:

> ... the capacity to develop a coherent narrative about emotional experiences, as seen in adults with secure autonomous styles in the Adult Attachment Interview, requires both the capacity to tell a coherent, consistent story, for which the left hemisphere and language centres are crucial, and the ability to take in and process emotional experiences via the right.

Hannah Segal, a Kleinian psychoanalyst [24], described how the ability to use words in an imaginative, symbolic manner required an emotional development from the Paranoid-Schizoid position to the Depressive position as described by Klein [25]. Thus, the capacity to use words to communicate and describe our emotional experiences is predicated on the capacity to recognise the other as a separate human being and to mourn the losses this separation entails. It necessitates the recognition of ambivalence and one's own aggression, and the toleration of guilt and regret. If this is not possible, and Paranoid-Schizoid functioning predominates, then Segal suggests words become symbolic equations. Trauma inevitably disrupts the capacity to use words in this way, rendering them instead as something more concrete and confused with what they are meant to describe. As an example, a traumatised woman who had been assaulted with a knife could no longer use that word – knife – as when she did, she physically felt the knife once again on her neck.

Trauma and Repetition

Traumatised patients, especially when feeling threatened or anxious, may well move into more paranoid-schizoid functioning [25] with projective identification acting as a powerful defence against these overwhelming life and death anxieties. Projective identification is an unconscious phantasy in which the patient expels what are usually disturbing contents of the mind into the other. This has an impact on the other and in a therapeutic setting may lead to enactments. One particular form they may take is best understood through Freud's concept of the Repetition Compulsion.

> If a person does not remember, he is likely to act out, he produces it not as a memory but as an action; he repeats it, without knowing, of course, that he is repeating, and in the end we understand that this is his way of remembering [26].

For Karen, the repetition compulsion may be seen in the history of abusive relationships in her early adult life reflecting the abuse she experienced at the hands of her father. One may also wonder about the repetition of her own mother turning a blind eye to the abuse having some link to Karen's own daughter being abused by a family friend.

Traumatised patients may also unconsciously construct a theatre within the therapeutic encounter in which the traumatic scenario may be endlessly repeated with the different roles of victim, perpetrator, witness and rescuer offered to others who may be drawn in. Psychiatrists may, almost inevitably, find themselves repeatedly and unconsciously drawn into such re-enactments of the traumatic scenario in its various forms.

In the service of the repetition compulsion, the pull to take part in an enactment where one is invited to be the powerful, distancing authority figure (the perpetrator) must be balanced against the pull to be the helpful, unassuming and non-threatening figure (the rescuer), and means the psychiatrist has to struggle to maintain a stance that is not simply moving back and forth between these two extremes. And of course, the invitation to be the victim may leave the doctor feeling helpless, overwhelmed and flooded. It is not that these states can be avoided – they are an inevitable part of the countertransference experiences – more that it is vital that reflection on what is happening is possible. This requires the doctor to find a third position whereby perspective on what is occurring in the therapeutic dyad can be viewed. Often this is what makes supervision, team meetings and other reflective spaces within the institution of such vital importance.

Trauma inevitably leads to a loss of trust, and this is particularly true when the trauma has been caused by an attachment figure. Coupled with this, the push to engage in enactments of the repetition compulsion, with powerful countertransference experiences, necessitates the therapist being aware of the importance of boundaries, especially when there is also often a need to be attending to external realities outside the therapeutic frame. It is therefore especially important in this work that boundaries in relation to the start and end time of the session, extra-session contact such as emails or phone calls and so on are clearly negotiated at the beginning and held firmly but not rigidly. Giving adequate notice for breaks and absences is also vital in establishing trust and continuity. Often these details require thought and attention in supervision and team meetings to understand some of the enactments that may occur around boundary issues.

Trauma Treatment

The International Society for Traumatic Stress Studies have produced recommended guidelines for the treatment of C-PTSD based on best available evidence to date [27]. Clearly with a formal diagnosis still pending, the research evidence base is small. However, most experts recommend a phase-based approach to treatment to include:

1. Phase one: stabilisation (establishing safety, symptom management, improving emotion regulation and addressing current stressors)
2. Phase two: trauma processing (focussed processing of traumatic memories)
3. Phase three: reintegration (re-establishing social and cultural connection and addressing personal quality of life)

Engagement / Safety and Stabilisation

This initial phase has the following aims:

1. Attending to safety
2. Trauma psychoeducation
3. Specific interventions – emotion regulation skills, stress management, grounding and relaxation, social and relational skills building, cognitive restructuring
4. Building therapeutic alliance

If one considers the many reasons why engagement in a therapeutic alliance may be difficult – a narrow window of tolerance, loss of trust in the good object, powerful persecutory anxieties and excessive use of projective identification, disorganised attachment, a history of problematic encounters with services (often in a kind of repetition compulsion manner) – it is understandable that more active attempts to engage may be necessary.

In the initial consultation period one may need to more actively attend to the capacity to work within the Window of Tolerance and if necessary, introduce simple psychoeducation measures to help the patient manage their fight/flight/freeze responses. This may be outlining simple breathing techniques for fight/flight or suggesting grounding techniques if freeze (dissociation) is problematic.

The pressure on the therapist at this point in the work is often best understood in relation to Wilfred Bion's description of container/contained [28]. The active containment is a considerable task and will also require containment of the therapist to support their capacity to think under pressure through supervision and reflective practice.

What is important in this engagement phase is the continuity of the therapist and the strengthening of the therapeutic alliance. Other therapeutic work – both practical and external and more internal resourcing – is all in the service of preparing for phase two.

Remembrance and Mourning/Active Trauma Work

All trauma involves loss – some losses may be obvious and easily seen. There is also the loss of one's view of the world as essentially safe, loss of a belief in one's immortality, the loss involved in facing the extent of human destructiveness among others. It is in the process of mourning these various losses, allowing oneself to feel and acknowledge the pain, guilt, sadness, despair and anger, that the work of the second phase occurs.

While the evidence base remains limited, general guidelines for phase two interventions encourage the use of PTSD best evidence modalities in the second phase, while acknowledging that other modalities such as mentalisation-based therapy and psychodynamic therapy may also be useful.

Psychological interventions having the best evidence for the treatment of PTSD are the trauma-focussed therapies of trauma-focussed Cognitive Behavioural Therapy (tf-CBT) and eye movement desensitisation and reprocessing therapy (EMD-R). Both are individual treatments usually provided over a course of up to 12–16 sessions [29].

The cognitive behavioural approach to treatment has a number of intervention models that focus to a greater or lesser degree on the behavioural and cognitive components [30]. More behavioural emphasis suggests that the original traumatic event results in a learned association of the emotional trauma that has occurred with the stimuli of the event. Future encounters with these triggers activate the traumatic experience resulting in increased anxiety. Thus, exposure with response prevention is necessary, where exposure involves re-experiencing the images for long enough that the patient habituates to the fear response and avoidance is prevented [31]. Cognitive techniques address the dysfunctional beliefs that have arisen through the episode and work on cognitive restructuring. Ehlers and Clark describe a tf-CBT model that incorporates a number of specific interventions reflecting three targets of treatment [30]: elaborating and integrating the trauma memory; modifying problematic appraisals; and dropping dysfunctional behavioural and cognitive strategies.

EMD-R was developed by Shapiro [32] and it requires the patient to evoke an image of events causing them anxiety, while tracking the therapist's finger as it is moved rapidly and rhythmically from side to side (or other forms of bilateral stimulation such as sound or tapping). At the same time, they generate cognitive coping statements. EMD-R is said to facilitate rapid adaptive, associative information processing by integrating sensations, affects and self-attributes.

Van der Kolk describes research on using yoga as an adjunct to trauma therapies [15]. This seems to enhance patients' capacity to be in their bodies, in touch with their own bodily states and more in the present.

Psychodynamic therapy with C-PTSD attends closely to the transference, using Freud's notion of the repetition compulsion to understand the inevitable enactments that occur. However, whatever modality is being employed, this understanding of the therapeutic relationship can be vital.

If we consider Davies description of a therapeutic enactment [33]:

A collapsing of past and present; a co-constructed organization of the transference–counter-transference matrix that bears such striking similarity to an important moment in the past that patient and analyst together have the unique opportunity to exist in both places at the same time.

Davies' description highlights the way in which the transference and the enactments that occur within the transference field bring the trauma alive and into the room. In this way they are actively available for work in the present moment through the recreation of the emotional experience of the original trauma through the repetition compulsion. Implicit in the way of working on trauma through the transference is the notion that what is repeated is not only the trauma itself but the interaction between the external trauma and the internal pre-existing and reactive phantasies. This enables an exploration within the therapy of the unconscious factors that gave meaning to the trauma.

What this may also highlight is the impact that this work has on the therapist. Pines in describing her work with Holocaust survivors [34] speaks of unbearable countertransference experiences that the analyst may wish to turn away from. Working with traumatised individuals requires the therapist to bear witness to what has happened to them. This can be particularly important when their reality has been denied – often seen in child sexual abuse when the child discloses and is not believed or the other turns a blind eye. The unbearableness may be linked to acknowledging the extent of human aggression and destructiveness, even sadism, the misuse of power and authority or even the communal guilt we may be required to feel that such terrible things have happened in our society to vulnerable individuals.

In acknowledging aggression and destructiveness, it is also vital to recognise this in the room. There can be a pull to see the patient as only a victim but in denying their aggression and potential to be the aggressor, there is also an invalidation of their assertiveness and their capacity to move forwards in the world. This can be a profoundly difficult area of the work and requires considerable training, tact and sense of timing.

It is often a difficult judgement as to when the third phase is reached as inevitably much of the work of mourning will already have been part of the second phase. At some point, ending the therapy will start to become more of the focus of the work. However, even before then, each holiday break or absence will have already brought the issue of separation to the fore and again mourning is required.

Reintegration/Endings

The final phase of therapy in C-PTSD involves the work of ending the therapy and reintegrating with life externally. As with the other phases, the boundaries of when these tasks commence is fluid.

Mourning the loss of the safe, trustworthy relationship that has been established in therapy is clearly no easy task. It is likely to lead to a resurgence of grief linked to the original traumas and losses but is part of the important work in this final phase. To begin to develop a more realistic acknowledgement of one's own guilt may pave the way for reparative acts. For many this leads to altruistic activities, sometimes linked to the original traumas. For one patient who had experienced multiple traumas and losses in his life, working as a volunteer in a charitable organisation for abused children was clearly reparative and healing. This also links in with the notion of reintegration; finding a way to reconnect with the world after trauma that acknowledges what has happened and yet allows for life to continue.

Ways to reconnect or to connect with the world in a different way will vary for each individual. There may need to be a transition phase such as attending a self-help group or establishing some form of peer support within the community. A strengthening of the social support network is essential to this process.

Recovery is a word that may be used by patients and therapists alike in this context. However, the notion of recovery is linked to a fantasy that one can go back to how things were before the trauma occurred. Letting go of this fantasy allows for further mourning and the recognition that life is forever changed by what has occurred. This links with the description of Post-traumatic Growth [35], which describes how traumatic events may lead to a changed sense of self, of relationships and of philosophy in life.

References

1. Herman J. Part 1: Traumatic disorders. In *Trauma and Recovery*. London: Pandora. 1992; pp. 7–129.

2. Wolf E, Miller M, Kilpatrick D et al. ICD–11 complex PTSD in US national and veteran samples: prevalence and structural associations with PTSD. *Clin Psychol Sci* 2015; 3(2): 215–29.

3. Karatzias T, Cloitre M, Maercker A et al. PTSD and complex PTSD: ICD-11 updates on concept and measurement in the UK, USA, Germany and Lithuania. *Eur J Psychotraumatol* 2017; 8(sup 7): 1418102.

4. Cloitre M, Garvert DW, Weiss B, Carlson EB, Bryant RA. Distinguishing PTSD, complex PTSD, and borderline personality disorder: a latent class analysis. *Eur J Psychotraumatol* 2014; 5: 25097. doi: 10.3402/ejpt.v5.25097.

5. Porges SW. *The Polyvagal Theory: Neurophysiological Foundations of Emotions, Attachment, Communication and Self-Regulation*. New York: W. W. Norton & Company, 2011.

6. Palombo DJ, McKinnon MC, McIntosh AR et al. The neural correlates of memory for a life-threatening event: an fMRI study of passengers from flight AT236. *Clin Psychol Sci* 2016; 4(2): 312–19. doi:10.1177/2167702615589308.

7. Anderson SL, Tomada A, Vincow ES et al. Preliminary evidence for sensitive periods in the effect of childhood sexual abuse on regional brain development. *J Neuropsychiatry Clin Neurosci* 2008; 20(3): 292–301.

8. Metha MA, Golembo NI, Nosarti C et al. Amygdala, hippocampal and corpus callosum size following severe institutional deprivation: the English and Romanian adoptees study pilot. *J Child Psychol Psychiatry* 2009; 50(8): 943–51.

9. Felitti VJ. The relationship between adverse childhood experiences and adult health: turning gold into lead. *Perm J* 2002; 6: 44–7.

10. Van Niel C, Pachter LM, Wade R Jr, Felitti VJ, Stein MT. Adverse events in children: predictors of adult physical and mental conditions. *J Dev Behav Pediatr* 2014; 35(8): 549–51.

11. Gonzales A. The impact of childhood maltreatment on biological systems: implications for clinical interventions. *Paediatr Child Health* 2013; 18(8): 415–18.

12. Klein M. Notes on some schizoid mechanisms. *Int J Psychoanal* 1946; 27: 99–110

13. Garland C (ed.). *Understanding Trauma: A Psychoanalytic Approach*. London: Tavistock Book Series, 1998.

14. Siegel DJ. *The Developing Mind: How Relationships and the Brain Interact to Shape Who We Are*. New York: Guilford Press, 1999.

15. Van der Kolk B. *The Body Keeps the Score: Brain, Mind, and Body in the Healing of Trauma*. New York: Penguin, 2014.

16. Main M, Solomon J. Procedures for identifying infants as disorganized/disoriented during the Ainsworth strange situation. In MT Greenberg, D Cicchetti, EM Cummings, eds., *Attachment in the Preschool Years: Theory, Research and Intervention*. Chicago: University of Chicago Press. 1990; pp. 121–60.

17. Fonagy P. *Attachment Theory and Psychoanalysis*. New York: Other Press, 2001.

18. Lyons-Ruth K. The two person construction of defences: disorganized attachment strategies, unintegrated mental states and hostile / helpless relational processes. *Psychologist Psychoanalyst* 2001; 21(1): 40–5.

19. Schore A. *Affect Dysregulation and Disorders of the Self*. New York: W. W. Norton & Company, 2003.

20. Howell E. *Understanding and Treating Dissociative Identity Disorder: A Relational Approach*. New York: Routledge, 2011.

21. Liotti G. Attachment disorganization and the clinical dialogue: theme and variations. In J Solomon, C George, eds.,

Disorganisation of Attachment and Caregiving. New York: Guilford Press. 2011; pp. 383–413.

22. Allen JG. *Traumatic Relationships and Serious Mental Disorders.* New York: Wiley, 2001.

23. Music G. *Nurturing Natures: Attachment and children's emotional, sociocultural and brain development.* London: Routledge, 2017.

24. Segal H. Notes on symbol formation. *Int J Psychoanal* 1957; 38: 391–405.

25. Klein M. Mourning and its relation to manic-depressive states. *Int J Psychoanal,* 1940; 21: 125–53.

26. Freud S. Beyond the pleasure principle. In J Strachey, ed., *The Standard Edition of the Complete Psychological Works of Sigmund Freud, Volume XVIII (1920–1922): Beyond the Pleasure Principle, Group Psychology and Other Works.* London: Hogarth Press. 1955; pp. 1–64. (Original work published 1920)

27. Cloitre M, Courtois CA, Ford JD et al. The ISTSS Expert Consensus Treatment Guidelines for Complex PTSD in Adults. 2012.

28. Bion WR. *Learning from Experience.* London: Karnac Books, 1962.

29. Bisson J, Andrew M. Psychological treatment of post-traumatic stress disorder (PTSD). *Cochrane Database Syst Rev* 2005; 2: CD003388.

30. Ehlers A, Clark DM. A cognitive model of post traumatic stress disorder. *Behav Res Ther* 2000; 38: 319–45.

31. Foa EB, Rothbaum BO, Molnar C. Cognitive behavioural therapy of post-traumatic stress disorder. In: MJ Freidman, DS Charney, AY Deutch, eds., *Neurobiological and Clinical Consequences of Stress: From Normal Adaptation to PTSD.* Philadelphia: Raven Press. 1995; pp. 483–94.

32. Shapiro F. Efficacy of the eye movement desensitisation procedure in the treatment of traumatic memories. *J Trauma Stress* 1989;2: 199–223.

33. Davies JM. Dissociation, therapeutic enactment, and transference-countertransference processes; a discussion of papers on childhood sexual abuse by S. Grand and J. Sarnat. *Gender Psychoanal* 1997; 2: 241–57.

34. Pines D. Working with women survivors of the Holocaust. In *A Woman's Unconscious Use of her Body.* London: Virago. 1979; pp. 178–204.

35. Calhoun LG, Tedeschi RG (eds.). *The Handbook of Posttraumatic Growth: Research and Practice.* Manwah, NJ: Lawrence Erlbaum Associates Publishers, 2006.

Chapter

17

Psychological Approaches to Medically Unexplained Symptoms

Simon Heyland

Introduction

Sorrow which finds no vent in tears may make other organs weep

Sir Henry Maudsley, 1835–1918

Since antiquity it has been postulated that emotions can produce or interact with physical illnesses. That statement in its broadest sense describes the field of psychosomatic medicine, which concerns itself with the multitude of ways that psychological and physical factors intersect – for example depression and myocardial infarction. The subject of this chapter is somewhat narrower – the issue of medically unexplained symptoms (MUS), defined below. A detailed account of the broader field of psychosomatics is given by Schoenberg [1].

In a sense psychotherapy as a formal discipline began with MUS; it was during his clinical practice as a neurologist that Freud observed patients with neurological symptoms which could not be explained by structural lesions or other disease processes of the nervous system. His interest in what might be causing these symptoms led him towards an exploration of psychological factors, and culminated ultimately in the development of psychoanalysis. However, in the century since then psychotherapeutic interest has not reflected the key role that MUS played in the origins of the discipline. This chapter will give a brief overview of MUS as a clinical topic and then focus on contemporary psychotherapeutic theory and practice.

Terminology

The phrase 'medically unexplained symptoms' (MUS) refers to physical symptoms which after medical investigation cannot be accounted for by organic disease or physiological disturbance. This implies in a general (and unhelpful) sense that there is no medical explanation for the patient's symptoms, but perhaps it would be more accurate to think of the implication being that there is no *biomedical* explanation. MUS is not a diagnosis but an umbrella term, loosely defined, which gives shelter to processes such as conversion, somatisation and dissociation. It encompasses somatoform disorders and functional somatic syndromes, and is sometimes extended to include hypochondriasis (health anxiety) and body dysmorphic disorder. The latter two conditions, however, are characterised by *concern about* the body rather than *symptoms in* the body. A medical psychotherapist is most likely to encounter patients who have been diagnosed with one or more functional somatic syndromes.

Functional Somatic Syndromes

Functional somatic syndromes are collections of symptoms described primarily according to a specific bodily system, for example the gastrointestinal system. See Table 17.1 for a list of common functional syndromes. The degree to which these syndromes truly represent discrete conditions is questionable – they frequently co-occur but the organisation of secondary acute care into specialties promotes 'salami-slicing' of patients' problems. MUS then become defined more by which specialists the patient is assessed by than presence of separate illnesses [2]. For example, a patient with abdominal, chest and jaw pain may be assessed by a gastroenterologist, a cardiologist and then an ENT surgeon, and end up diagnosed with IBS, non-cardiac chest pain and temporomandibular joint dysfunction. This unfortunate iatrogenic process leaves the patient treated as if they have three separate diseases in three separate body parts. At this point the opportunity for intervening in a way which considers the patient as a whole is remote, unless efforts are made to integrate the various medical perspectives.

As Table 17.1 illustrates, such syndromes are likely to have been diagnosed by GPs or acute care specialists. Discrete diagnostic labels for different forms of MUS are rarely generated by psychiatrists, probably because these diagnoses relate to physical symptoms, are often unattractive to patients and do not usefully indicate to the psychiatrist what treatment(s) to recommend. The most obvious exception to this is non-epileptic attack disorder (NEAD), which may be first diagnosed by a neuropsychiatrist. In acute hospital settings the input of a liaison psychiatrist may be essential for management of complex MUS. This will include careful assessment and casenote review in order to rule out malingering and factitious disorder. MUS are not exaggerated or fabricated symptoms – neuroimaging studies have demonstrated that patients with MUS show heightened activation in cortical regions associated with pain when a painful physical stimulus is applied

Table 17.1 Functional somatic syndromes

Syndromes	Key symptoms	Medical specialty
Chronic pelvic pain	Pelvic pain	Gynaecology
Non-epileptic attack disorder (NEAD) also known as dissociative convulsions	Abnormal movements which resemble epilepsy	Neurology, neuropsychiatry
Irritable bowel syndrome (IBS)	Bloating, constipation, loose stools, abdominal pain	Gastroenterology
Non-cardiac chest pain	Chest pain, palpitations	Cardiology
Chronic fatigue syndrome (CFS) also known as myalgic encephalomyelitis (ME)	Fatigue	Rheumatology, infectious diseases, endocrinology
Hyperventilation	Shortness of breath	Respiratory
Temporomandibular joint (TMJ) dysfunction	Jaw pain, teeth grinding	Oral medicine, ENT, dentistry
Fibromyalgia	Pain and tender points	Rheumatology

[3, 4]. In other words, pain (the most common type of MUS) is a demonstrable physical experience.

In addition to the complexities outlined above, there is a long tradition of terminology in this area of medical practice being repeatedly abandoned and replaced. Terms such as hysteria would now be seen as pejorative, but despite multiple attempts it has not yet proved possible to find a diagnostic label that is both accurate and culturally acceptable. This search may perhaps mirror the deeper issue of how we struggle to conceptualise problems that defy the division between physical and mental symptoms created by Cartesian dualism. Currently the preferred term in the UK is MUS, but newer diagnostic entities such as 'bodily distress syndrome' and 'somatic symptom disorder' may supersede it for a time in the near future.

A further consideration for psychiatrists is co-morbidity with personality disorder, particularly more severe forms of MUS co-occurring with histrionic and borderline personality disorders [5]. It has been argued that modern diagnostic systems have split up the syndrome of hysteria arbitrarily into personality disorder, somatisation, conversion and dissociation subsyndromes [6, 7]. These are interesting and important debates in their own right. The main task of an assessing psychotherapist, however, is to ensure that all physical *symptoms* are discussed in the assessment, regardless of diagnoses made elsewhere in the health system.

MUS in Primary and Secondary Acute Care

Although not often referred to psychotherapy services, MUS are extremely common, with a wide spectrum of severity [8], and patients are found in all areas of the healthcare system. Around a fifth of new symptoms presented to GPs are MUS [9], although over half of these resolve spontaneously within 12 months [10]. In secondary care MUS tends to be more persistent and severe, accounting for 35–50 per cent of new outpatients at specialist medical clinics [11, 12] and 20–25 per cent of all frequent attenders at medical clinics [13, 14]. Furthermore, frequent attenders with MUS get investigated more than other frequent attenders at acute hospitals [15].

It is clear from the data that MUS is costly in healthcare terms. The magnitude of the cost is staggering – annual NHS costs of MUS in England have been estimated to be around 10 per cent of total NHS expenditure in adults of working age [16]. This is roughly comparable to the cost of caring for diabetes, yet service provision for MUS is scanty in the NHS [17], and MUS remains a neglected topic in medical education.

Perhaps unsurprisingly, MUS are experienced as difficult to manage by many doctors. Studies of GPs and acute hospital doctors report finding MUS stressful [18–20] and hard to help [21], and feeling psychologically deskilled in this area [22]. There is a common medical view that MUS patients pressurise doctors to perform tests, but research findings suggest the opposite – GPs frequently suggest physical investigations for MUS even when patients are not demanding them, possibly in attempts to end psychologically difficult consultations [23]. The advanced consultation skills needed are not taught to acute care specialists at any stage of medical education [24]. There is an overwhelming case for medical schools and royal colleges to revise their curricula to make teaching about MUS a priority, for the sake of both patients and doctors.

Predictably, perhaps more than with any other group of patients seen by psychotherapists, the input of medical colleagues in other parts of the healthcare system has a huge impact on the success or otherwise of psychotherapeutic treatment. The struggle to manage MUS medically should always be borne in mind sympathetically; support for colleagues is a central activity for specialist liaison psychotherapy services in GP practices and acute hospitals. Some of the key medical tasks which need to precede psychotherapy assessment are described later in this chapter.

The Origins of Psychotherapy for MUS

As we noted at the start of this chapter, psychotherapy in Western medicine began with Freud's clinical work with unexplained neurological symptoms. At the time in Europe there was interest in understanding and treating *hysteria*, a condition characterised by histrionic behaviour and MUS in women. The name derived from the Greek word for uterus and had been thought to be due to abnormal movements of that organ. Freud and others however attempted to understand the psychological causes of hysteria. Taking inspiration from the famous French neurologist Charcot, Freud initially tried using hypnosis but found its effects to be short-lived. He then began to explore new methods for treating this group of patients, which ultimately culminated in the discipline of psychoanalysis.

Freud theorised that hysterical patients' symptoms were the consequence of painful repressed memories linked to childhood abuse. He believed that unconscious sexual conflicts (e.g. between *guilt* and *excitement* aroused by incestuous behaviour) were unbearable and so were rendered unconscious and converted into physical symptoms which symbolised the conflict in a disguised form. The concept of conversion comes from this source. From this perspective, the mind and the body are seen as related but separate entities; problems arising in the mind are passed down, as it were, to a physical body which receives them and expresses them.

At around the same time, Pierre Janet developed a different psychological theory of physical symptoms. He postulated that rather than acquiring symbolic meaning, traumatic experiences can cause a kind of 'disintegration' of the mind, with one possible consequence being disturbances of bodily functions in ways which are dissociated from higher cortical functions. From this perspective, mental trauma can affect the body without being processed by thought.

These two views can be regarded as complementary or conflicting; symptoms are symbolic representations of psychic conflicts and/or symptoms are pre-symbolic sequelae of traumatic experiences. For most of the twentieth century the Freudian view came to dominate psychotherapeutic approaches to MUS; however, in recent decades there has been a resurgence of interest in the Janetian perspective. Freud and Janet are key figures whose ideas substantially inform psychotherapy in this field today, and some consequences of their differing theoretical views will be explored in a later section when we consider the defence and dissociation models of MUS in use currently. Prior to discussing psychotherapy, we turn our attention to considering how MUS arise.

Developmental Theory

Modern theories of MUS are informed by developments in psychoanalysis, neurology and neuroscience, as well as a convergence of psychodynamic and cognitive-behavioural concepts. There is less emphasis nowadays on the separateness of body and mind. One key theoretical advance has been the elucidation of the view of the self as a mind–body entity, as suggested by Winnicott [25] and subsequently many other psychotherapists. This is a very large topic indeed and beyond the scope of this chapter. A very brief summary statement with regards to MUS would be to say that thinking psychoanalytically about what constitutes selfhood paved the way for appreciating that humans are not born with fully integrated minds and bodies. From this perspective, we can view the integration of mind and body in adulthood as a *developmental achievement*, made up of a series of milestones en route to a healthy sense of self in adulthood.

This is a complex area conceptually, but worth grappling with in the effort to understand MUS. If not present from birth, how does our sense of self arise? And what is it made up of? It may help to imagine a small baby when considering these questions. That baby probably does not have a sense of self as we would understand it in adult terms, but certainly does have a level of self-awareness. For example, the baby can have non-conscious awareness of its own hunger or thirst, without a cognitive process occurring which says 'I am hungry/thirsty'. We might think of this as an embryonic mind–body connection, an example of the biological process of interoception – our conscious and non-conscious sense of the internal state of the body – which can in turn be viewed as the fundamental basis of selfhood [26].

Possessing interoception, the baby can then eventually begin to discern not just basic biological experiences (e.g. hunger) but also the sensorimotor phenomena that form the basis of its emotions. These phenomena, the physical components of emotions, do not need to be imagined by us – we all experience emotions as powerfully physical. But our hypothetical baby at this stage does not *recognise* those phenomena for what they are. He experiences them bodily but cannot think about them. It is only later that the baby gradually achieves the milestone of recognising certain sensorimotor experiences as 'belonging' to, being part of, certain emotions.

The ideas summarised above (and the empirical and observational studies of humans and other mammals that support them) inform the psychodynamic idea that affect development follows a sequence from body to emotion to thought, with all three elements present and intricately intertwined in healthy adult functioning. Research now supports this idea – the modern discipline of affective neuroscience has shown that emotions are embodied phenomena which form a foundational level of the mind both preceding *and* underpinning cognition [27].

As we noted above, the human starting point – the normal state of the infant – is theorised as one of undifferentiated sensations, in which emotions are primarily experienced as bodily, as sensorimotor phenomenon. In other words, it can be argued that humans begin emotional life in a state of somatisation. Affect development is from this perspective a process of *desomatisation* [28]. We have to learn how not to somatise our feelings. How do we achieve this milestone? Not on our own. From a psychodynamic perspective, in early life we require considerable nurture in order to recognise, differentiate and begin to verbalise our feelings. Protective caring relationships with adults are essential. *Knowing what we feel* (physically and mentally) and *being able to say what we feel* are not innate characteristics. Adverse childhood experiences such as misattunement, neglect or abuse can damage this process, leaving the person vulnerable to ongoing somatisation as a major aspect of a damaged sense of self [29]. Early childhood adversity is a known risk factor for adulthood MUS [30]. There are some important similarities here to developmental theories of affect dysregulation in personality disorders, and the theoretical overlap between MUS and personality disorder has been noted by some psychiatrists and psychotherapists [7, 31, Mace, personal communication, 2008].

In both types of disturbance it is often necessary psychotherapeutically to help the patient learn to recognise *what* they feel as well as express it verbally, before exploring *why* they feel what they feel. This kind of therapeutic effort (a demanding and painstaking one for both patient and therapist) may need to start by aiming to rebuild or repair the very foundations of the sense of self.

Defence and Dissociation Models

As noted earlier, Freudian theory and Janetian theory represent two distinct ways of understanding MUS. Psychotherapists in the present day are more likely to think in terms of defence and dissociation models rather than whose ideas they spring from. Both models can be useful for psychotherapeutic formulation. Loosely speaking, the defence and dissociation models map onto the concepts of conversion and somatisation respectively[1].

Defence Model

MUS can be seen as a consequence of the need to defend against unbearable emotional conflict as described by Freud with regard to incestuous abuse. From this perspective physical symptoms are a symbolic representation of that conflict, a coded expression of unconscious wishes and fears. This approach is still valuable; however, we would no longer exclusively view sexual conflicts as the prime cause – other types of emotional conflicts can also produce MUS.

Vignette 1

A 50-year-old man presented to his GP with slurring of speech, muscle weakness and unusual hand movements. Neurological conditions were excluded, and a stressful family life was described which led to a referral for psychotherapy. In therapy he revealed that his first wife had died of Huntingdon's disease. The patient had nursed her throughout her final illness, unflinching in the face of her escalating violence and then her physical disability. He had subsequently established a good relationship with a kindly woman, but when her children reached adolescence, he struggled to set boundaries for them. It seemed that angry feelings aroused in him, and the need for him to show these feelings, were in massive conflict with a fear of becoming his violent former wife. Both his extreme passivity and his identification with his dead wife were being expressed in physical form – slowed down and weak, unable to speak or act violently (exactly as she had been in the final phase of her illness). He was surprised to realise that his symptoms were exactly like his wife's.

The conflict here is about aggression, and possibly loss too. The symbolic nature of the neurological symptoms is clear, but not consciously perceived by the patient. The conversion of repressed affect into symbolically meaningful somatic symptoms is key to understanding this patient's presentation.

---

[1] For medical psychotherapists there is a risk of confusion with diagnostic terminology here. Symptoms regarded as dissociative within the International Classification of Diseases system (e.g. fugue, amnesia, convulsions) would usually be regarded psychodynamically as caused by the defence of conversion. This is distinct from the use of the term dissociation as a theoretical model of MUS.

Dissociation Model

Dissociation-based models of MUS, following Janet, suggest that the mind is overwhelmed by an experience to such an extent that thinking (a high-level brain function) is not possible. The mind has in a sense 'fallen apart' [32], that is, dissociated, and brain processing of the experience occurs only at a primitive level – emotional and/or physical. From this perspective, the patient is literally unable to make meaning of their experience and so their physical symptoms do not carry symbolic significance for them.

Vignette 2

A 29-year-old woman was seen for psychodynamic assessment. She had multiple problems due to a complex personality disorder and years of physical pains in her head, her joints and her abdomen. She would frequently present to A&E departments in agony, having gained no relief from analgesic medications and in fear of having some terrible stomach condition such as cancer. Her childhood was spent in terror of her violent father, whom her mother largely failed to protect her from. As she recounted her history the patient repeatedly wept and clutched at her abdomen and her head as waves of pain overwhelmed her. As the assessment proceeded the therapist was struck by the extreme levels of distress that this woman suffered and how undifferentiated her bodily experience seemed from her psychological anguish. No material emerged which suggested a symbolic link between mind and body.

Cognitive Model

It is worth mentioning cognitive models of MUS alongside psychodynamic approaches. Numerous cognitive processes have been implicated as predisposing, precipitating and/or perpetuating factors in MUS. Patients may have restrictive assumptions about health and body functions, learnt from family members. They may anxiously overinterpret physical symptoms as signs of physical disease, and engage in symptom catastrophising. Memory bias for illness-related stimuli makes it more likely that symptoms will cause concern and lead to care-seeking behaviours. Autonomic arousal in anxiety states often adds to the physical symptom burden for the patient. Harmful effects of inappropriate self-management can be severe – for example excessive rest leading to weakness and immobility due to loss of muscle mass and tone. Standard models of cognitive behavioural therapy can be used to try to address maladaptive behaviours and cognitions, and/or hyperarousal in a structured and strategic way.

Psychotherapy Technique

As with theory, this is a complex area and can be confusing for any inexperienced MUS therapist. The evidence base for psychodynamic psychotherapy suggests that a range of approaches are effective [33], but the main issue is often lack of familiarity and therefore confidence. There is no general agreement regarding modifications of psychodynamic technique despite the fact that working with MUS psychotherapeutically poses some unique challenges. In part this lack of agreement may be due to the breadth of the MUS concept, as noted earlier. A multitude of symptoms and diverse processes such as conversion and somatisation can all fall under the general rubric of MUS. While their definitions are not universally agreed by experts (as is often the case

Table 17.2 Therapeutic implications of distinguishing somatisation from conversion

Process	Developmental level	Primary difficulty	Therapist task	Therapeutic aim
Somatisation	More primitive e.g. pre-verbal	Unsymbolised emotions i.e. sensorimotor phenomena	Facilitate emotional expression	Integrate bodily and emotional aspects of experience
Conversion	Less primitive	Symbolised psychic conflicts	Interpret significance	Resolve conflicts

with psychoanalytic terms), if we consider conversion and somatisation as distinct processes then it follows that different approaches to psychotherapy may be needed for them (Table 17.2) [34].

Taylor has suggested that if somatisation is a more primitive process which involves unsymbolised emotions then it follows that the therapist needs to focus on emotional expression, to facilitate the somatising patient's capacity to link bodily and mental experiences [34]. There is some empirical evidence to support this assertion – one such approach (psychodynamic-interpersonal therapy, also known as the conversational model) is a NICE-recommended treatment for IBS [35]. If conversion is a higher-order process involving symbolised psychological conflicts, then interpretive techniques may be appropriate for this group of patients [34]. Hypothetically a 'classical' psychoanalytic technique could be used when working with the latter patient group.

Unfortunately, the above makes things sound neater and more binary than is usually the case! In practice, establishing whether a patient's symptoms are due to conversion or somatisation can be very difficult (assuming that one accepts the distinction at all). Some patients will have both. To complicate matters further, some patients who appear to have a somatisation 'picture' will have sought and found meaning for their symptoms. This is known as secondary symbolism. In addition, a simplistic equation (symbolic symptoms = interpretive technique) does not account for the capacity that a particular patient has for exploratory psychotherapy. In other words, a more relevant question may be 'What is tolerable by this patient?'. Patients with MUS can be highly sensitive to premature psychological explanations for their symptoms. Common fears are that the clinician is telling them that the symptoms are not real and all in their head, or that they are making it up, or are mad. Very careful attention and a degree of caution is needed by the therapist. Below is an example of the therapist progressing too quickly to psychological issues.

Vignette 3

A 42-year-old man attended the first session of a psychotherapy assessment. He had developed multiple MUS soon after a routine vaccination. The assessor took a very detailed history of the visit to the GP surgery for the injection, and of the patient's childhood. As a boy he had been severely sexually abused by his older brother, and the assessor was struck by the similarity in how the patient described the two physical experiences – the sexual abuse by his brother and the injection (by a male nurse). The assessor made an interpretation linking the two events, which the patient found revolting. He did not return for further assessment and sent a somewhat angry reply when asked by letter if he wanted to continue.

In this example the symbolic meaning of the vaccination needle seems clear, and we can formulate that the ensuing MUS symbolically represent physical damage done by the sexual abuse. However, none of this was acceptable to this patient, and as a result he disengaged from assessment. The assessor reflected in supervision on his mistake, which highlighted the need to establish a more empathic alliance with the patient before making such a challenging suggestion.

Assessment and Psychotherapy

Psychotherapy assessment of MUS is a complex task. Most commonly, patients will be referred for mental health problems with no mention of their physical symptoms. Under such circumstances, the assessor has little opportunity to anticipate what may arise in the assessment. On occasion, a patient will be referred specifically for therapy for MUS. Then it is essential to carry out a thorough casenote review, which may not be limited to the psychiatric notes. Critical issues to clarify at the referral stage are shown in Table 17.3.

Failure to consider the medical issues can significantly complicate or delay psychotherapy assessment. If incomplete medical issues are detected by the psychotherapy assessor then they should be addressed as a matter of priority. This will often require liaison with the referrer and/or further casenote review. If medical questions remain unanswered then the patient will understandably be reluctant to engage with any exploration of mind–body issues; for instance someone awaiting the results of a colonoscopy needs to be free of the fear of cancer before being able to engage psychologically in an exploration of their bowel symptoms. It is better to suspend or extend the assessment than proceed at this point. If ignored, medical issues can adversely affect the prognosis for therapy (see Vignette 4).

Table 17.3 Key pre-assessment issues

Medical issue	Problem for psychotherapy
Has the doctor completed relevant investigations? Or are more planned?	The patient will understandably still be concerned about the possibility of organic physical illness
Has the patient received all necessary opinions from specialists?	The patient will not have received adequate reassurance that their symptoms are not dangerous
Has the patient had an explanation that their symptoms are not due to a physical illness?	Unless offered an alternative explanation (by a doctor) then many patients will maintain the belief that their symptoms are due to physical illness
Is the patient aware that they are being referred for psychotherapy assessment?	The patient may feel deceived or regarded as 'making it up' or crazy

Vignette 4

A 35-year-old man with a history of non-epileptic seizures was referred to a psychotherapy service by a neuropsychiatrist. No other physical symptoms were mentioned in the referral and the assessor did not ask. He felt that he had made emotional contact with the patient and a formulation of the symptoms was possible, so psychodynamic psychotherapy was offered. Early progress was made in exploring the patient's history of being an invulnerable carer prior to the start of his symptoms. Then when his disavowed feelings of rage and hatred began to be talked about, the patient began to miss sessions. He had a regional pain syndrome (missed by the referrer and the assessor) which began to flare up. He did not consider this relevant to psychotherapy as it had not been discussed at the start, and therefore was reluctant to talk about it with his therapist. With each successive session the pain got worse, until the patient disengaged entirely from psychotherapy.

The therapeutic alliance in MUS depends on the patient believing that you take their physical experiences seriously. Many patients will be highly sensitive to any suggestion that you think their symptoms are psychological in origin. Signs of ambivalence about psychotherapy should be looked for, and proactively addressed. The assessor may need to emphasise that the purpose of assessment is to see if the patient can be helped to cope with their symptoms – not to remove them.

Assessment may need to be prolonged in order to gain a full picture of the patient's physical and mental experiences – some experts recommend an extended session of 2–3 hours to achieve this [36]. The priority initially is to engage the patient in an exhaustive exploration of their physical experiences. Careful listening to the patient's description of their physical life will usually give clues regarding key intra and interpersonal themes in their mental life. If a good-enough alliance has been formed then it may become possible to tentatively comment on how the physical symptoms embody the story of the patient's life more broadly.

Vignette 5

A 28-year-old woman with irritable bowel syndrome (IBS) described in psychotherapy assessment how she felt ruled by her bowels. Themes of self-disgust, humiliation and panic were prominent as she talked about the noise and mess she produced and her attempts to conceal her symptoms from other people. As the discussion broadened to her interpersonal world it was evident that the same themes were present in her relationships. The patient was not consciously aware of any similarities, but the assessment was going well overall and so the assessor very tentatively drew attention to the ways in which the patient's physical and interpersonal worlds resembled each other. The patient was able to agree that some of her words and feelings applied to both aspects of herself. A therapeutic conversation had begun, one in which seemingly unconnected experiences of herself could start to be drawn together and looked at in the presence of another.

As implied at the end of the vignette, an assessment can lead to fruitful exploration of psychological difficulties in relation to physical symptoms, but no assumptions should be made regarding the psychological meaning of physical symptoms at this early stage. It is far better to leave that step until much later, when the patient is ready to make that link themselves. In addition to the risk of proceeding too quickly and alienating the patient, there is the diametrically opposite risk of creating an iatrogenically compliant patient; some people with MUS will attune very quickly to the mindset of a psychotherapist and skim over their physical symptoms to produce 'psychological talk'. This can be appealing for psychotherapists, believing that they have a psychologically minded person in front of them who is ready to work and does not need their body attending to. This sort of countertransference should be taken as a warning sign of a pseudo-psychological alliance being formed, which is likely to result in a failed therapy.

Conclusion

From promising beginnings in late nineteenth century Vienna, psychotherapy for MUS failed to become a widely practised mainstream activity in the twentieth century. That an effective treatment is not made widely available to those who suffer from MUS is a great shame. In fact, MUS remains largely in the shadows across the whole of health care – in part due to the pervasive impact of Cartesian dualism, the philosophical mind–body split which still dominates Western medicine. As long as mind and body continue to be regarded as separate 'things' we will struggle to help this group of patients. Technical medical language for MUS remains contentious, unsettled and unsatisfactory. Personal language is hard to find; it seems to be difficult for any of us to fully appreciate the unity and disunity of our own mental/physical experiences, and to express those experiences to someone else.

However, if a positive alliance has been formed and physical/mental experiences thoroughly attended to, then psychotherapy can become a unique space in which these patients can begin to develop an emotional language and start to understand how their mind and body interact and affect each other. It cannot be emphasised enough that genuine progress depends on painstaking attention to potential links between mind and body, and proceeding at the patient's pace. This does not mean letting the patient fill the therapy hour with bodily complaints, but neither must the body be forgotten once conversation turns to emotional and relational issues. The ultimate aim of psychotherapy for MUS is to help the patient to better integrate their physical and mental experiences – to develop their sense of self, to become more whole, to acknowledge and even resolve conflicts which are not confined to their mind. It is arguably a bigger task than psychotherapy for mental disorders, and can be both daunting and hugely rewarding in equal measure.

References

1. Schoenberg P. *Psychosomatics: The Uses of Psychotherapy.* Basingstoke: Palgrave Macmillan, 2007.

2. Guthrie E. Medically unexplained symptoms in primary care. *Adv Psychiatr Treat* 2008; 14: 432–40.

3. Hobson AR, Furlong PL, Sarkar S et al. Neurophysiologic assessment of esophageal sensory processing in noncardiac chest pain. *Gastroenterology* 2006; 130: 80–8.

4. Perez DL, Barsky AJ, Vago DR, Baslet G, Silbersweig DA. A neural circuit framework for somatosensory amplification in somatoform disorder. *J Neuropsychiatry Clin Neurosci* 2015; 27(1): e40–50.

5. Bornstein R, Gold S. Comorbidity of personality disorders and somatization disorder: a meta-analytic review *J Psychopathol Behav Assess* 2008; 30: 154–61.

6. North C. The classification of hysteria and related disorders: historical and phenomenological considerations. *Behav Sci (Basel)* 2015; 5(4): 496–517.

7. Meares R. *A Dissociation Model of Borderline Personality Disorder*. New York: W. W. Norton & Company, 2012.

8. Edwards TM, Stern A, Clarke DD, Ivbijaro G, Kasney LM. The treatment of patients with medically unexplained symptoms in primary care. *Ment Health Fam Med* 2010; 7(4): 209–21.

9. Simon GE, Von Korff M. Somatization and psychiatric disorder in the NIMH Epidemiologic Catchment Area study. *Am J Psychiatry* 1991; 148: 1494–500.

10. Khan AA, Khan A, Harezlak J, Tu W, Kroenke K. Somatic symptoms in primary care: etiology and outcome. *Psychosomatics* 2003; 44: 471–8.

11. Nimnuan C. Rabe-Hesketh S, Wessely S et al. How many functional somatic syndromes? *J Psychosom Res* 2001; 51(4): 549–57.

12. Creed F, Henningsen P, Fink P. *Medically Unexplained Symptoms, Somatisation and Bodily Distress: Developing Better Clinical Services*. Cambridge: Cambridge University Press, 2011.

13. Fink P. The use of hospitalisations by persistent somatising patients. *Psychol Med* 1992; 22: 173–80.

14. Reid S, Wessely S, Crayford T, Hotopf M. Medically unexplained symptoms in frequent attenders of secondary health care: retrospective cohort study. *BMJ* 2001; 322(7289): 767–9.

15. Reid S, Wessely S, Crayford T, Hotopf M. Frequent attenders with medically unexplained symptoms: service use and costs in secondary care. *Br J Psychiatry* 2002; 180: 248–53.

16. Bermingham SL, Cohen A, Hague J, Parsonage M. The cost of somatisation among the working-age population in England for the year 2008–2009. *Ment Health Fam Med* 2010; 7: 71–84.

17. Chew-Graham C, Heyland S. *Joint Commissioning Panel for Mental Health guidance for commissioners of services for people with MUS*. London: JCP-MH, 2017.

18. Ringsberg KC, Krantz G. Coping with patients with medically unexplained symptoms: work-related strategies of physicians in primary health care. *J Health Psychol* 2006; 11(1): 107–16.

19. Dowrick C, Gask L, Hughes JG et al. General practitioners' views on reattribution for patients with medically unexplained symptoms: a questionnaire and qualitative study. *BMC Fam Pract* 2008; 19(9): 46.

20. Yon K, Nettleton S, Walters K, Lamahewa K, Buszewicz M. Junior doctors' experiences of managing patients with medically unexplained symptoms: a qualitative study. *BMJ Open* 2015; 5: e009593.

21. Carson AJ, Stone J, Warlow C, Sharpe M. Patients whom neurologists find difficult to help. *J Neurol Neurosurg Psychiatry* 2004; 75: 1776–8.

22. Salmon P, Peters S, Clifford R et al. Why do general practitioners decline training to improve management of medically unexplained symptoms? *J Gen Intern Med* 2007; 22(5): 565–71.

23. Ring A, Dowrick CF, Humphris GM, Davies J, Salmon P. The somatising effect of clinical consultation: what patients and doctors say and do not say when patients present medically unexplained physical symptoms. *Soc Sci Med* 2005; 61(7): 1505–15.

24. Salmon P, Humphris GM, Ring A, Davies JC, Dowrick CF. Primary care consultations about medically unexplained symptoms: patient presentations and doctor responses that influence the probability of somatic intervention. *Psychosom Med* 2007; 69: 571–7.

25. Winnicott DW. Mind and its relation to the psyche-soma. In DW Winnicott, *Through Paediatrics to Psycho-Analysis. The International Psycho-Analytical Library*, 100. London: The Hogarth Press and the Institute of Psycho-Analysis, 1975; pp. 243–54. (Original work published 1949)

26. Damasio A. *The Feeling of What Happens: Body, Emotion and the Making of Consciousness*. San Diego: Harcourt Press, 2000.

27. Panksepp J, Biven L. *The Archaeology of Mind: Neuroevolutionary Origins of Human Emotion.* New York: W. W. Norton & Company, 2012.

28. Krystal H. Desomatization and the consequences of infantile psychic trauma. *Psychoanal Inq* 1997; 17: 126–50.

29. Krueger DW *Integrating Body Self & Psychological Self: Creating a New Story in Psychoanalysis.* New York: Taylor & Francis, 2002.

30. Adshead G, Guthrie E. The role of attachment in medically unexplained symptoms and long-term illness *BJPsych Adv* 2015; 21: 167–74.

31. Bass C, Murphy M. Somatoform and personality disorders: syndromal comorbidity and overlapping developmental pathways. *Journal Psychosom Res* 1995; 39: 403–27.

32. Gottlieb RM. Psychosomatic medicine: the divergent legacies of Freud and Janet. *J Am Psychoanal Soc* 2003; 51: 857–81.

33. Abbass A, Kisely S, Kroenke K. Short-term psychodynamic psychotherapy for somatic disorders. Systematic review and meta-analysis of clinical trials. *Psychother Psychosom* 2009; 78: 265–74.

34. Taylor GJ. Somatization and conversion: distinct or overlapping constructs? *J Am Acad Psychoanal* 2003; 31: 487–508.

35. National Institute for Health and Clinical Excellence. *Irritable bowel syndrome in adults: diagnosis and management of IBS in primary care.* London: NICE, 2008.

36. Guthrie E, Creed F, Dawson D, Tomenson B. A controlled trial of psychological treatment for the irritable bowel syndrome. *Gastroenterology*, 1991; 100: 450–7.

Chapter 18

The Psychodynamics of Self-Harm

Rachel Gibbons

Introduction

He remembered the sensation, the satisfying slam of his body against the wall, the awful pleasure of hurling himself against something so immovable. . . .

. . . he soon grew to appreciate the secrecy, the control of the cuts. . . . When he did it, it was as if he was draining away the poison, the filth, the rage inside him.

Hanif Kureishi – A Little Life [1]

The act of harming oneself, causing pain, injury and scarring, can in a similar way to suicide appear deeply puzzling. It stands in stark contrast to more acceptable and seemingly understandable urges to protect and care for oneself. Yet violence directed against the self is common, and when an individual is in a disturbed and less rational state of mind, as described in the quote above from *A Little Life*, this action can seem reasonable. This chapter will explore the motivation, theoretical understanding and management of self-harm, with the aim of increasing understanding and improving outcomes.

Self-harm encompasses a broad spectrum of behaviour that is the 'final common pathway' [2] of many different emotional difficulties. Although it is most frequently associated with Emotionally Unstable Personality Disorder (EUPD) the majority of self-harm does not occur in those who have been diagnosed with mental illness of any sort, and as much as 80–90 per cent may not come to the attention of professionals [3]. For some patients, the behaviour is comparatively brief and discrete during a stressful time of life; for others, it is chronic and intertwined with the way they perceive themselves.

Definition

Self-harm is a term that serves as a catch all for a wide range of self-destructive behaviour that even in a single individual can mean different things at different times. Psychological and psychiatric professional bodies use different definitions of self-harm and apply a variety of exclusion criteria. For example, NICE defines self-harm as [4]:

> *an expression of personal distress, usually made in private, by an individual who hurts him or herself. The nature and meaning of self-harm, however, vary greatly from person to person. In addition, the reason a person harms him or herself may be different on each occasion, and should not be presumed to be the same.*

The terms 'intentional' and 'deliberate', which were previously used as part of the definition, are rarely used now. They are not favoured by patient groups or professional bodies, as they imply purposeful, conscious, rational determination. This implication can interfere with the therapeutic alliance, and contribute to the stigma suffered by those who have self-harmed.

Self-harm describes a spectrum of behaviour that includes apparently non-suicidal self-injury and serious attempts to die by suicide. Views differ as to whether these two groups indicate discrete aetiologies and should be considered separately [5]. Two of the UK's leading academics on self-harm, Professors Keith Hawton and Nav Kapur, believe that dividing the group creates a false dichotomy and can lead to a dangerous underestimation of suicidal risk [6]. What is agreed is that a degree of dissociation, or temporary disconnection from reality needed to cross the body boundary in order to harm oneself is the strongest indicator for future death by suicide [7]. The risk of dying by suicide in the 12 months following a presentation of self-harm is around 30 times higher than the expected rate in the general population [8, 9]. Almost half of those who end their life by suicide have previously harmed themselves [6, 10] and the more violent the method of self-harm, the greater the chance of completed suicide [11].

There are two international manuals used to classify mental disorders; the Diagnostic and Statistical Manual (DSM), and the International Classification of Diseases Manual (ICD). A diagnosis of non-suicidal self-injury is included in the 2013 version of the former under the section: Conditions for further study. This provides a somewhat limited framework for diagnosis; however, it does recognise the need to identify self-harm as separate and distinct from other mental disorders.

Types and Methods

Self-harm encompasses a wide range of activities that include:

- Those conducted in a less acutely dangerous manner that can be habitual such as cutting, burning, asphyxiation, poisoning, head banging, inserting, bloodletting and swallowing
- The severe and bizarre such as disembowelling
- The clearly life-threatening and suicidal, including overdosing, stabbing and hanging

The method used will have an unconscious meaning for the patient. Self-cutting and self-poisoning with medication are among the most common methods of self-harm in high-income countries such as the UK [12].

Epidemiology

Self-harm largely occurs in the community so accurate epidemiological figures are hard to establish, with the majority of incidents never coming to the attention of services. Research has shown that 10 to 20 percent of people worldwide report having self-harmed at least once and it is three times more common in women than men [12, 13]. There is evidence over recent years of a threefold increase in reported self-harm across the population of young people in general, and women in particular. The reason for this increase is not clear and could represent an increase in self-harm or an increase in reporting [8].

Motivation

It can be challenging to make sense of the motivation that underlies self-harm. It can be helpful to recognise the variety of unconscious intentions that include:

1. **A means of communicating:** the ability to put feelings into words, to 'mentalise' [14], is a developmentally complex task. A feeling usually starts as a somatic response to an internal or external event. This bodily experience can be very painful and frightening. To create a mental representation in a word for this embodied experience requires symbolic transformation. This experience can then be contained linguistically and expressed. So, for example if someone experiences their heart beating very fast, their chest as tight and a sense of constriction around their throat, they may recognise this as anxiety. When identified as anxiety this state can be identified as familiar and expressed both to the self and others. This process is cathartic and frees up the internal world. It also allows the experience to be stored in semantic memory where it remains located in time and place. If there is a difficulty in symbolising emotions (alexithymia) then mentalising is compromised and an individual is left easily overwhelmed by feeling states that are physically and psychologically painful. In these circumstances a way to communicate this pain to oneself and to others is through self-harm.

   Case example:

   Alan was admitted to a psychiatric ward after presenting to A&E. He had taken a life-threatening overdose after an argument with his partner. He was a young man who seemed very composed and articulate. He shocked the team by coming into his first ward round in a T-shirt exposing bright red cuts and old scars interweaving up both arms.

   In this case Alan both communicated and projected his distress into the ward team and in this way let them know how cut off he was from his own emotional experience. These scars also served to warn the staff, who were exposed to the full force of the disturbance through their countertransference, not to be deceived by his apparently self-possessed facade.

2. **To regulate overwhelming emotions and regain a sense of control:** individuals who have a reduced capacity to mentalise can displace and transform their emotional pain, when overwhelmed, into physical pain. This physical pain is then contained in a primitive way by the body and the mind is freed of fragmentation and mental control is regained.

3. **To contain traumatic memories:** self-harm often occurs when individuals become overwhelmed by deep undigested traumatic memories from childhood [15]. A recurrence of this 'original pain' [16] is triggered in the present by less substantial events. This existential pain can be substituted and temporarily released by the self-harm, the pain of which also resolves the numbness and dissociation that accompanies these disturbing memories. This allows a past traumatic event where individuals previously felt powerless and helpless to be re-enacted in the present with subjective control.

4. **A dysfunctional method of eliciting care:** self-harm can be triggered by fear of abandonment or neglect in relationships. The self-harming behaviour then performs the function of eliciting care from others. If successful in extracting care in this dysfunctional and perverse manner, damaging spirals can ensue where the violence and frequency of the self-harm increases.

5. **As an addictive behaviour:** recent literature suggests that repeated self-harm can be understood as an addictive behaviour that has features in common with other addictions such as gambling and substance misuse. The self-harm itself is thought to release endogenous opioids and stimulate the dopamine reward pathway. This explains why

self-harming can become compulsive, entrenched and prevent more functional methods of communication being developed [17]. Some authors also comment on the masochistic excitement resulting from the cruelty inflicted on the body and describe how there can be 'a frenzy of self-harm not unlike sexual satisfaction in some cases' [16].

6. **Protection both of the self and others:** Some people suggest that self-harm is a mechanism by which they reduce the intensity and impulse to act on suicidal thoughts [18, 19]. Various analysts perceive self-harm as a manifestation of the defence 'anger turned against the self' and, when managed in this way, prevents an attack on others [16, 20].

7. **Defence against intimacy:** those who have been traumatised and/or abused can have a terror of intimacy. Evidence of self-harm can serve to keeps others at bay.

8. **Maintaining coherence:** Anna Motz, a consultant clinical and forensic psychologist who has worked with women who are perpetrators of violence, argues that self-harm reflects a *split and divided self* [21]. When the ego becomes overwhelmed by 'toxic' thoughts and starts to fragment, a way of retaining coherence is for it to split into 'good' and 'bad'. The 'bad' is projected into the body where it can become *other to the self*, attacked and punished for its aggressive and violent feelings. Motz emphasises that nursing the wounds often plays an important role in the ritual of self-harm. She argues that as well as protecting the ego from disintegration self-harm allows for *a reunion where the attacking self then becomes the caring, nursing self.*

Theoretical Understanding

Emotional dysregulation

Neuroscience

Early trauma has been found to affect the development of the brain by modifying the neural structures that underly emotional regulation. The result is an emotional system which, when triggered, responds to stimuli with greater speed and strength than in those who have not been traumatised [22–24]. This leads to emotionally overload and a dynamic change in the brain functioning where the more mature left hemisphere of the brain shuts down leaving the more primitive right side of the brain to respond.

The left and right sides of the brain develop at different speeds and have different functions. Different rates of development of the hemispheres mean that memories are stored differently at different times of life. The right side, active from birth, functions in a less developmentally mature way. It is responsible for emotional and sensory memory. The left side, responsible for language and temporal memory, develops around the age of three and it is only after this time that memories can be stored linguistically and sequenced in time (see Chapter 16). Before the age of three, memories tend to be housed in body memory in a sensory form, without mental representation. When overwhelmed in the here and now, the left side of the brain can turn off and the right side be turned on. The capacity for language, mediated by the left hemisphere, needed for emotional regulation, is blocked. Individuals are then left to relive childhood memories in the present as a bodily experience mediated by the right hemisphere [15]. This increases the experience of emotional overload and emotional dysregulation. Self-harm is the method on hand to acutely manage this psychological pain.

Attachment, Attunement and Symbolisation

The quality of early childhood attachment is vital for the later capacity to mentalise and regulate emotions. Language development depends on having an attuned carer who can recognise and put into words the child's emotional experience. These words can then be learned by the child and used to store this experience in memory. Difficulties in this primary relationship can lead to an incapacity to put feelings into words. This inability to mentalise is related to insecure attachment. This is illustrated by research that shows that over 70–75 per cent of those who self-harm has an insecure attachment style compared to 15–20 per cent in the group that do not. [2, 25, 26].

Attachment System Activation

For those with insecure attachment objectively minor events in the present can elicit strong emotionally dysregulated responses. These 'trigger' events elicit unconscious memories of past trauma and therefore may be perceived as overly abandoning or rejecting. A delayed reply to an email or text can be the spark that lights an emotional fire and causes activation of the attachment system. When stimulated, the attachment system generates a powerful drive to seek care and closeness to the primary attachment figure '. . . *at highest intensity, when distressed and anxious, nothing but a prolonged cuddle will do*' [27]. This works well in securely attached individuals but less well with insecure attachment where proximity can be sought to the source of the maltreatment. In later life clinging, controlling (perceived manipulative) or panicked behaviour can elicit re-enactments of the original trauma and a vicious cycle ensues.

Case example:

> *Ellen had been seriously neglected as a child, and was removed from her mother's care and placed with foster parents. She had a history of self-harm and had recently been referred to her local mental health team for depression. She met for the first time with her new keyworker, Claudia, who had little experience of self-harming behaviour. She found Ellen appealing and during this meeting Ellen felt especially understood and cared for. Ellen found it very difficult to leave the appointment and go home to an empty flat. She felt anxious and abandoned. She tried phoning Claudia to seek reassurance. When Claudia did not answer her calls, Ellen's emotions overwhelmed her. She cut her arms very deeply and sought care for these wounds at the A&E department. Claudia had thought that she had a good session with Ellen and was surprised to get a call from the mental health team in A&E. She felt confused, let down and angry. She did not want to talk to Ellen next time she called and gradually withdrew from contact. Ellen felt rejected and abandoned, her self-harm increased and she had a brief hospital admission.*

In this case Ellen's attachment system was activated by the intimacy with Claudia, leading to emotional dysregulation and self-harm. Claudia's difficulty in fully formulating the case left her ill-equipped to manage her own feelings of rejection and disappointment and she withdrew.

Anthony Bateman and Peter Fonagy, leading academics in the treatment of emotional instability and borderline personality disorder (BPD) and pioneers of the development of Mentalization-Based Treatment (MBT), describe how a lack of attunement and inaccurate mirroring in the early caregiving relationship leads to an '*internalisation of representations of the parents' state rather than of a usable version of the child's own experience*'. They call this internalisation '*the alien self*'. This 'alien self' is an incongruent aspect of the child's identity that has been projected into them by their caregiver. This is experienced as part of the self but does not seem to belong, and disrupts the sense of coherence '*which can only be restored by constant and intense projection of this alien self onto another*'. This keeps a fragile equilibrium. When the recipient of the projection is absent, temporarily or permanently, the equilibrium breaks down and can be restored only by projection of this alien self onto the body. This act is carried out in the mode of '*psychic equivalents*', which means that symbolic capacity has broken down and the body is experienced as '*isomorphic with the alien parts of the self*'. The hatred felt towards the abandoning attachment figure can then be externalised and violence enacted. They comment that the sense of despair is not from the loss of the object, who normally would not have been a genuine attachment figure in the first place, but the anticipated loss of self-cohesion [22].

Case example:

George, a psychiatric nurse, was accompanying Amy on a home visit. They were on the bus. Amy was calm and chatty, and George was wondering why she had been admitted to hospital. She was smiling and looked very relaxed. She looked down at her phone having received a text. Within a second something profoundly changed. She opened her mouth in a silent scream, grabbed the back of the seat in front of her and shook herself backwards and forwards, she then started scratching the back of her wrists with her nail and gradually calmed down. This happened so quickly that George was shocked and frightened. He felt he could not manage with Amy by himself and they returned to the hospital. He found out later that the text was from Amy's mother telling her that she could not visit that afternoon.

In this case Amy received a trigger that she perceived as abandoning and rejecting. Her equilibrium was lost, her alien self returned and she was emotionally overwhelmed with aggressive feelings. She then functioned in the mode of 'psychic equivalence' and was only able to re-establish some stability by projecting onto her body and becoming the recipient of her own aggression. The distress and shock projected into George felt overwhelming and he lost confidence in his capacity to manage Amy on the home visit.

Psychoanalytic Theory

Persecutory Superego, Underdeveloped Ego and Primitive Defences

Contemporary psychoanalytic writers such as David Bell, John Malzberger, Rob Hale and Don Campbell emphasise the role of the persecutory superego, the weak ego, and primitive defences in self-harm. They propose that childhood difficulties result in an inability to successfully individuate and become differentiated as separate from the caregiver. This leads to an internal world that remains underdeveloped and barren. The individual then lacks the healthy and helpful internal objects that would be installed following a successful separation process. A primitive 'ego destructive' superego remains, dominating a vulnerable and frail ego. This superego inflates '*quite ordinary faults and failures, turning them into crimes that must be punished*' [16]. There is '*a psychic claustrophobia*' and terror of disintegration when left alone. Due to the lack of psychic development, the only way to cope with this torment is to use primitive, immature defences including projection, splitting and denial. The weak ego is divided, and the part identified with the hated abandoning object gets located in the body, and then attacked. The violence serves two functions, to punish the abandoning, and therefore, hated other, and to provide a self-punishment for the hatred and cruelty. A vicious circle then can occur. The more attacks, the more guilt for the attacks, the more punishment needed and so on.

The Role of the Skin

Esther Bick, a psychoanalyst who promoted the importance of observing babies with their mothers as part of psychotherapeutic training, wrote a seminal and very short paper on the importance of the skin as the physical and psychic container of the self [28]. She described how problems with separation and individuation can be expressed by and on the skin. Bell emphasises that the skin itself may be concretely felt to be the prison where the ego is trapped and tortured relentlessly by the persecutory superego [16].

Case example:

Jessica worked as a successful lawyer. At the weekend when not working she habitually harmed herself. She secretly 'blood let' via small tubes she inserted into her arms, she then hid the blood. She was admitted to hospital after a collapse and was found to have a low haemoglobin. During this hospital admission, she admitted to this self-harm and was transferred to a psychiatric ward. She said that when working she felt fine, was capable and on top of things but at the weekend, she felt abandoned and left alone, terrified. She heard a voice that she knew was located somewhere within her, yet she felt as 'other', telling her she was 'bad through and through' and she 'deserved to die'. She felt hopeless. There was no escape and the self-harm was the only relief and release from this terrible experience.

In this case, Jessica's apparently bizarre behaviour can be understood with reference to the described theory. She felt imprisoned by her skin and tortured by her sadistic primitive superego. The only way to escape was by identifying herself with her blood, which she then furtively helped to flee.

Enactment of the Internal World

The internal torturous experience can be projected into the outside world and enacted in the external environment. This is unfortunately still an all too common experience in psychiatric settings. Relationships between those that self-harm and the providers of their care can break down and instead of improvement there can be a decline in the mental health of all involved. This is much more likely to happen where staff lack a both a psychological model for their work and reflective spaces to process and think about their experiences.

Case example:

Chloe was admitted to an adolescent mental health unit because her parents were struggling to cope with their anxiety, after a shocking and unexpected overdose where she nearly died. They felt they could not trust her to stay alive. In the adolescent unit Chloe would say she was fine, and then when she was given some independence would overdose. The restrictions increased and the self-harming behaviour also increased. Chloe started putting shoelaces and belts around her neck repeatedly. The team that had been caring for her seemed exhausted and had lost all confidence in her capacity to improve. They became focussed only on trying to prevent Chloe from self-harming, neglecting other patients. They became very frightened of Chloe. What would happen to them if she died? They were sure they would be held responsible and punished. Chloe's level of observation and restriction increased, and she was eventually transferred to a secure adult inpatient facility.

In this case there was an escalation and a re-enactment of Chloe's disturbed inner state. A helpful quote from Bell follows [16]:

Such situations can result in a particularly deadly scenario. The patient recruits more and more people to become responsible for his own life. But the more individuals allow themselves to feel so responsible, the more the patient dissociates himself from the wish to live, now located in others. Further, as the patient becomes increasingly taken over by the cruel inner organisation, the sanity and concern now located in external others becomes the object of scorn and derision.

Management

The management of self-harm varies depending on the underlying aetiology. Those who receive a diagnosis of EUPD often get referred to personality disorder services where certain models or psychological treatment, such as MBT and Dialectical Behavioural Therapy (DBT) are offered. Some basic principles of management follow.

Management Principles

- Have time and space to think about what the self-harming means for this patient at this particular time. Accept the self-harm and help the patient to think through the consequences of their actions
- Recognise and validate the patient's pain
- Maintain separateness and agree to disagree
- Avoid confrontation and consider oneself as a travelling companion who is trying to view the world from a similar vantage point
- Work within a group or a team, ensuring decisions are not taken in isolation
- Ensure there are regular structured reflective spaces including supervision and case discussion groups
- Develop alternative means of recognising and managing distress
- Develop a safety plan with the patient (see Figure 18.1).

Challenges in the Countertransference

Self-harm is an acting out behaviour and powerfully projects distress into others resulting in strong countertransference experiences. These projections provide important and meaningful information, but also, through the countertransference responses elicited, which can be a dangerous barrier to effective treatment. The first step is to recognise the countertransference effects, think about the meaning and resist immediate action.

Countertransference responses include:

1. **The promise of omnipotent mothering**: the projection of early infantile distress by those who self-harm communicates powerfully and primitively and can reciprocally activate the attachment system of the professional. '...*The diagnosis "borderline" describes an enmeshed clinical dyad in which at least the inner experience of both participants can begin to meet the criteria for the disorder*' [29]. This can elicit an idealised maternal response in the caregiver, increasing rather than decreasing risk, and obstructing a helpful and reality based therapeutic intervention. '*Borderline patients take the promise of mothering as seriously as they do the promise of a magic pill*' [30].

MY SAFETY PLAN

My name:	Date:

Step 1: Warning signs that things are difficult for me

2. Things I can do to take my mind off my difficulties - what have I done in the past that will help me now? (Coping strategies – e.g. relaxation)

Step 3: Things I can do to keep myself safe and reduce my distress (e.g. environment)

Step 4: Friends and family I can call

Name:	Number:	Do they know I might call?	Will they have a copy of this plan?

Step 5: What can they do to help?

Step 6: Professionals or Agencies I can call in a crisis?

Name:	Number:

Other helpful numbers

Name	Number
Samaritans (24hr)	116123

Figure 18.1 Example of a safety plan.

Case example:

In the evening when the personality disorder service was closed, Marie felt lonely and anxious. She phoned the mental health trust and asked to be put through to one of the wards. Mark, a new care assistant, picked up the phone. 'I wonder if you can help me?' she asked Mark in a childlike manner. Mark wanting to be helpful and activated by her childlike tone became drawn into the discussion. He offered Marie advice and suggestions of support that were not within the boundaries of his normal role. He felt pleased, Marie initially seemed grateful and helped by his suggestions. Marie felt less lonely and close to Mark. In time, Mark realised that he needed to get on with his job; as soon as he indicated to Marie that he needed to finish the call she became distressed, and her fear of abandonment was activated. She tried to hold onto Mark and became agitated and aggressive. The last words Mark heard Marie say were 'I am going to kill myself and it will be your fault!' This left Mark shaken and frightened. To alleviate his anxiety about Marie and the role he had played in any self-harm that might ensue he called the emergency services. It was only the next day that he was told by other team members that Marie had done this many times before and ambulances attended her home at least three times a week.

2. **Helplessness, confusion and uncertainty:** self-harm communicates undigested distress. There is usually no clear indication of the cause, or the way it can be alleviated. Those that work in health services often want to feel effective and useful in lessening distress. This can lead to a need to 'do' something, in large part, to reduce their own feelings of helplessness. This can interfere with a reality-based therapeutic response. It can also lead to an inappropriate certainty about diagnosis and treatment.

3. **Repulsion:** self-harm can communicate the patients experience of an undigested abusive boundary violation through projection, for example in genital mutilation, very deep cutting or disembowelling. This frequently elicits aversive responses in others.

4. **Hatred:** this is a very important countertransference response. Self-harm can be a violent and aggressive act, driven by hatred. To deny this can lead to reciprocal disavowed violence.

When Dr Freeland was the psychiatric doctor on call for the hospital, he was frequently called to the A&E department to assess patients. The doctor or nurse who called him would often start off the referral with words laced with contempt and hatred: 'Is that the on-call psychiatrist? We have PD for you down here. One of yours'. Frequently the patients had been ignored while they were waiting. They had rarely been treated with parity to other patients who were seen to be more deserving of care.

5. **Frustration and anger:** self-harm can be a communication of a complaint about the care provided. Taking this personally is a mistake because it is not directed primarily at the care provided in the here and now, but a historical grievance maybe rooted in profound mistrust of the primary attachment figure [20].

6. **Pain and fear:** Powerful identification can occur with the projection of early separation anxiety, loss, and the fear of disintegration leaving care professionals in pain and distress.

Clinical Role and Realistic Responsibility

Responsibility is explained as the obligation to perform duties, tasks or roles using sound professional judgement and being answerable for the decisions made in doing this [31].

The responsibility of a clinician is to work within their role, and to give advice and make decisions using their expertise within their clinical field. Working with those who self-harm challenges clinical and personal boundaries and the concept of responsibility is easily distorted. The reproduction of the early caregiving situation can trigger inappropriate and omnipotent responses. Responsibility cannot be taken for someone else's thoughts or behaviour. It is important to differentiate whether someone has or has not got capacity, for example if the self-harm is in the context of psychosis capacity may be limited. If someone has capacity and is going to harm themselves, this is unlikely to be controlled and prevented by others in a coercive manner. It is important to work together with the patient and to see them as an equal and responsible adult in the development of their management plan. This is where safety plans are very useful (see Figure 18.1). The clinician's role is to provide containment enabling the patient to think through the symptoms and signs of their distress, to take responsibility for their own well-being and welfare, and to plan for the future.

Endings and Transitions

Endings and transitions can bring up early trauma and fears of abandonment. The risk can be particularly high when patients are struggling with dependent personality traits or a dependent personality disorder, an over-represented but underidentified group within health services. These patients need to project onto others for self-coherence and are terrified of being left on their own. There is an unconscious fear and threat that lies under their relationships with other – 'that if you leave me, I will not survive and I will therefore have to kill myself'. This vulnerability can be hidden and only emerge overtly at discharge.

> The mental health team realised that Gloria had been a patient of the mental health services where she had been transferred from one team to another for the last 20 years. There had not been any apparent improvement in her functioning and in fact some deterioration seemed to have occurred. Whereas she had paid work prior to her initial contact with services she had not worked since. They discussed discharge from services with Gloria who was normally compliant. She became very angry and told the team that 'they were nothing but rubbish and had given her nothing, that they had made her worse rather than better'. After discharge she took a life-threatening overdose and was admitted to the Intensive Care Unit.

In this case Gloria had a realistic complaint to the team. They had avoided the challenging developmental work of engaging with her immature dependence on services because they were frightened of eliciting Gloria's anger when she was confronted with reality. The more challenging aspects of the team's countertransference towards Gloria, that of hatred and fear, had not been acknowledged. They had found it much more ego-syntonic to discuss their positive feelings. They finally acted out their countertransference feelings by enacting the total abandonment Gloria feared.

Conclusion

Patients who have self-harmed need to be treated with compassion. This is not always easy because of the intense countertransference responses that self-harm elicits. Those who have recently self-harmed are in a vulnerable emotional state and are particularly sensitive to accepting or rejecting responses from professionals. To meet those who self-harm with an open heart requires: an understanding of the nature of the act, thoughtful and containing team structures, a therapeutic model that includes reflective spaces, and thoughtful compassionate leadership. When these conditions are met clinicians have greater confidence and less fear and uncertainty when approaching those who express their distress in this way. This leads invariably to a more reparative and therapeutic outcome.

References

1. Buchanan B. *Hanif Kureishi*. Basingstoke: Palgrave Macmillan, 2007.

2. Adshead G. Written on the body: deliberate self-harm as communication. *Psychoanal Psychother* 2010; 24(2): 69–80.

3. Madge N, Hewitt A, Hawton K et al. Deliberate self-harm within an international community sample of young people: comparative findings from the Child & Adolescent Self-Harm in Europe (CASE) study. *J Child Psychol Psychiatry* 2008; 49: 667–77. doi: 10.1111/j.1469-7610.2008.01879.x.

4. National Institute for Clinical Excellence. Self-harm: short-term treatment and management. 2004. www.nice.org.uk/guidance/cg16/resources/selfharm-shortterm-treatment-and-management-189900253 [Accessed 30/11/2020]

5. Muehlenkamp JJ. Self-injurious behavior as a separate clinical syndrome. *Am J Orthopsychiatry* 2005; 75(2): 324–33.

6. Kapur N, Cooper J, O'Connor RC, Hawton K. Non-suicidal self-injury v. attempted suicide: new diagnosis or false dichotomy? *Br J Psychiatry* 2013; 202(5): 326–8.

7. Hawton K, Zahl D, Weatherall R. Suicide following deliberate self-harm: long-term follow-up of patients who presented to a general hospital. *Br J Psychiatry* 2003; 182(6): 537–42.

8. McManus S, Gunnell D, Cooper C, et al. Prevalence of non-suicidal self-harm and service contact in England, 2000–14: repeated cross-sectional surveys of the general population. *Lancet Psychiatry* 2019; 6(7): 573–81. doi:10.1016/S2215-0366(19)30188-9.

9. Chan MK, Bhatti H, Meader N et al. Predicting suicide following self-harm: systematic review of risk factors and risk scales. *Br J Psychiatry* 2016; 209(4): 277–83.

10. Geulayov G, Kapur N, Turnbull P et al. Epidemiology and trends in non-fatal self-harm in three centres in England, 2000–2012: findings from the Multicentre Study of Self-harm in England. *BMJ Open* 2016; 6(4): e010538.

11. Beckman K, Mittendorfer-Rutz E, Waern M et al. Method of self-harm in adolescents and young adults and risk of subsequent suicide. *J Child Psychol Psychiatry* 2018; 59(9): 948–56.

12. Bergen H, Hawton K, Waters K, et al. Premature death after self-harm: a multicentre cohort study. *Lancet* 2012; 380(9853): 1568–74.

13. Muehlenkamp JJ, Claes L, Havertape L, Plener PL. International prevalence of adolescent non-suicidal self-injury and deliberate self-harm. *Child Adolesc Psychiatry Ment Health* 2012; 6(1): 10.

14. Fonagy P, Target M, Gergely G, Allen JG, Bateman AW. The developmental roots of borderline personality disorder in early attachment relationships: a theory and some evidence. *Psychoanal Inq* 2003; 23(3): 412–59.

15. Van der Kolk B. *The Body Keeps the Score: Mind, Brain and Body in the Transformation of Trauma*. London: Penguin UK, 2014.

16. Bell D. Who is killing what or whom? some notes on the internal phenomenology of suicide. *Psychoanal Psychother* 2001; 15(1): 21–37.

17. Blasco-Fontecilla H, Fernández-Fernández R, Colino L et al. The addictive model of self-harming (non-suicidal and suicidal) behavior. *Front Psychiatry* 2016; 7: 8.

18. Nock MK. Why do people hurt themselves? New insights into the nature and functions of self-injury. *Curr Dir Psychol Sci* 2009; 18(2): 78–83.

19. Weinberg A, Klonsky ED. Measurement of emotion dysregulation in adolescents. *Psychol Assess* 2009; 21(4): 616–21.

20. Scanlon C, Adlam J. Why do you treat me this way? Reciprocal violence and the mythology of 'deliberate self harm'. In A Motz, ed., *Managing Self-Harm: Psychological Perspectives*. Hove: Routledge. 2009; pp. 55–6.

21. Motz A. Self-harm as a sign of hope. *Psychoanal Psychother* 2010; 24(2): 81–92.

22. Bateman A, Fonagy P. *Psychotherapy for Borderline Personality Disorder: Mentalization-Based Treatment.* Oxford: Oxford University Press, 2004.

23. Zanarini MC. Childhood experiences associated with the development of borderline personality disorder. *Psychiatr Clin North Am* 2000; 23(1): 89–101.

24. Paivio SC, Laurent C. Empathy and emotion regulation: reprocessing memories of childhood abuse. *J Clin Psychol* 2001; 57(2): 213–26.

25. Cicchetti D, Beeghly M. Symbolic development in maltreated youngsters: an organizational perspective. *New Dir Child Adolesc Dev* 1987; 1987(36): 47–68.

26. Shuk-Ching C. A case control study of attachment style in deliberate self harm patients: A systemic perspective (Doctoral dissertation, University of Hong Kong).

27. Bowlby J. Disruption of affectional bonds and its effects on behaviour.

Canada's Mental Health Supplement 1969; 59: 12.

28. Bick M. The experience of skin in early object relations. In M Harris Williams, ed., *Collected Papers of Martha Harris and Esther Bick.* Strathtay: Clunie Press, 1968.

29. Vaillant GE. The beginning of wisdom is never calling a patient a borderline; or, the clinical management of immature defenses in the treatment of individuals with personality disorders. *J Psychother Pract Res* 1992; 1(2): 117–34.

30. Groves JE. Taking care of the hateful patient. In G Adshead, C Jacob, eds., *Personality Disorder the Definitive Reader.* London and Philadelphia; Jessica Kingsley Publishers. 2009; pp. 52–63.

31. Nursing and Midwifery Board of Ireland. Considerations in determining scope: responsibility, accountability & autonomy. www.nmbi.ie/Standards-Guidance/Scope-of-Practice/Considerations-in-Determining-Scope/Responsibility,-Accountability-Autonomy [Accessed 13/11/2020]

Psychodynamic Aspects of Suicide and Homicide

Rachel Gibbons and Gwen Adshead

This chapter will be divided into two parts. The first on suicide will look at the current epidemiology of suicide, the psychodynamic understanding of the pathway to a death of this nature and the effect the suicide of a patient can have on the clinician and teams working with them. The second part will describe the psychodynamic understanding of homicide. The suicide section is written by Dr Rachel Gibbons and the homicide section by Dr Gwen Adshead.

Suicide

Introduction

there is only one serious philosophical question, that is suicide
Camus [1, p. 5]

Suicide stands as the single most powerful action any individual can make in terms of its finality and the devastation it leaves for others. Yet it is a constant and unchanging aspect of human behaviour, across history and cultures. This chapter will explore this paradox and both the unthinkable and the familiar in the suicidal act.

One of the ways we can seek to make sense of suicide is to see it as the result of mental illness or madness; this does not however fit with the data. The National Confidential Inquiry into Homicide and Suicide [2] has repeatedly found 70–80 per cent of deaths by suicide occur in those without a diagnosis of mental illness and with no recent contact with mental health services. This challenges assumptions and necessitates a closer examination of the nature of suicide. Nevertheless, working with the suicidal and experiencing deaths of our patients through suicide is a central issue in psychiatry and anxiety about it permeates all areas of mental health work.

Suicide frequently follows significant loss events such as bereavement, loss of a job, a role, a home or a relationship [3]. In many cases there is little warning and those that are truly suicidal can, and often do, hide it from those around them [4]. Those bereaved following the suicide of a loved one often report that the act came 'out of the blue' as the example below shows.

> *A couple who had been happily married for 15 years sat down to dinner. Neither had any noted history of mental distress. They shared a bottle of wine. They went to bed together. In the morning the husband woke to find his wife had taken her life in the bathroom overnight.*

This example and the others related in this part of the chapter are composites of cases taken from clinical practice, those recounted by relatives and other survivors of suicide, data from suicide audits and coroners record examination.

Epidemiology

There are globally around 800 000 deaths by suicide per year [5]. In England it is around 10 per 100 000 population, giving a total of around 6000 deaths in the UK and Republic of Ireland per year with men outnumbering women by 3 to 1 [6]. The rate, nationally and locally has remained reasonably constant over the last 10 years. The data on suicide are unreliable and the true rates may be around 30–50 per cent higher than those reported. There are several reasons for this. Firstly the level of proof needed for the coroner to give a suicide verdict, until June 2018, had to reach that required by criminal law and to be 'beyond reasonable doubt' [7]. In cases of suicide this is difficult to provide because often there is no clear record of intent. Secondly coroners have different attitudes towards suicide and some generally try to avoid suicide verdicts in an attempt to lighten the burden on families. Thirdly there has been a recent rise in narrative verdicts, a longer verdict based more on a description of the circumstance of the death, rather than a briefer suicide verdict. This can make the deaths harder to code as suicide for official statistics [8].

It is likely that suicidality resides within us all and can emerge more clearly at times of emotional difficulty. Fleeting suicidal thoughts may be universal, occurring as a natural human response to life's stresses and losses. At any one time around 50 per cent of the population report having had suicidal thoughts [9]. In some people these thoughts become persistent and compulsive. Suicidal thoughts are a primary diagnostic symptom of different types of mental disorder including depression and personality disorder [10]. Even though self-destructive thoughts are frequent, suicide is rare, so very few people with suicidal ideation go on to take their life and those that do are hard to predict. There is now a general consensus that risk assessment tools do not predict the risk of suicide [11, 12], and the most recent risk assessment of those that die is often low [13]. This is the 'low risk paradox' [14]. This picture is further complicated because the majority of people who die by suicide denied having suicidal thoughts when last asked before their death [15]. Suicide prevention therefore cannot rely on prediction. The best evidence relates to population prevention of access to mean and indicates a fundamental role for public health [15].

Pathway to Suicide

There is a growing literature on suicide and suicide prevention, but little has been written about the complex internal mental processes that lead an individual to take their own life. Psychoanalysts are the group that have addressed this challenging issue and Donald Campbell and Rob Hale, from the Portman Clinic, have made a recent major contribution in their 2017 book on suicide, *Working in the Dark* [4]. In this publication they describe what they believe to be the mental pathway to suicide derived from their extensive work with suicidal patients. The author of this part of the chapter (RG) has been researching completed suicide for over a decade, which has included the close examination of 39 Coroners' records of completed suicides. Through the analysis of these records, she builds on the work of Campbell and Hale to shine more light on why people kill themselves.

Stage 1: EARLY DEVELOPMENTAL DIFFICULTY AND RESULTING SPLIT IN THE INTERNAL WORLD

In psychoanalytic theory the ability to mourn loss is seen as key from very early development onwards. It is this process that allows separation of the baby from the mother and the development of an individual identity (individuation). The baby has ambivalent feelings towards the mother, both loving her presence and nurturing, while hating her absence and perceived neglect due to her other preoccupations. Through the mourning process this ambivalence is resolved, and the hated feelings accepted and integrated with the love enabling the baby to develop a more realistic picture of the mother. How this path is negotiated at this early stage of life sets the template for the individual's capacity to deal with loss thereafter. Each time a loss occurs mourning is repeated and reworked, and the internal world and ego matures [16].

The majority of individuals who go on to take their own life are thought to have some temperamental or early developmental difficulty with separation and individuation that renders them profoundly vulnerable when confronted with later losses. These events are not experienced as sad events but as 'a catastrophic blow to self-esteem and psychic integrity' [4]. The response to these losses can therefore be destructive and result in suicidal thoughts, self-harm and completed suicide.

Freud described how this destructive response to loss occurs in his 1917 paper, Mourning and Melancholia [17]. He said that ambivalent feelings towards what has been lost, referred to as the lost object, have not been resolved. Splitting is used in the internal world to protect the loving feelings by separating them from the hatred which is taken up by the 'critical agency' or superego. Fuelled by this hatred, the superego sadistically attacks the ego that has identified itself with the lost object. This identification is a normal stage of mourning but if it cannot be resolved it may result in a division in the internal world between the superego, and the ego.

> ... but the free libido was not displaced onto another object, it was withdrawn into the ego. There, however, it was not employed in any unspecified way, but served to establish an identification of the ego with the abandoned object. Thus the shadow of the object fell on the ego, and the latter could henceforth be judged by special agency, as though it were an object, the forsaken object. In this way an object loss was transformed into an ego loss and the conflict between ego and the loved person, into cleavage between the critical activity of the ego and the ego as altered by identification.   Sigmund Freud, 1917 [17, p. 249]

This process is unconscious, and the individual is unaware of both the loss, and of the resultant internal split in the ego. The effect is the development of a duality in the personality with two distinct sides, each with its own way of engaging with others. One side apparently copes well, is detached, can be ruthless and is identified with a primitive superego. The other side carries the vulnerability, is identified and projected into the body. This body/ego part is perceived by the superego/ego as the source of the current pain.

A clinical example of this split functioning follows:

> Christine functioned very well as a barrister. She worked compulsively. She had no obvious problems at work and was seen by her colleagues as somewhat overly dedicated and responsible. She found it very difficult to take holiday from work feeling overwhelmed by terror and desperation when she did. She consulted her GP reporting intense suicidal thoughts during a holiday when she was feeling very disturbed. Her GP referred her urgently to mental health services. By the time she was seen in secondary care a week later she was back at work and denied any concern about herself. She said that she had just attended the meeting with the mental health team to make her GP happy. She did not know what her GP was so worried about and did not want to engage with the crisis team as she could see no need. The mental health

team were concerned but felt they could not do anything. Christine went on to take her life when not working while at home the following weekend.

In this case there were two sides to Christine split off from each other. One side was vulnerable and knew that she was overwhelmed, in distress and at risk. It was this side that was contacted to by her GP. The other side was disconnected, impenetrable and dissociated from this vulnerability. It was this latter side that came to the meeting with the mental health team and would not allow any contact. In this meeting she projected this concerned side into the mental health team and was then able to treat it dismissively.

This split in the ego provides the dangerous territory needed for the pathway to suicide. We all have some degree of split in our ego functioning; however, in the group that go on to kill themselves this splitting is profound. Even within this latter group many will not go on to take their life. The description of this process can be helpful in explaining how the individual can become so detached and alienated from their own body as to see it as separate, and its death as the solution to distress and a way to preserve the good relationship with the lost object.

. . . while in committing suicide the ego intends to murder its bad objects, in my view at the same time it also aims at saving its loved objects, internal and external . . .. the phantasies underlying suicide aim at preserving the internalized good objects and that part of the ego which is identified with good objects, and also at destroying the other part of the ego which is identified with the bad objects and the id. Klein, 1935 [18, p. 160]

Stage 2: TRIGGER OF PATHWAY TO SUICIDE: First Loss Event

The role of loss and an inability to tolerate the feelings this evokes therefore seems key to understanding suicide. The pathway to suicide is triggered by an initial loss event that can occur weeks, months and occasionally years before the death.

For the individual to process this loss event there needs to be a capacity to mourn. However, in this vulnerable group the capacity to mourn is compromised. According to Campbell and Hale [4, p. 34] this event is then not experienced as loss but as a ruthless intentional abandonment or betrayal. The intense emotional pain and aggressive energy released by this loss cannot be discharged and instead fuels and increases the split in the psyche. The detached superego part of the individual gains destructive energy and power and starts to plan the death of the vulnerable body ego part as the only method of relief. This then becomes the pre-suicidal state. It is important to say that we all may have the capacity to develop a pre-suicidal state if we are faced with a loss too great for us to mourn.

This first loss event could be seen in all the 39 Coroners' records examined. The commonest examples were bereavement (20%), a relationship breakdown (33%), business failing (6%), loss of home (10%) or diagnosis of a serious health problem (6%).

Stage 3: THE PRESUICIDAL STATE

Campbell and Hale [4, p. 36] describe the 'Presuicidal State' as a quasi-delusional psychic retreat from unbearable anxiety. This means a transitory breakdown in reality testing which serves to detach the individual from unbearable pain. In this retreat suicidal phantasies start to dominate mental life. Phantasy is the term used for unconscious fantasies that are not known to the conscious mind. At no point does the individual really think that they will stop existing following the planned suicide. There is a phantasy, which is not fully consciously realised, that a 'survival self' will continue life in a pain-free 'bodiless way' [4, p. 27]. The death will provide a phantasised resolution, an opportunity to start again, to be reborn and reunited with those that are lost. In some cases, the individual aims to enact revenge for betrayal and imagines that they will witness the aftermath of this retribution.

These phantasies can be seen on occasion by the symbolic nature of the suicidal acts themselves. For example, people travel from all over the world to jump from the Golden Gate Bridge in America (or Beachy Head in the UK), in a bid to transition through a portal or 'Golden Gate' to a pain-free heavenly world where their life can begin again.

Stage 4: FINAL TRIGGER: Second Loss Event

It seems likely that individuals enter into the pre-suicidal state as described but most do not progress to suicide. In the group that go on to die the pre-suicidal state does not abate and continues either consciously or unconsciously. A final trigger [4] or 'Second Loss Event' is awaited by the suicidal part of the personality.

This final event can seem apparently small or trivial but is experienced by the individual as penetrating proof of lack of care and functions as permission to act [4, p. 35]. An eloquent account of this process has been described by Kevin, a young man, and one of the very few people to survive jumping from the Golden Gate Bridge; there was no doubting his suicidal intent and his survival was down to chance, as he discussed on the BBC2 Horizon documentary 'Stopping Male Suicide'. He said that he was feeling ambivalently suicidal and had gone to the Bridge to think about jumping. He met a passerby on the bridge:

> A woman from my left approached me and pulled out a camera. She asked me to take her picture. She posed, I took her picture quite a few times and then she walked away. That is when I said absolutely nobody cares. A voice in my head said, 'jump now' and I did. The milliseconds my hands left the rail I had an instant regret for my actions and the recognition that I had just made the greatest mistake of my life, but it was too late. Kevin – Horizon documentary BBC2

There was evidence of this 'Second Loss Event' just before the suicide in 38 of the 39 Coroners' records examined. Examples included; receiving various painful letters or emails including evictions warnings, demand for rent or being chased for debt repayment. There were difficulties career-wise including rejection following an interview, a reprimand from work, exam results and letters from solicitors. There were many cases of relationship difficulties including arguments, rejection or being told that romantic unions were at an end. There were arguments with friends and family, and interactions with the police such as parking tickets and other minor offences. There were frustrations such as losing a wallet or a phone, and not being able to renew a passport. Such loss events are a normal part of life and would be hard to avoid.

> Ellen, a doctor, was presenting the death of a patient by suicide in a reflective practice group. She said that for a few months before the death she had been receiving out-of-hours emails (to her work email address) by her vulnerable patient. She did not know how to stop this because she was concerned, wanted to do the right thing and didn't want the patient to feel rejected. She was very conscientious and anxious about her work and would sometime check her work emails in the evenings and weekends, on a rare occasion replying to her patient when she did so. She went away for a weekend during which she did not check her inbox. When she returned to work on Monday, she found an email from her patient, sent on Sunday, saying that she was going to kill herself. Ellen was very concerned and phoned her home number: her patient's mother

answered the phone and told Ellen that her daughter had taken her life in the early hours of that morning.

This case is an amalgam of several. In this case the doctor may have unconsciously been set up by the ruthless part of the patient to provide the 'Second Loss Event' and proof of lack of care by letting her down. The result was that Ellen felt deeply implicated in the death and found it very difficult to recover. She later left the service where this death occurred.

Stage 5: SUICIDAL ACT CONFUSION AND DISSOCIATION

The experience of betrayal and being let down after 'Second Loss Event' is the 'straw that breaks the camel's back' and conditions for the enactment of suicide are reached. The ambivalence and repeated switching between different parts of the mind, one associated with life and one with death, means that a period of confusion precedes the suicidal act.

George was seen on CCTV cameras on the platforms of different train stations walking up and down for 12 hours before finally jumping in front of a train.

This dissociation, or disconnection with life-seeking aspects of the self, can be reinforced by use of alcohol, which also reduces inhibition. There is then a primary engagement with the suicidal phantasy. This is often seen as a period of calm. The decision is made, it is highly determined and hidden from others, who can believe that everything has improved, and they can reduce their vigilance. It is at this point that all attempts to communicate stop and others are often reassured that nothing is wrong [4].

This dissociation continues until the point of no return – where there are many reports of a sudden resolution and re-engagement with reality. This can be seen in Kevin's recounting of his suicide attempt above, which is consistent with previous reports from survivors of serious suicide attempts.

When my hand left the handrail I suddenly realised that everything in my life was fixable apart from the fact I had jumped. Ken Baldwin, 2003, *New Yorker* [19]

After the Suicide

Those of us who work with patients who have died by suicide or have had personal experience of this type of loss ourselves know how intensely complex and painful these deaths can be. The projection through 'acting out' of the very primitive and unresolved, angry, blaming, stage of mourning into the survivors leaves intense feelings of guilt and regret. On occasion those left behind can feel accused of murder themselves. Acting out is a defence mechanism and occurs when psychological pain cannot be put into words. The effect of this acting out is to get rid of the pain by expelling it from inside the mind of the individual, 'out' and 'into' others minds who are in close physical or emotional proximity.

... the dead person is the apparent victim, but the true victim is the one that stays alive, for he or she has to live with what they feel but they might have caused . . .. The dead person has achieved immortality in the survivor's mind . . .. It seems as though the act suicide freezes the relationship at the zenith of its sadism, and that the survivor directs enormous resistances to any change working through this state, almost as a memorial to the dead *[4, p. 40].*

These powerful aggressive projections of guilt and blame are almost impossible to bear and inhibit the capacity to mourn the death. This make the time afterwards dangerous for the survivors whom are at a higher risk of suicide themselves in the aftermath [20]. There is daily newspaper evidence of society's identification with these projections with clear assumptions of who, or what, is to blame after the death.

In mental health, the suicide of a patient can become a dominating preoccupation and a daily dread. When it does occur, it can have a profound effect on those clinicians involved with the patient [21]. The uncertainty about the pathway to the death is unbearable. Therefore, clear narratives, however uncertain, are quickly derived and adhered to with absolute conviction. The search for someone to contain this blame who could be held to be accountable for the death is overwhelming. This denies the reality that the only person who can reasonably give an account, or some rational for the death, is no longer present.

Current research shows that the distress left with clinicians after the suicide of a patient can have a profound effect on their personal and professional life [21]. The majority of mental health clinicians will have at least one experience of a patient suicide during their career [22, 23], with many experiencing more. In one study [24], 53 per cent of the psychiatrists responding reported stress levels in the weeks following a suicide comparable to those reported in studies of people seeking treatment after the death of a parent. The intensity of this experience can result in a combination of post-traumatic stress disorder symptoms, shame, guilt, anger, isolation, fear of litigation and fear of retribution from the psychiatric community [25, 26]. Intense feelings of distress, anxiety and persecution can be exacerbated by organisational responses including serious incident enquiries and the pressure of attending the Coroner's Court [4, 21]. Those suffering a severe stress reaction often consider retirement [22] or change in career [27]. The results of a survey of psychiatrists indicated a serious unmet need for support and information after these tragic and traumatic deaths [21]. Intervention at this point would seem important in order to mitigate distress, effects on clinical practice and career change.

Final Thoughts on Suicide

Suicide is an act that defies conscious rational understanding and leaves survivors with a level of uncertainty as to the cause that is beyond the human capacity to process. The human mind compulsively organises uncertain experiences into a narrative [28]. Stories are made up very rapidly following a death, about why it has occurred, and then can be held with passionate certainty.

The assumption of a fundamentally constant causal link between mental illness and suicide is repeatedly disproved by data. This leaves us facing the possibility that suicide or a drive to self-destruction is a part of the human condition, and not only a part of mental health condition. This is the view of some psychoanalysts, including Freud [29, p. 231], who saw suicide as a manifestation of the death instinct or 'Thanatos', which works in conflict with the life instinct or 'Eros', as a force that 'seeks to lead what is living to death' [30, p. 46]. It is important to say that we all have some degree of splitting of our ego and it is likely that for all of us there would be a loss too great to mourn that could propel us to take our own life. There is a significant ongoing debate about end of life suicide (often called Assisted Suicide) which can be seen as a means of gaining control for those whom are terminally ill and in pain. Suicide in this group, may be more acceptable to society then a death earlier on in life. Freud himself may well have died as a result of suicide at the end of his life following the diagnosis of terminal illness.

If suicide is a part of the human condition then it might touch us personally, affecting those close to us without warning, including friends and family. We may even be vulnerable to dying in this way ourselves. The most suitable psychiatric diagnosis, if one is wanted, for those who die by suicide would generally be that of an Adjustment Disorder F43.2 9. An Adjustment Disorder is something we all might suffer with as life events are universal, uncontrollable and inevitable.

Suicide can be prevented by finding words for the pain and distress that underlies the need to act out in this profoundly self-destructive manner. To talk openly, without stigma, about suicide and to find words for the pain reduces risk. This chapter aims to contribute to this open discourse with the hope of increasing general confidence in facing these relieving and transformative discussions.

Homicide

Background and Context

Homicide is a much rarer event than suicide; however, in a similar way a development and psychodynamic approach can help to elucidate factors that contribute to a homicidal state of mind. Like suicide homicide is an aspect of human behaviour that has occurred throughout history and transcends cultures. This part of the chapter will focus on the type of homicide that involves mental health services.

Epidemiology

The rate of homicide is 11 per million population in the UK (650–700 homicides annually). Similar to suicide this rate has been pretty constant over time even with the abolition of capital punishment in 1967.[1] The majority (60–70 per cent) involve the perpetrator killing someone to whom they have, or have had, close relational bonds: partners, ex-partners, parents, family members, children. Occasionally one intoxicated person will kill another in a fight; however, homicides of strangers by strangers are comparatively rare. Homicides by the mentally ill are very rare [31]; however, those that have killed, who do have mental illness, will spend a long time in psychiatric services, usually within secure institutions. Many psychiatrists will come across patients who express homicidal ideation and this does form part of the risk assessment.

Legal Process

When an individual is arrested for a homicide they are charged with murder; and will get a psychiatric assessment by a prison psychiatrist. If the defence solicitors opt to present a psychiatric defence, then a psychiatrist will be instructed by both the defence and the prosecution to assess whether the criteria for diminished responsibility or insanity are met. If the experts for both sides agree that the defendant has a psychiatric defence, then the court will agree to accept a plea of 'guilty of manslaughter' and proceed to sentencing. Those who

---

[1] The exception is in 2003 when the Crime Survey for England and Wales statistics show a highly unusual peak of 900 homicides; this was due to the findings of the Smith Inquiry which 'convicted' Dr Shipman of over 200 homicides.

kill when mentally ill will be detained in a secure hospital under Section 37 of the Mental Health Act; usually also under a Section 41 restriction order, which means that the Ministry of Justice must be involved in decisions about their care.

The Psychodynamics of Homicide

An act of homicide is complex both in intention and its effects; and the origins are multifactorial [32]. Although it is probably true that, like suicide, all humans have the potential to commit a homicide, it is also true that most will never act on homicidal thoughts or feelings. Psychologically healthy individuals develop psychological defences during their childhood and early adulthood which enable them to contain and process psychological pain. Defences therefore make up a kind of psychological 'lock' in the mind which keeps potential violence contained and secure; and which will only open if the right 'lock numbers' are in place. The commonest 'numbers' are:

- The actuarial ones for violent crime generally: male sex, youth and substance misuse
- Willingness to use violence (e.g. previous violence perpetration and antisocial attitudes
- Problems with reality testing (which is where mental illness may play a role)
- The final 'number', which unleashes the homicidal violence and is the most important, is highly idiosyncratic; and usually has personal, unconscious meaning and significance for the perpetrator. It may be something the victim says or does; or it may be a traumatic memory has been triggered that generates intolerable unresolved distress. The existence of the victim becomes unbearable and what they have come to represent to the perpetrator must be got rid of

The pathways to homicide and suicide bear some similarities. As with suicide the perpetrator moves into a state of mind that make homicide seem real, necessary and inevitable. There is an overlap in the emotional states that underly both suicide and homicide, especially in the relational context. Just like the pre-suicidal states referred to above, homicide perpetrators also often describe a long period of intense turmoil and agitation about their homicidal ideas; which is then replaced by a kind of calm. Perpetrators also phantasise that life will continue in a pain-free way, with all conflicts resolved; they use reality distorting defences to exclude from awareness any ideas of arrest, trial or detention. However, like Kevin on the Golden Gate Bridge, who realised just as he let go how wrong he was, so most people who kill (especially those with a mental illness) realise after the death that they have made a dreadful error:

Mr Jenkins (72) was found in the garden of his house in a London suburb. He was dressed in pyjamas and covered with blood. He said to the paramedics and police when they arrived 'I have done the wrong thing again'. Inside the house, the police found the body of Mrs Jenkins, dead from multiple head wounds. Mr Jenkins was having treatment for agitated depression; his medication had been changed two weeks before the homicide. The psychiatrist who saw him made a diagnosis of an acute confusional state at the material time; but also wondered what 'wrong thing' Mr Jenkins had done before, and what 'wrong thing' had happened before the killing. It was later found that Mr Jenkin's had a disturbed childhood where his mother had frequently criticised him and Mr Jenkin's had repressed his aggression under a meek and compliant exterior. Just before the homicide Mr Jenkin's wife, like his mother, had told him that he had taken the wrong bins out again.

As discussed above, the final event that triggers a homicide often has deep symbolic significance for the offender; and may be linked to unresolved childhood distress associated with betrayal, loss or fear. Personal reality is distorted by the use of psychotic defences such as projection, concrete thinking, denial and splitting; and can be exacerbated by the use of substances. Dissociation is also common in the perpetrators of homicide; which can lead legal examiners to mistake psychotic dissociation for 'absence of mental disorder', because the perpetrator appears so calm and rational. Like with suicide once the reality of the homicide is established, the dissociation tends to evaporate, and perpetrators (especially of domestic homicide) experience extreme distress. The murderousness that was projected into the victim is now internalised; and the suicide risk escalates with sometimes fatal consequences [33]. This suicide risk is especially high for homicides involving a child or a parent; and the suicide risk can be hidden under a mask of cheerful 'normality': perpetrators who kill themselves in this context are often later described as 'model' prisoners or patients.

> Linda killed her two-year-old son and three-month-old daughter in the context of a post-natal psychosis. She was found guilty of manslaughter on the grounds of diminished responsibility and was sent to hospital for treatment. Her psychotic illness improved at once; and the main focus of psychotherapy was her enduring sense of guilt, grief and pathological bereavements; including flashbacks of the index offence. Linda complied with all therapies; and insisted that she would not kill herself because of the effect on her elderly parents and her ex-husband (who divorced her and remarried). Linda was having leave from the secure hospital and there was a plan to rehabilitate her into the community near her supportive family. However, on what would have been her fifteenth wedding anniversary, she put herself in front of a train while on unescorted leave and died.

Treatment

The psychotherapeutic treatment of people who have killed needs to address both the unconscious motivations; and the conscious experience of the killing and its aftermath. Psychodynamic psychotherapy is particularly helpful in these cases because it allows a focus on the relational and attachment disturbance, most commonly ambivalent, that has contributed to the enactment. Psychodynamic group therapy with a mentalising perspective is frequently used because it reduces shame and social isolation; and also facilitates taking up different perspective on the previously fixed 'cover story' for the killing [34]. Treatment presents challenges because of the need to retain the psychotic state as a retreat and prevent awareness of the reality of what they have done.

Impact on Psychiatrists following the Homicide of a Patient

Although rare many psychiatrists will come across a small number of patients who have perpetrated a homicide. Like suicide, homicide involves powerful projections of painful emotions; such as rage, guilt, shame and fear which frequently leave those connected with the perpetrator; such as family members, or staff in mental health teams where the perpetrator is known in intense distress. It is common for media to focus on either the perpetrator's 'evil madness' or the 'madness' of medical professionals who did not predict the homicide. Even in cases where perpetrators are not found to have been mentally ill at the material time, psychiatrists can find themselves the object of blame and persecution.

In a current study exploring the impact on psychiatrists of a homicide by a patient under their care [35], 78 per cent of responders said that the homicide had a major impact on both their personal and professional lives. As in the suicide impact study illustrated above, professionals describe a lack of support and negative consequences for their mental health and professional career. Many commented that the legal and institutional inquiry processes that followed the death had been major stressors. Although these inquiries were presented as inquisitorial, many psychiatrists described a highly adversarial 'feel' to these processes, where they were identified as a 'bad' doctor and 'offender'.

Homicides by patients are rare and highly publicised cases generate considerable fear in psychiatrists that they are expected to prevent homicides; which, like suicide, are rare and highly unpredictable events.

References

1. Camus A. *The Myth of Sisyphus* (Penguin Modern Classics). London: *Penguin Books Ltd*, 1955. Kindle Edition.

2. Healthcare Quality Improvement Partnership. National Confidential Inquiry into Homicide and Suicide: Report 2018. HQIP, 2018. https://sites.manchester.ac.uk /ncish/ [Accessed 1/12/2020]

3. Coope C, Donovan J, Wilson C et al. Characteristics of people dying by suicide after job loss, financial difficulties and other economic stressors during a period of recession (2010–2011): a review of coroners' records. *J Affect Disord* 2015; 183: 98–105.

4. Campbell D, Hale R. *Working in the Dark: Understanding the Pre-suicide State of Mind*. Abingdon: Routledge, 2017.

5. World Health Organization. Disease burden and mortality estimates: cause-specific mortality, 2000–2016. www .who.int/healthinfo/global_burden_di sease/estimates/en// [Accessed 13/11/2020]

6. Samaritans. Suicide facts and figures. https://www.samaritans.org/scotland/ about-samaritans/research-policy/suicide-facts-and-figures/ [Accessed 1/12/2020]

7. Pritchard C, Hansen L. Examining undetermined and accidental deaths as source of 'under-reported-suicide' by age and sex in twenty Western countries. *Community Ment Health J* 2015; 51(3): 365–76.

8. Hill C, Cook L. Narrative verdicts and their impact on mortality statistics in England and Wales. *Health Stat Q* 2011; 49(1): 81–100.

9. Rudd MD. The prevalence of suicidal ideation among college students. *Suicide Life Threat Behav* 1989; 19(2): 173–83.

10. World Health Organization. *The ICD-10 Classification of Mental and Behavioural Disorders: Clinical Descriptions and Diagnostic Guidelines*. Geneva: World Health Organization, 1992.

11. Quinlivan L, Cooper J, Meehan D et al. Predictive accuracy of risk scales following self-harm: multicentre, prospective cohort study. *Br J Psychiatry* 2017; 210(6): 429–36.

12. Rahman MS, Kapur N. Quality of risk assessment prior to suicide and homicide. *Psychiatr Bull* 2014; 38(1): 46–7.

13. Windfuhr K, Kapur N. Suicide and mental illness: a clinical review of 15 years findings from the UK National Confidential Inquiry into Suicide. *Br Med Bull* 2011; 100(1): 101–21.

14. Berman A. Risk factors proximate to suicide and suicide risk assessment in the context of denied suicide ideation. *Suicide Life Threat Behav* 2018; 48: 340–52.

15. Appleby L, Hunt IM, Kapur N. New policy and evidence on suicide prevention. *Lancet Psychiatry* 2017; 4(9): 658–60.

16. Klein M. Envy & gratitude. *Psyche* 1957; 11(5): 241–55.

17. Freud S. Mourning and melancholia. In J Strachey, ed., *The Standard Edition of the Complete Psychological Works of Sigmund Freud, Volume XIV (1914–1916): On the History of the Psycho-Analytic Movement,*

Papers on Metapsychology and Other Works. London: Hogarth Press. 1957; pp. 243–57. (Original work published 1917)

18. Klein M. A contribution to the psychogenesis of manic-depressive states. *Int J Psychoanal* 1935; 16: 145–74.

19. *New Yorker* Letter from California October 13, 2003 Issue Jumpers.

20. Pitman AL, Osborn DP, Rantell K, King MB. Bereavement by suicide as a risk factor for suicide attempt: a cross-sectional national UK-wide study of 3432 young bereaved adults. *BMJ Open* 2016; 6(1): e009948.

21. Gibbons R, Brand F, Carbonnier A et al. Effects of patient suicide on psychiatrists: survey of experiences and support required. *BJPsych Bull* 2019; 43: 236–41.

22. Alexander DA, Klein S, Gray NM, Dewar IG, Eagles JM. Suicide by patients: questionnaire study of its effect on consultant psychiatrists. *BMJ* 2000; 320(7249): 1571–4.

23. Courtenay KP, Stephens JP. The experience of patient suicide among trainees in psychiatry. *Psychiatr Bull* 2001; 25(2): 51–2.

24. Chemtob CM, Hamad RS, Bauer G, Kinney B, Torigoe RY. Patients' suicides: frequency and impact on psychiatrists. *Am J Psychiatry* 1988; 145(2): 224–8.

25. Ruskin R, Sakinofsky I, Bagby RM, Dickens S, Sousa G. Impact of patient suicide on psychiatrists and psychiatric trainees. *Acad Psychiatry* 2004; 28(2): 104–10.

26. Gitlin MJ. A psychiatrist's reaction to a patient's suicide. *Am J Psychiatry* 1999; 156(10): 1630–4.

27. Dewar I, Eagles J, Klein S, Gray N, Alexander D. Psychiatric trainees' experiences of, and reactions to, patient suicide. *Psychiatr Bull* 2000; 24(1): 20–3.

28. László J. *The Science of Stories: An Introduction to Narrative Psychology.* Hove: Routledge, 2008.

29. Freud S. Contribution to a discussion on suicide. In J Strachey, ed., *The Standard Edition of the Complete Psychological Works of Sigmund Freud, Volume XI (1910): Five Lectures on Psycho-Analysis, Leonardo Da Vinci and Other Works.* London: Hogarth Press. 1957; pp. 231–3. (Original work published 1910)

30. Freud S. Beyond the pleasure principle. In J Strachey, ed., *The Standard Edition of the Complete Psychological Works of Sigmund Freud, Volume XVIII (1920–1922): Beyond the Pleasure Principle, Group Psychology and Other Works.* London: Hogarth Press. 1955; pp. 1–64. (Original work published 1920)

31. Nielssen O, Bourget D, Laajasalo T et al. Homicide of strangers by people with a psychotic illness. *Schizophr Bull* 2011; 37(3): 572–9.

32. Yakely J, Adshead G. Locks, keys and security of mind: psychodynamic approaches to forensic psychiatry. *J Am Acad Psychiatry Law* 2013; 41(1): 38–45.

33. Liettu A, Mikkola L, Saavala H et al. Mortality rates of males who commit parricide or other violent offense against a parent. *J Am Acad Psychiatry Law* 2010; 38: 212–20.

34. Adshead G. The life sentence: using a narrative approach in group psychotherapy with offenders. *Group Anal* 2011; 44(2): 175–95.

35. Mezey G, Rowe R, Adshead G. Impact of homicide by a psychiatric patient on forensic psychiatrists: national survey. *BJPsych Bull* 2020; 0: 1–7. doi:10.1192/bjb.2020.96.

Chapter 20

Forensic Psychotherapy

Jessica Yakeley

What Is Forensic Psychotherapy?

Forensic psychotherapy is the application of psychological knowledge to the assessment, treatment and management of mentally disordered offenders and patients who commit violent or destructive acts against others or themselves. Forensic psychotherapy creates a bridge between forensic psychiatry with its main focus on mental illness and risk, and psychoanalytical psychotherapy which aims to understand the conscious and unconscious motivations of offender or forensic patient [1]. Forensic psychotherapy emerged from a psychoanalytic theoretical framework, which continues to be its predominant influence, although its remit has widened to encompass other psychodynamic approaches, including group psychotherapy and therapeutic community approaches, and it is also influenced by the related disciplines of psychology, criminology, sociology, ethology, neuroscience, philosophy and ethics.

History of Forensic Psychotherapy

Forensic psychotherapy developed as a specialty in its own right from the pioneering work of psychoanalysts in forensic mental health and prison settings in the 1930s. Although a huge psychoanalytic literature has been established on the nature of aggression since Freud's initial writings, psychoanalytic treatment was not traditionally thought suitable for violent and antisocial patients. Nevertheless, there were a few early innovative clinicians interested in expanding the boundaries of classical psychoanalysis by attempting to treat violent patients, such as Karl Menninger [2] in the United States. But it was in the UK that forensic psychotherapy was established with inception of the Portman Clinic in London, originally founded in 1931 as the Psychopathic Clinic, the clinical arm of the then Institute for the Scientific Treatment of Delinquency, by Grace Pailthorpe, a gifted psychiatrist and psychoanalyst. The Portman Clinic developed as a centre of expertise in treating patients with violent, antisocial, delinquent and perverse behaviours, and notable psychoanalysts and psychiatrists such as Edward Glover, Mervyn Glasser, Adam Limentani and Estela Welldon who worked there have been influential in advancing psychoanalytic theories on the aetiology and treatment of violence and perversion. Their clinical work inspired other psychoanalytically trained psychiatrists such as Murray Cox, Leslie Sohn and Arthur Hyatt Williams in their treatment of violent individuals in forensic hospitals and prisons in the UK, and laid the foundations for forensic psychotherapy to develop and expand into an international multidisciplinary field of clinicians from different professional backgrounds, including psychiatry, psychology, nursing, art therapies, social work, probation and law. The International Association for Forensic Psychotherapy (IAFP) was formed by Estela

Welldon and a small group of European psychiatrists trained in psychoanalytic psychotherapy working within forensic settings in 1991 whose aim is to promote the health of offenders and victims through the use of psychotherapeutic understanding, risk assessment and treatment techniques, and has grown into an international society with members from all disciplines, including service users, in Europe, the United States, South America and New Zealand.

In 1995 the first Consultant Psychiatrist in Forensic Psychotherapy was appointed in the UK at Broadmoor High Secure Hospital, and in 1999, forensic psychotherapy was approved by the General Medical Council and the Royal College of Psychiatrists to become a formal sub-specialty of higher psychiatric training. In 2007, the Forensic Psychotherapy Special Interest Group was established within the Royal College of Psychiatrists, which aims to promote and support practice, training and research in forensic psychotherapy within psychiatry and other disciplines.

Principles of Forensic Psychotherapy

Psychoanalytic Principles

Forensic psychotherapy is based on certain fundamental tenets of psychoanalysis – the existence of a dynamic unconscious of fantasies, feelings, conflicts and motivations; psychic determinism whereby one's conscious choices are influenced by these unconscious processes; a developmental approach which understands that the adult personality is shaped by significant events in childhood; and the notion that behaviours and symptoms have unconscious symbolic meaning, so that violent and antisocial acts may be understood as a form of 'acting out' – a meaningful communication of unconscious wishes, needs and conflicts.

Violence as Communication

In his paper 'Remembering, repeating and working through' Freud writes, '. . . the patient does not remember anything of what he has forgotten and repressed, but acts it out. He reproduces it as not as a memory, but as an action: he repeats it, without, of course, knowing that he is repeating it. For instance, the patient does not say that he remembers that he used to be defiant and critical towards his parents' authority; instead, he behaves that way to the doctor.' [3, p. 150]. Freud went on to show how acting out represented a resistance to psychoanalytic progress – an unconscious repetition of the patient's past in action that occurred in the relationship, or transference, with the analyst, that could not be thought about consciously but acted out instead.

The concept of 'acting out' has since widened to include a range of impulsive, risky and antisocial behaviours of patients, not solely arising from the clinical context, but as an inherent part of how the person habitually relates to himself and others, where certain thoughts and feelings, stemming from adverse childhood experiences, cannot be represented and processed in the conscious mind, and are therefore expelled in action. One of the tasks of forensic psychotherapy is to help the patient tolerate the disturbing thoughts and feelings, often associated with vulnerability, shame and humiliation, that underlie their violent behaviours, and understand their traumatic origins in the patient's early childhood. However, forensic psychotherapy is as much aimed at helping the professionals who manage such patients or offenders in understanding that their offences and crimes may not be immoral actions committed by people who are inherently bad, but have arisen within a developmental context as pathological defences against experiences of neglect, trauma and abuse from people responsible for their care.

Understanding Not Condoning

However, professionals, as well as the general public, may be resistant to an approach that pathologises antisocial and illegal behaviours and suggests that the offender may be suffering from a mental disorder, such as antisocial personality disorder, which may be amenable to treatment, particularly when the offender does not appear to suffer, but makes other suffer, and may be reluctant to think of himself as a 'patient' or engage in treatment at all. This highlights the historical and ongoing tensions between legal and medical approaches, often played out within the court arena, over whether 'treatment' is really a disguise for moral re-education, particularly for people who are not voluntarily seeking help themselves [4]. Confusion arises because the offender attacks the outside world – other people and society – who then understandably focus on that person's actions which are deemed worthy of punishment. This may indeed be the correct response, as the offender needs to know that his actions damage others and have consequences, but from a psychodynamic viewpoint it is only a partial response. From this perspective, attention is erroneously focussed on the offender's external actions, rather than his internal world, and any attempt to understand that his offences against others arise from his own self-destructive internal and compulsive needs is equated by the public with condoning them [1]. Forensic psychotherapy does not operate within a condoning–condemning axis but seeks to enable the offender to take responsibility for his actions and choices through a greater understanding of himself. Indeed, treatment and punishment are not diametrically opposed but may be both necessary for rehabilitation where the legal process of proportionate justice – by imposing imprisonment or a community sentence – may establish an essential external boundary without which therapeutic work could not take place.

Three Parties in Forensic Psychotherapy

As with all psychoanalytically oriented psychotherapy, forensic psychotherapy focusses on exploring the internal world of the patient, but the therapist also needs to be aware of what is actually happening in his external life and the potential risks that he poses. In this respect, forensic psychotherapy differs from more traditional psychoanalytic psychotherapy where the relationship between patient and therapist remains private and confidential. In forensic psychotherapy the dyadic relationship between patient and therapist is not sacrosanct as there is always a third party – the criminal justice system – involved in the therapeutic endeavour which brings in the external reality of the patient's actions, their consequences and management. This third party may be a professional or agency currently involved in the patient's/offender's management, such as his probation officer or the court, or may be represented by the patient's contact with criminal justice or forensic services in the past. However, the therapist needs to have some independent knowledge of the patient's offending history and risk to others, rather than solely relying on sources of information arising within the therapy from the patient themselves or from the therapist's countertransference. This triangulation of the therapeutic process alters the nature of confidentiality – on the one hand, confidentiality needs to be protected as much as possible to facilitate engagement in treatment, but on the other hand, where there is a serious risk of harm to others it may be necessary to disclose information to third parties, and not to do so may be unconsciously experienced by the patient as a dangerous collusion on the part of the therapist who is not protecting the patient from his dangerous impulses. Negotiating this triangular situation successfully by managing the competing demands of confidentiality and risk opens up a containing space where a therapeutic process can develop safely. The bringing in of a third perspective or 'paternal function' – in contrast to the more 'maternal function' of the therapist – parallels the way in which a good 'parental couple' will promote the best interests of their child, an experience many offenders never had. When therapy takes place in a forensic setting, the lines of communication and duties of care of different members of the team should be clearly defined [5].

In view of the complexities of risk, security, confidentiality and disclosure inherent to forensic work, forensic psychotherapy should take place in the public sector in an institutional setting that can provide the appropriate governance structures and multidisciplinary team support to ensure the necessary containment for individuals who pose a significant risk to themselves and others. Forensic psychotherapy is ideally located at the juncture of two institutional systems in the UK: the National Health Service (NHS) and the criminal justice system. This ensures that the work between therapist and patient/offender is not carried out in isolation, but is subject to the regulatory frameworks and institutional boundaries needed to protect both parties in the therapy dyad. While the forensic psychotherapist must be constantly mindful of the tensions arising from the different ethos and agendas – therapeutics versus public protection – of the respective institutions, being able to work within the rules of the institutional settings is a vital part of facilitating the offender's eventual transition back into the wider society from which he has been excluded.

Theoretical Contributions to Forensic Psychotherapy

Unconscious Sense of Guilt, the Superego and Primitive States of Mind

Freud described in his paper 'Some character-types met with in psycho-analytic work' [6] individuals whom he referred to as 'criminals from a sense of guilt' who were drawn to committing forbidden antisocial deeds to relieve an unconscious sense of guilt, which preceded the crime, and which Freud linked to unresolved forbidden Oedipal wishes and led to the need for punishment. Freud later attributed the unconscious sense of guilt to the existence of the death instinct [7].

Although Freud believed that the superego was absent in psychopaths, Klein furthered these ideas in proposing that by contrast, their superego was present but overly harsh and punitive, which led to an internal sense of persecution between the superego and ego and unconscious sense of guilt that could only be alleviated via violent or antisocial actions [8]. Klein believed that violence was the result of innate envy and destructiveness that were manifestations of the death instinct and predominated in early life, giving rise to the primitive anxieties, defences, unconscious phantasies and archaic superego which characterised the 'paranoid-schizoid' position [9]. Klein's ideas are helpful in conceptualising violent and antisocial states of mind as being governed by primitive defence mechanisms such as splitting, denial, omnipotence and projection, with a lack of more mature defence mechanisms such as repression and sublimation. Similarly, primitive emotions such as envy, shame, boredom, rage and excitement predominate, whereas more mature affects such as guilt, fear, depression, remorse and sympathy which involve an appreciation of whole objects and are characteristic of the 'depressive position' [10] are missing.

Violence as a Defence against Trauma and Disorders of Attachment

Klein's belief that aggression and violence were primarily instinctual were opposed by Winnicott, who viewed aggression as a creative force necessary for healthy development, facilitated by a 'good enough mother' by enabling individuation and separation [11]. He proposed that pathological aggression and antisocial behaviour arose as a defensive reaction to early deprivation and trauma [12, 13]. Bowlby coined the term 'affectionless psychopaths' for children whose apparent indifference to others hid their anxiety of 'the risk of their hearts being broken again' [14].

Influenced by these ideas of Winnicott and Bowlby, more contemporary authors (e.g. De Zulueta [15], Gilligan [16], McGauley [17], Meloy [18]) highlight the high frequency of early abuse and loss in the histories of antisocial and forensic patients, and view adult antisocial behaviour as a defence against early trauma which interferes with the normal development of attachment between the infant and mother or primary caregivers. Such pathological attachment relationships in early childhood may lead to later difficulties in affect regulation, impulse control and a deficient capacity for representation and mentalisation. Gilligan [16] proposes that all violence is a defence against experiences of shame and humiliation, which has its roots in the person's early abusive experiences of being shamed and humiliated. Such painful affects are associated with anxieties of vulnerability and dependence, which cannot be tolerated or mentalised within the fragile defensive structure of the person's mind and instead are converted into the excitement of violence or projected into others.

These ideas are illustrated in the case of Mr B, who was physically abused by his mother and stepfather, his own father having disappeared when he was a baby. Mr B was initially a very anxious child with persistent bedwetting, which further enraged his mother and made him feel terribly ashamed. As a teenager he became aggressive and delinquent, getting into fights, stealing cars and drinking heavily. In early adulthood Mr B became closer to his mother after she divorced from his stepfather, but had a series of relationships in which he was domestically violent to female partners, culminating in a conviction for grievous bodily harm and a custodial sentence. In prison he commenced a group treatment programme for intimate partner violence, but was soon excluded due to his argumentative behaviour resulting from his sensitivity to feeling slighted and humiliated by the female group facilitators.

These failures in mentalisation and poor impulse control may be seen to be the result of Mr B's early childhood history of trauma and neglect, in which his mother was unable to foster the development of a secure attachment, but instead violently intruded upon his mind and body. His experiences of being abandoned by his biological father, and violently abused by his stepfather offered him no opportunities for developing a healthy male identification, nor any respite from the pathological relationship with his mother. However, Mr B was not consciously aware of his anger towards his mother, but unconsciously projected this in the violence towards his girlfriends, making them feel humiliated and powerless, as he himself did as a child.

Perversions

Forensic psychotherapy has also been concerned, since its inception at the Portman Clinic, with the origins and psychotherapeutic treatment of perverse sexual fantasies and behaviours. Although the term perversion has assumed pejorative connotations, and has been replaced by the diagnostic category of paraphilias and paraphilic disorders in the DSM-5, certain psychoanalytic concepts of perversion retain utility in how we might think about and help individuals whose sexual desires and practices cause distress to themselves and/or others, particularly in the realm of intimate relationships [19].

Freud originally proposed that perversions were due to infantile sexual instincts that had escaped repression, and later as a defence against castration anxiety [20]; later psychoanalysts shifted the aetiological roots of perversion, as with those of violence, to earlier in the person's development, locating them in the primary relationship between the mother and baby, where perverse fantasies and behaviours arise as a sexualised defence against primitive anxieties and aggression towards a narcissistic, abusive or neglectful mother. Sexualisation, however, is a more mature defence than the primitive defences of projection, splitting, idealisation and denigration which characterise the mental states of individuals who are more overtly violent, whose aggression may be understood as a more primitive defence against disturbances and related anxieties in the early mother–infant relationship. As described above, when these anxieties become overwhelming, they are no longer kept in check within the mind but are projected into others in overt violence. By contrast, in people with perversions, violence is inhibited by the sexualisation of their aggressive impulses towards the mother in early development into fantasies and behaviours that provide gratification and preserve the relationship with the mother, but in which sadomasochism takes the place of care and love.

Stoller described perversion as 'the erotic form of hatred' [21], where hostility, hidden behind overt sexualisation, was the primary motivation in perversion and represented a fantasy of revengeful triumph over childhood trauma and a pathological relationship with the mother. Extending Stoller's ideas, Glasser proposed, in his theory of the core complex, that sexual perversion in adulthood arose from a constellation of primitive anxieties, sadistic sexual fantasies and denigratory defences [22], which he called the core complex, originating in infancy as a defence against fears of aggression, separation, abandonment and helplessness in relation to the mother. For both Stoller and Glasser, the father is absent or ineffectual, and thus unable to protect the child from an engulfing relationship with the mother. In adulthood, true emotional intimacy is avoided by keeping the other person at a distance within a paradigm of sexual dominance and control, where the aggression may be openly manifest, as in sadomasochistic sexual practices, or more hidden, as in the secret triumph of voyeurism or the omnipotence of exhibitionism, where hostility towards the other person is concealed within an envelope of sexual excitement [19].

These interpersonal dynamics may be seen in a patient, Mr M, who was referred for therapy for his 'addiction' to sadomasochistic sexual practices such as bondage, which left him feeling increasingly isolated and depressed. He was the only child of a single mother and remembered feeling suffocated by his mother's attention and control. He exhibited aggressive and disruptive behaviour in primary school, but as an adolescent withdrew into a fantasy world of violent video games, which were gradually replaced by internet pornography of an increasingly sadistic nature. As an adult he could only become sexually excited in aggressive encounters with his partners, and although these sexual relationships were initially consensual, he became increasingly aroused the more his partners resisted his violent behaviours, and finally sought treatment when he feared that his aggressive and sadistic impulses could no longer be contained.

Although Stoller and Glasser focussed on the early relationship with the mother, patients with perversions and paraphilic disorders often have pervasive histories of childhood traumas, abuse or rejection in later childhood or adolescence and may have been prematurely sexualised via experiences of overt childhood sexual abuse, or more covertly sexualised such as being prematurely exposed to pornography. Normal psychosexual developmental is hijacked and sexual impulses may become confused with aggressive impulses arising from prior experiences of maltreatment or neglect. Such individuals frequently describe a very disturbed sense of self in which feelings of self-disgust, shame and humiliation predominate.

Female Violence and Perversion

The forensic psychotherapy patient or offender has been referred to as male throughout the chapter as the majority of violent and sexual offences are carried out by men. Women, of course, can also exhibit violent and perverse behaviour, as well as break the law in other ways such as theft, fraud and prostitution, but their profile of violent and offending behaviour tends to be different in that they are more likely to direct their aggression towards themselves, by self-harm, than towards others. Welldon challenged the traditional psychoanalytic view that perversions did not exist in women [23]. She believed that the genesis of female perversions, as Glasser proposed was the case for male perversions in his concept of the core complex, was based on the struggle to separate from a terrifying and overwhelming maternal object, but unlike male perversions where the aggression was overtly sexualised, located in the genitals and directed at an external object or person, Welldon proposed that in perverse women the perverse act was in the form of an aggressive attack on their own bodies, or the bodies of their children. Welldon suggested that sometimes women unconsciously choose motherhood for perverse purposes, using their own bodies, including their reproductive systems, as vehicles for the expression of unconscious conflict, often stemming from a neglectful or abusive relationship with their mothers.

Motz extended Welldon's work on female perversions to considering the psychology of female violence in general [24], and described how the baby can become the receptacle for the mother's unconscious violent impulses and toxic feelings directed towards her own mother, leading to transgenerational patterns of abuse. Both Welldon and Motz posit that such women are not able to view their children as separate individuals but experience them as narcissistic extensions of themselves, using them for the expression of their own unconscious needs and unresolved conflict, which may result in violence towards the child. Infanticide and Munchausen's syndrome by proxy (fabricated or induced illness) may be seen as extreme examples of female perversions where the woman's murderous fantasies towards herself and her own mother are split off and not available to her conscious mind.

What Does the Forensic Psychotherapist Do?

Working in Forensic Settings

Forensic psychotherapists work in a variety of forensic settings within both the NHS and the criminal justice system including high secure institutions and prisons, medium secure units, community forensic teams and the courts to promote psychotherapeutic work. Although this is informed primarily by a psychoanalytic or psychodynamic perspective, the forensic psychotherapist must have the capacity to work as part of a multidisciplinary team where a variety of modalities of treatment are offered.

The forensic psychotherapist can contribute to the therapeutic work within the forensic team or setting in a number of ways. Direct clinical work involves the assessment of patients to see if they might be suitable for psychodynamic therapy, or to provide a psychodynamic formulation to enhance the patient's overall treatment and risk management plan. He or she may treat patients themselves in individual or group psychoanalytic or psychodynamic psychotherapy or supervise others in doing so, as well as attending ward rounds, case conferences and other meetings to provide psychoanalytically informed opinions regarding patients' treatment.

Consultation to Forensic Institutions

One of the most important roles of the forensic psychotherapist is to provide supervision or consultation to the institution. The propensity of violent and antisocial individuals to project their anxieties and aggression into those around them inevitably has an emotional impact on staff tasked to care for or manage them, who may unconsciously defend themselves against these projections in unhelpful or unhealthy ways, such as overly punitive responses to patients, interprofessional disputes and rivalries, or sickness and burnout. The institution as a whole may become dysfunctional and fragmented as a result of the staff group unconsciously employing pathological group defences and maladaptive solutions to protect themselves against the intense anxieties generated by working with highly disturbed patients. The task of the forensic psychotherapist is to facilitate and promote reflective forums aimed at restoring the healthy cohesion of the group – whether this comprises members of the ward, the multidisciplinary team or the whole institution – where staff can come together in a non-threatening way to think about their conscious and unconscious countertransference feelings and responses to their patients and clients and how these are enacted within the service or organisation in which they work. Such meetings may be case discussion groups which revolve around discussion of a particular patient, or reflective practice groups which look more explicitly at the dynamics within the group which may reflect those of the institution as a whole.

Risk Assessment

Consideration of clinicians' countertransference feelings towards their patients also constitutes an important contribution of psychoanalytic thinking towards risk assessment. Inadequate analysis of the clinician's emotional responses to the patient can contribute to subjective judgements that interfere with more objective evaluations of risk, and may in themselves increase risk. Certain offences, such as the abuse of children, may provoke anxiety, outrage or disgust in professionals which may elicit unconscious punitive or sadistic responses, so that the risk of the patient to others is exaggerated and interventions may be instituted which are unwarranted such as prolonged incarceration or physical restraint. On the other hand, clinicians' empathic responses to their patients' abusive histories and experiences as victims in childhood may cloud their recognition of the patient's aggression such that the risk he poses to others is underestimated.

Working with the Courts

Forensic psychotherapists are increasingly active in medico-legal work, in providing expert opinions in both criminal and family courts, where judges often welcome a more nuanced psychodynamic understanding of the defendant's behaviour linked to their personality and developmental history than more traditional forensic psychiatric court reports which focus solely on mental illness. However, when a therapist's patient becomes involved in legal proceedings it may be in the patient's best interest if an independent clinician assesses the patient for any reports required by the courts, to mitigate against interference in the therapeutic alliance and the patient's motivation for therapy by protecting the confidential nature of the therapeutic process.

Forensic Psychotherapies

The majority of psychological treatments available for forensic patients and offenders within both health and criminal justice settings derive from a cognitive-behavioural framework such as relapse prevention programmes, anger and violence management programmes, sex offender treatment programmes, and treatments based on risk–need–responsivity principles. The availability of psychodynamic or psychoanalytic psychotherapies is less widespread, although there is some provision within prisons and in secure and community forensic mental health settings within the NHS in the UK. Moreover, psychological treatments for offenders are often mandatory, as part of a licence condition, or for patients detained under the Mental Health Act, and therefore genuine engagement in psychotherapy may be hampered by the individual not coming of their own free will. Many offenders are distrustful and resistant to thinking of themselves as patients in need of help, as this is associated with vulnerability and abusive experiences of care from those originally tasked to look after them. Ideally, forensic psychotherapy should be long term given the degree of psychopathology and entrenched nature of the patients' problematic behaviours. At the same time, the aims of treatment should be realistic, as long-term therapy is not readily available within today's NHS given its financial constraints and investment in shorter-term therapies that have been able to establish more of an evidence base than forensic psychotherapy to date.

Individual Psychoanalytic Psychotherapy

Even if they are seeking therapy voluntarily, forensic patients and offenders, who often have difficulties in mentalising, emotional instability and poor impulse control, may not fulfil conventional suitability criteria for traditional individual psychoanalytic psychotherapy such as psychological mindedness, the capacity to tolerate anxiety and the ability to make links between past and present and so many forensic psychotherapists advocate lowering of the threshold for acceptance for psychotherapy as well as flexibility in psychotherapeutic technique. This would include the therapist avoiding encouraging free association or the use of long silences as these may be perceived as persecutory; interpretations should be worded simply and focus on the here and now rather than reconstructions of the past; early interpretations of unconscious conflicts and fantasies should be avoided as the patient may find this strange and disturbing; and similarly premature interpretations of the transference should be avoided, especially the negative transference, as this may be perceived by the patient as critical and retaliatory. The therapy should be more focussed on the patient's preconscious thoughts and feelings, helping him to connect his internal states of mind to his behavioural actions, particularly focussing on the role of affect, especially negative affects, such as anxiety, shame and humiliation, that underlie the offending behaviours. A balance, which is often precarious, needs to be found in order to engage the person in a meaningful therapeutic process, between fostering in the patient a sense of curiosity, exploration and self-awareness into the workings of his mind, and ensuring that his defences are not prematurely breached so that he becomes overwhelmed with disturbing memories, feelings, thoughts and impulses which become impossible to contain and are acted out in destructive behaviours. The patient's risk of harm to others may be at the forefront of people's minds but the risk of self-harm and suicide should not be overlooked.

Although direct interpretations of the transference may not be tolerated, the therapist's awareness and monitoring of transference and countertransference dynamics between patient and therapist and their meaning is essential, particularly in providing insight into disturbances in the patient's internal object relationships, how these have been shaped by their early experiences, and how these in turn influence their relationships with others. The therapist should be alert to how the patient's offending behaviour and underlying conflicts might become enacted within the transference to the therapist: for example, a violent patient might behave in an overly compliant way as a defence against his fear of losing control and becoming aggressive towards his therapist; a more perverse patient may alternate between seeming emotionally available and open to exploration followed by states of being more distant and missing sessions, reflecting his struggle with core complex anxieties in becoming too close to and dependent on the patient; sessions may become overtly sexualised with the patient flirting with the therapist and pushing the boundaries of the therapeutic frame; or the patient may experience the therapist as overly critical reflecting a projection of his harsh superego onto the person of the therapist.

The therapist's countertransference should be closely monitored, and as with professionals working in forensic institutions, as described above, the importance of the role of ongoing supervision should not be underestimated in providing a protected space to reflect on and explore the therapist's unconscious reactions to the patient. For example, the therapist may be unwittingly drawn into colluding with the patient in minimising the seriousness of their offences, or into a sadomasochistic relationship mirroring the patient's external relationships, where the therapist finds herself being 'abused' by the patient in him missing sessions or being denigratory or contemptuous, and then responding in a punitive, critical or humiliating way, such as giving the patient complex transference interpretations that he cannot grasp.

Forensic Group Psychotherapy [25]

For many violent, antisocial and sexually perverse patients, group therapy may be the treatment of choice. For patients who fear losing control of their impulses, group therapy can be less anxiety provoking than individual therapy where the intensity of the relationship with the therapist may feel overwhelming. In a group the multiple transferences between the different group members and the therapist offer each patient potentially more than one target for their aggression, which may paradoxically diffuse their levels of anxiety and arousal. Group therapy may also provide relief in being with others struggling with similar difficulties; offers more opportunities for mentalisation than in individual therapy, in there being several other minds in the room; and facilitates the modelling of more appropriate behaviour and interpersonal interactions. The group can act as a socio-familial microcosm in which the offender's interactions with other group members can be understood as reflecting the pathological dynamics of their original familial experiences [26] and the perpetuation of these difficulties in their current relationships. As with individual therapy, the patients' offending behaviours will become manifest within the group: for example, the exhibitionist may dominate and excite the group with lurid stories of his offending, then not attend subsequent sessions, leaving the group feeling that he has 'flashed' to them and disappeared; or at the other extreme, the patient convicted of voyeurism who silently observes others in the group and is experienced as secretive and violating of their privacy. Patients whose activities involve secretiveness and deception, such as the perpetration of sexual abuse, can be more effectively challenged in a group in penetrating pervasive patterns of evasiveness and deception.

Other Therapeutic Interventions

Forensic psychoanalytic psychotherapy has been developed for the treatment of child, adolescents, their families and carers [27] and also for individuals with intellectual learning disabilities [28].

Specific psychological psychotherapies that were originally developed from a psychoanalytic model for the treatment of borderline personality disorder have been in the past decade increasingly applied to forensic patients. In the UK, mentalisation-based treatment (MBT) has been adapted for the treatment of individuals with antisocial personality disorder (ASPD) [29] and its efficacy is currently being evaluated in a large multisite randomised controlled trial for male violent offenders with ASPD under the supervision of the National Probation Service, as part of the Offender Personality Disorder Pathway. MBT groups are also currently offered in several prisons in the UK. In Germany, transference-focussed therapy has been used for some years in the treatment of offenders.

Therapeutic community approaches have been used for many years in the treatment of offenders and patients diagnosed with ASPD. In the UK, the first prison therapeutic community was established at HMP Grendon Underwood in Buckinghamshire in 1962. Several other therapeutic communities in different British prisons have also been established since, including the world's only prison democratic therapeutic community for women at HMP Send, in Surrey.

The Offender Personality Disorder Pathway [30] was initiated in 2011, jointly commissioned by the UK NHS and criminal justice system to identify, assess, manage and treat high risk male and female offenders with personality disorder in prisons, secure hospitals and the community, and is specifically underpinned by a psychoanalytically informed developmental model of personality disorder. It promotes education of the workforce about personality disorder towards the goal of creating more therapeutic environments in prisons and secure hospitals, with an expansion in democratic therapeutic communities and the creation of psychologically informed planned environments. It also offers a range of specialised psychotherapeutic interventions for offenders with personality disorder, including MBT.

Training in Forensic Psychotherapy

Until recently, formal training pathways to specialise in forensic psychotherapy were limited to medically qualified professionals. Forensic psychotherapy was formally recognised as a sub-specialty of psychiatry in 1999 and involves a five-year higher specialty dual training which integrates the two psychiatric sub-specialties of medical psychotherapy and forensic psychiatry. Eight training posts currently exist in forensic psychotherapy in the UK.

Non-medical psychotherapists did not have a well-defined clinical training route to qualify in forensic psychotherapy until 2014, when the British Psychoanalytic Council formally approved a new clinical training in forensic psychotherapy: the Forensic Psychodynamic Psychotherapy course (D59 F) at the Tavistock and Portman NHS Foundation Trust. This course last two years and require trainees to see patients under supervision as well as having their own personal psychotherapy.

References

1. Welldon E. Definition of forensic psychotherapy and its aims. *Int J Appl Psychoanal Stud* 2015; 12: 96–105.

2. Menninger KA. *The Crime of Punishment.* New York: Viking, 1968.

3. Freud S. Remembering, repeating and working through (further recommendations on the technique of psycho-analysis II). In J Strachey, ed., *The Standard Edition of the Complete Psychological Works of Sigmund Freud, Volume XII (1911–1913): Case History of Schreber, Papers on Technique and Other Works.* London: Hogarth Press. 1958; pp. 145–56. (Original work published 1914)

4. Yakeley J, Williams A. Antisocial personality disorder: new directions. *Adv Psychiatr Treat* 2014; 20: 132–43.

5. Yakeley J. *Working with Violence – A Contemporary Psychoanalytic Approach.* London: Palgrave Macmillan, 2010.

6. Freud S. Some character-types met with in psycho-analytic work: III Criminals from a sense of guilt. In J Strachey, ed., *The Standard Edition of the Complete Psychological Works of Sigmund Freud, Volume XIV (1914–1916): On the History of the Psycho-Analytic Movement, Papers on Metapsychology and Other Works.* London: Hogarth Press. 1957; pp. 311–33. (Original work published 1916)

7. Freud S. Beyond the pleasure principle. In J Strachey, ed., *The Standard Edition of the Complete Psychological Works of Sigmund Freud, Volume XVIII (1920–1922): Beyond the Pleasure Principle, Group Psychology and Other Works.* London: Hogarth Press. 1955; pp. 1–64. (Original work published 1920)

8. Klein M. Criminal tendencies in normal children. *Br J Med Psychol* 1927; 7: 177–92.

9. Klein M. Notes on some schizoid mechanisms. In M Klein, ed., *Envy and Gratitude and Other Works.* London: Vintage. 1946; pp. 1–24.

10. Klein M. A contribution to the psychogenesis of manic depressive states. In M. Klein, ed., *Love, Guilt and Reparation and Other Works 1921–1945.* London: Vintage. 1935; pp. 262–89.

11. Winnicott DW. *Playing and Reality.* London: Tavistock, 1971.

12. Winnicott DW. The anti-social tendency. In *Through Paediatrics to Psychoanalysis.* London: Hogarth Press, 1984; pp. 306–15.

13. Winnicott DW. *Deprivation and Delinquency.* London: Tavistock, 1986.

14. Bowlby J. Forty-four juvenile thieves: their characters and home life. *Int J Psychoanal* 1944; 25: 1–57.

15. De Zulueta F. *From Pain to Violence.* London: Wiley, 2006.

16. Gilligan J. *Violence: Our Deadliest Epidemic and its Causes.* New York: Grosset/Putnam, 1996.

17. McGauley G, Yakeley J, Williams A, Bateman A. Attachment, mentalization and antisocial personality disorder; the possible contribution of mentalization-based treatment. *Eur J Psychother Couns* 2011; 13: 1–22.

18. Meloy JR. *Violent Attachments.* Northvale, NJ: Jason Aronson, 1992.

19. Yakeley J Psychoanalytic perspectives on paraphilias and perversions. *Eur J Psychother Couns* 2018; 20: 164–83.

20. Freud S. Three essays on the theory of sexuality. In J Strachey, ed., *The Standard Edition of the Complete Psychological Works of Sigmund Freud, Volume VII (1901–1905): A Case of Hysteria, Three Essays on Sexuality and Other Works.* London: Hogarth Press. 1953; pp. 125–248. (Original work published 1905)

21. Stoller RJ. *Perversion.* New York: Pantheon, 1975.

22. Glasser M. Aggression and sadism in the perversions. In: I Rosen, ed., *Sexual Deviation*, 3rd ed. Oxford: Oxford University Press. 1996; pp. 278–305.

23. Welldon E. *Mother, Madonna, Whore: The Idealization and Denigration of Motherhood.* London: Karnac Books, 2004.

24. Motz A. *The Psychology of Female Violence: Crimes Against the Body*, 2nd ed. London and New York: Routledge, 2008.

25. Woods J, Williams A (eds.). *Forensic Group Psychotherapy: The Portman Clinic Approach*. London: Karnac Books, 2014.

26. Welldon E. Group-analytic psychotherapy in an out-patient setting. In C Cordess, M Cox, eds., *Forensic Psychotherapy: Crime, Psychodynamics and the Offender Patient*. London and Philadelphia: Jessica Kingsley Publishers. 1996; pp. 63–83.

27. Music G (ed.). Special forensic issue. *J Child Psychother* 2016; 42: 257–384.

28. Corbett A. *Disabling Perversions: Forensic Psychotherapy with Children and Adults with Intellectual Disabilities*. London: Karnac Books, 2014.

29. Bateman A, Fonagy P. *Mentalization-Based Treatment for Personality Disorders: A Practical Guide*. Oxford: Oxford University Press, 2016.

30. NHS England. *Offender Personality Disorder Strategy* 2015.

Chapter

The Effect on Staff and Organisations of Working with Patients with Psychotic Illness

Rachel Gibbons

Introduction

Clinical work with patients who have psychotic illness is rewarding; however, it is also psychologically demanding. The more challenging side of this work is not often emphasised in routine psychiatric practice. There are powerful unconscious processes present in psychosis that have strong countertransference effects that need to be understood and worked with.

This chapter links with Chapter 14 and highlights relevant aspects of psychoanalytic theory. Case examples are used to illustrate the countertransference effects of this work, on individual clinicians, teams and the care organisation itself. Interventions that reduced the impact, alleviate the risks and improve clinical care will be recommended. The novel clinical material is drawn from the experience of the author as psychiatric consultant, and psychoanalyst. Most of the case examples are composites drawn from inpatient work where these experiences can be seen most distinctly: they will hopefully be recognisable to those working in frontline services.

Theory

The Psychotic versus the Non-psychotic Part of the Personality

Wilfred Bion, one of the first psychoanalysts to analyse individuals in a psychotic state, described a universal division or split in the mind that results in two parts to the personality. On one side is the healthy developmental 'non-psychotic' part which strives to cope with emotional pain, engage with life, grow and develop: this part is able to make contact with others and ask for help when it is needed. On the other side is the 'psychotic' part of the personality which hates reality, and mounts 'sadistic attacks' on the thinking process, fragmenting thoughts which are then projected into the outside world: this 'psychotic part' attacks any connection with others and any need for help [1]. Each part functions separately, has little awareness of the other and fights for dominance of the mind.

Roger Money-Kyrle, a psychoanalyst with a background in philosophy who was analysed by both Freud and Klein, developed these ideas further. He portrayed the two parts as two sides, a 'sane side' 'painfully acquired' during development, and a 'chaotic side'. His opinion was that sanity may be 'no more than an island ... in a sea of chaos' which throughout life continues to exist unconsciously. In those that developed a psychotic illness the 'chaotic side' has ascendency; however, the 'sane side' is still there and available for contact [2].

Richard Lucas, an adult psychiatrist and psychoanalyst already mentioned in Chapter 14 who worked as an inpatient psychiatric consultant at St Ann's Hospital in North London, applied Bion's ideas to the reality and the challenges of working with psychotic illness on the front line of mental health. In his influential and unique book *The Psychotic Wavelength* [3] published just before his death in 2008, Lucas states that our 'normal' or 'neurotic' sensitivities can be likened to being on 'wavelength 1', while the psychotic patient may be operating on an entirely different radio frequency, 'wavelength 1,000'. If we want to be able to work effectively with patients suffering with psychotic illness we need to tune into 'this psychotic wavelength'. To do this requires us to continually bear in mind the two separate parts of the personality as described by Bion. We need to ask ourselves which part we are being confronted by at any particular moment in time. Lucas warns that if we are not aware of this risk we are in danger of missing underlying psychosis. If we are mindful of this, it means that 'there is always a part of the patient that we can talk to about the way that their psychotic part is operating' [3]. He was a great proponent of the use of humour in clinical work. He gives a lovely example where he and his patient's 'non-psychotic' part have a joke at the expense of 'the psychotic part'.

> *My patient on admission said that he was God's older brother, but smiled and joined me in the reflexive position when I said that he must have been really pissed off with his younger brother getting all the publicity.*   [3, p. 155]

In clinical settings the battle between the 'psychotic' or 'sane' versus the 'non-psychotic' or 'chaotic' is ongoing in staff and patients alike. Mutual and powerful projective processes go on all the time between both groups. The psychotic part of the staff's mind can be projected, located and attributed to the patients and the sane part of the patients can likewise be projected into the staff. This give the impression that there is a clear division between the staff, who are entirely sane, and the patients who are seen as entirely mad. This is not the case and this perception can be a barrier to understanding the patients. Sane communications from the patients may then be missed or dismissed.

> *William was admitted for the first time to the ward shortly after his 75th birthday. He was unwell with a depressive psychotic illness. He had a delusional belief that he was dead. He repeatedly told the ward team that he had to go home to look after his dead mother. The ward team assumed that this was a delusional belief. One of the Occupational Therapist's went with him to do a home visit and found a lady in her 90s living in an upstairs room.*

This feeling of walking a tightrope between 'psychosis' and 'non-psychosis' is further heightened by the level of 'psychotic' or 'primitive' anxiety that is ever present in clinical teams. 'Psychotic anxiety' is a term initially used by Bion to describe the anxiety that accompanies the ego disintegration in psychosis. This anxiety results from the unconscious awareness of the fragmentation of the mind. It is more severe than 'neurotic' anxiety where the ego remains intact. This primal terror can lead to unpredictable desperate and destructive behaviour, such as suicide or violence. Staff working in this environment have to tolerate this ever-constant feeling of threat which heightens their tension, leaving them close to their own psychotic functioning.

Countertransference

The primitive and powerful defences used by the psychotic part of the mind – denial, projection, splitting and rationalisation – are ubiquitous from very early in life. They are easily activated and have a strong countertransference and controlling effect on the unwary clinician.

Lucas makes a very strong argument for those working with psychotic illness to be constantly aware that the commonest symptoms of psychosis are not hallucinations, delusions or first rank symptoms, but in over 95 per cent of cases, denial and rationalisation dominate. These defences are used by the 'psychotic part' of the mind to try 'to cover up its murderousness' [3, p. 142]. It is murderous because it wants to totally destroy the sane part of the mind.

The Clinicians

Particularly potent countertransference responses to a patient with a psychotic illness include:

1. Denying or disregarding the patient's history
2. Accepting the rationalisation of the 'psychotic' part of the patient
3. Mental confusion
4. Concretisation of thinking
5. Overidentification with projected sadism

The risk of being overwhelmed increases if the clinician is seeing the patient for the first time, and/or on their own. Money-Kyrle said that enormous forces are used by the 'chaotic' part of the mind to 'convert, pervert or override' the threat of the 'sane' parts, not only of the patient themselves but also of others [2]. The risk of being overwhelmed is minimised when the clinician knows the patient and their history, and if a third person is present at the assessment. In this latter case each assessor can rely on the other to check the reality and likelihood of what they are being told and to take into consideration their countertransference responses.

Denying or Disregarding a Patient's History

Diagnosis in psychiatry is a complex and conflictual area. A reliable diagnosis is generally determined over a significant period of time. Psychiatrists are currently trained to follow a psychiatric diagnostic hierarchy which forms the basis for classification systems such as the International Classification of Diseases (ICD) and Diagnostic and Statistical Manual (DSM). Each level of the hierarchy needs to be ruled out before a diagnosis from a lower level can be confirmed. For example, an organic cause for illness needs to be ruled out before a psychotic illness can be diagnosed, a psychotic illness before a mood disorder and mood disorder before a personality disorder. A patient's psychiatric history is also very important in reaching a diagnosis – what has happened before is likely to happen again. Delusions that have been present in the past tend to emerge in a similar form in each episode of illness. If there has been a serious psychotic illness in the past a recurrence cannot be ruled out.

The powerful projective countertransference effects of psychosis that overwhelm the clinician frequently result in the disregarding or denial of the psychiatric diagnostic hierarchy and the history of the patient.

Catherine was brought in with contractures of muscles in her hands and legs from lack of mobility over several months. She had been lying on her sofa not moving, she had very poor self-care, and recently had not been eating, drinking or washing. She had had a diagnosis of psychotic illness earlier in her life, with two episodes with clearly recorded psychotic symptoms. She had been seen by a locum consultant in an outpatient clinic. At the time she was taking antipsychotic medication, but the consultant felt very provoked, frustrated and irritated in the clinical interaction with her and as a result decided she had a personality disorder. He stopped her medication and changed the diagnosis on her records to borderline personality disorder. Over the next nine months, she deteriorated physically and mentally. She was seen by the community team and even though there was clear evidence of a profound decline it was repeatedly put down to 'acting out'. No medication was given, and no admission offered. When Catherine was finally admitted she was close to death. She was started back on antipsychotic medication and recovered.

Although extreme, this scenario is seen frequently in a less severe form and illustrates how dangerous it can be when clinical management is powerfully influenced by unmetabolised countertransference reactions. The splitting, denial and rationalisation is projected, and a clinician who does not know the patient well changes the diagnosis due to their immediate countertransference experience. The history is discounted, and the psychotic diagnosis overwritten with a one lower in the hierarchy. The team can then become divided and entrenched diagnostically. Psychotic illness is higher up the psychiatric diagnostic hierarchy than a personality disorder. If psychosis cannot be ruled out it needs to be retained as a possibility. Personality disorder services can get frequent referrals of patients on high doses of antipsychotic medication with a clear history of psychosis over many years. It is also not uncommon for a very disturbed patient with a persistent diagnosis of personality disorder, who actually has an undiagnosed psychotic illness, to be admitted to an acute psychiatric ward and fully recover with antipsychotic medication.

Accepting the Rationalisation of the Psychotic Part of the Patient's Mind

In the following case Helen, a medical student, met with Philip, a recent admission to the psychiatric inpatient ward, for an assessment on her own. She presented Philip's history in the ward round to the team.

Helen seemed preoccupied and said she was puzzled as to why Philip was in hospital. Surely the ward staff should be more concerned with his neighbour who pursued him, listening to his every move, banging on the floor and walls wherever Philip was sitting so he had no peace. This neighbour would record him, Helen said, and would lie in wait to abuse him and tell him to kill himself when he left the flat. She said that Philip had discussed it with his mother, but he realised that she was conspiring with the neighbour. He said he had also tried reporting this to the police, but he became aware that they too were in this conspiracy. Helen asked why were the ward team not helping him get the appropriate prosecution started? As she was recounting this history out loud, she started to realise that the reality may not be quite as Philip had outlined it.

In this case Helen had been pulled into accepting the rationalising of the psychotic part of Philip and lost her own contact with reality. It was only when others were present, and she could see the doubt they expressed that she could reconnect. This experience is a frequent one because rationalisation is a very powerful defence. We often do not want to believe how unwell our patient is, or we may want to believe that they are getting better when they are not.

Mental Confusion

Another common countertransference response to psychotic illness is confusion. Lucas describes the reason for this:

The clinician's countertransference feelings will mirror the patient's state of mind. If they have projected feelings that they have experienced as totally unbearable and have murderously attacked, then the clinician's mind will be affected so that he or she feels deskilled, unable to think or have constructive associations [3].

In the following case example, the psychotic attacks on mental linking that have resulted in Edith's psychosis infiltrate the mind of Dr Ball, whose thoughts also lose coherence and fragment.

Dr Ball had returned from holiday refreshed and relaxed. His first job on returning to the ward was to review Edith a newly admitted patient. When he had been talking to her for a while, he realised he wasn't able to concentrate. He tried to pull his thoughts together but struggled and within a very short space of time he had lost track again. He couldn't remember the question he had asked, or quite grasp why Edith was saying what she was saying. This happened repeatedly. He found that his mind felt 'fuzzy' and he couldn't remember why he was meeting with Edith in the first place. Once he left the room his thinking recovered.

In this example Dr Ball recognised that his experience of confusion was a countertransference response because he was aware that it occurred specifically when he was sitting and talking to Edith. Before the assessment, and following a period of recovery after the meeting, his thinking was clear.

Concretisation of Thinking

In psychosis, symbolic function is lost and thinking becomes concrete. Concretisation of thinking is also a very common countertransference experience. A staff member may have a good thinking capacity in general but lose the capacity to think symbolically at times when in the working environment.

Dr Lee was generally a calm, containing and thoughtful clinician. She had a busy outpatient clinic and was reaching the end of the day. She was tired and running late. Eric was an older patient who had been referred by his GP for forgetfulness and suspected dementia. Dr Lee quickly tested Eric's mental functioning, which was reasonable. She grumbled to herself about the referral. She told Eric she need not see him again and wrote a reassuring discharge letter to the GP. However, later that evening when she had more space to think she started to feel uneasy and anxious: something had not been right in the consultation. She phoned Eric and asked him to return to the clinic the following day. On further questioning he reported significant delusional symptoms believing he was dead, and that suicide made perfect sense to him. His apparent memory difficulties were a symptom of depression.

In this case Dr Lee's mind had been concretised and she could only 'do' and not 'think'. Symbolic thinking could only return when she had space to reflect later that evening.

Overidentification with Projected Sadism

An aspect of the battle between the psychotic and non-psychotic parts of the personality is that the superego (conscious) can start to act in keeping with the psychotic part and become persecutory and sadistic. In this state the superego derives excitement from humiliating and threatening the ego which is trying to keep contact with reality. In this state the superego attacks thought processes, severing links and threatening the individual with psychic annihilation [4]. For the patient to have some respite from the destructive forces in the internal world and to allow psychic space to recover, the superego needs to redirect these sadistic attacks into the external environment for a period of time. This projection of sadism is unpleasant: recipients need to be resilient and take care not to overidentify and to start to believe that they are sadistic. It is important for the multidisciplinary team to be able to tolerate and recognise the countertransference experience of sadism in order to work in a healthy way with those struggling with a psychotic illness.

> *Otis was very unwell. He was deluded and self-destructive. He accused the staff of being abusers and cowered in his room terrified of them. The consultant and the team found it very difficult to give him medication because they would have to physically intervene to do so. They said this would make them feel like sadistic abusers, so they could not act, and Otis remained unwell. Eventually he had to be transferred to a psychiatric intensive care unit where the staff were more used to these painful projections. He returned to the ward having been established on an injectable form of medication given on a monthly basis, and far more stable in his mental state.*

The System

Some examples of the countertransference responses to the work with psychotic illness by the system include:

1. Splitting of the system around the patient. The Jigsaw
2. Rationalisation and denial of psychosis by the Mental Health Review Tribunal
3. Enactment of psychotic functioning by the whole staff team

Splitting of the System around the Patient. The 'Jigsaw'

In psychotic illness the mind becomes fragmented. The fragments are then projected into the external world, freeing the patient from painful awareness of mental disintegration. The multidisciplinary team, family and friends become containers for these fragments and so can pick up and identify with different conflicting parts of the patient's mind. This can result in splitting in the professional, social and family network around a patient. If recognised and worked with, this becomes a strength providing important information for the treating team. If this splitting is not engaged with it becomes a dangerous vulnerability and each faction can become hostile and dismissive of the others. Lucas describes the work of the review, or ward round, 'as like assembling the pieces of a jigsaw puzzle where you do not know who will bring the most important piece' [3, p. 147].

This fragmenting process can happen prior to admission when an individual becomes very unwell with a psychotic illness. Family and friends can fall out with each other and the patient.

> *Yasim was brought to the ward by the police. He was clearly very unwell and unkempt. He said he had no family, no friends and no home and wouldn't give a name. He was looked after on the ward and started taking antipsychotic medication. Gradually he gave the ward team some information about his brother whom the team then contacted. Yasim's brother was angry and said he did not want to hear from the ward. He said he could not cope anymore. He said their parents were ill and it was too much for all of them. He did, however, give contact details for their sister. She was concerned and came to the ward review to represent the family. Gradually as Yasim started to improve and the psychosis receded, the weekly meetings became more populated with family members, who re-engaged with each other and began planning the future with Yasim.*

This is a very common scenario. As the patient gets better the fragmented system around them reintegrates. This tends to be a reliable indicator of improvement and the recovery of the patient's mind. This concept is the driving force behind the 'Open Dialogue' model of care where the patient is seen as part of a network and the focus of intervention is the system (see Chapter 26).

The following example illustrates a relatively common example of where a whole team, in this case on a ward, identified with the rationalising 'psychotic part' of the patient.

> Zaheer wanted to be discharged home from the ward. Everyone in the ward team agreed with discharge as Zaheer appeared to be better than when admitted a month previously. The discharge was planned somewhat prematurely for that Friday afternoon due to Zaheer's apparent enthusiasm to go to a distant family member's birthday party at the weekend. Due to the fast planning, and counter to the team's usual practice, Zaheer's Care Coordinator/Key Worker had not been informed about the plan. The Key Worker phoned up alarmed, saying he had only been informed about the discharge by Zaheer that morning on the phone. He said that during the conversation Zaheer still seemed very unwell. The ward team initially wanted to hold onto the split from the Care Coordinator and dismiss his concerns, agreeing that he just was not keen for Zaheer's discharge because it was challenging to provide care for him in the community. However, to be on the safe side they postponed the discharge. Later that evening they found all the medication Zaheer had been given while in hospital hidden under his mattress. Once the team had found the medication Zaheer became manifestly acutely psychotic.

In this case the 'non-psychotic' part of Zaheer was letting the Care Coordinator know that he was still unwell and that the 'psychotic' part had tricked the team. Once Zaheer knew that the team were aware he was unwell he could relax his defences. In this case it was the Key Worker that held the key piece of the jigsaw.

Rationalisation and Denial of Psychosis by the Mental Health Review Tribunal

Rationalisation and denial of psychosis can be projected into Mental Health Tribunals. These Tribunals are a very important part of the legal and human rights process when someone is deprived of their liberty and detained under the Mental Health Act. These panels consist of a Lawyer, a Lay Member and an Independent Psychiatrist. During the hearing evidence about the need for detention is provided by the treating team whom are then cross-examined by the patient's solicitor who speaks on their behalf. The tribunal then make a decision as to whether the detention should continue or not. If they decide that the section is not warranted it is lifted there and then and the patient can leave hospital the same day. This is a situation where the legalistic approach and the lack of experience and understanding of the countertransference effects of psychosis can determine decision-making. The tribunal can at times align with the rationalising 'psychotic' part of the patient against the 'non-psychotic' part represented by the psychiatric team.

> Mark was a powerful city lawyer. He was admitted to the ward in a manic state. Immediately there were problems. He repeatedly said that he was going to sue the staff and report them to their professional bodies. They were then too intimidated and frightened to treat him. He was elated and manic. He intruded into everyone's space, propositioning them, took their things, and wanting to talk to all the visitors to the ward. He phoned the police and ambulance services 5 to 10 times a day complaining of being incarcerated and held against his will. He managed to get the private phone numbers of the ward consultant, whom he phoned repeatedly. He succeeded in

getting access to a computer and bought thousands of pounds worth of goods that were constantly being delivered to the ward. Mark appealed against his detention immediately after admission and had a tribunal after two weeks in the hospital.

Mark attended his tribunal presenting himself very well. He dressed in his suit and behaved like the lawyer he was when well. The tribunal allowed him to cross-examine the consultant, which was not normal practice. Although the consultant reported Mark's recent history of disturbance, the tribunal found him to be well and decided that he could be discharged from hospital. The following week the police returned Mark to the ward after he took his clothes off in a high-end restaurant in a popular part of London. On readmission, he was clearly in a poor state.

Enactment of Psychotic Functioning by the Whole Staff Team

Herbert Rosenfeld, an analyst who worked alongside Bion, likened the internal functioning of the disturbed part of the mind to a powerful gang dominated by a leader, very like the Mafia. This gang threatens the healthy part of the psyche when it tries to elicit help. This illustrated why it is so difficult at times to tip the balance to health from destructive functioning [5].

When the staff team are overwhelmed this ever-present and pervasive gang can be projected whole-heartedly into the team [6]. The whole environment can then function on 'the psychotic wavelength' without the staff realising that this is the case. The team then starts working to its own delusional rules disconnected from external reality. The effect can be profound, as in the following example.

One of the mental health wards had suffered a very serious inpatient death by suicide. The team were traumatised and had accessed no support to process the loss and shock. The consultant and ward manager had left the organisation following the internal inquiry. The team lost confidence and felt abandoned without the containment of clinical leadership. They were working with very unwell male patients and had become very frightened of taking any risks in treating them, fearing any intervention might lead to another death. There were no discharges and no admissions. The team were overwhelmed, there were frequent staff and patient assaults, they became fearful of the patients, and felt there was no point in asking their managers for help and instead reassured them that everything was OK. They took refuge in the nurses' station where they stuck paper up over the windows so they could not be seen and could not see out. A new doctor who went onto the ward to work said that the staff team on the ward felt like a 'gang' and she felt left out and paranoid. The Gym Instructor and the Ward Clerk, neither of whom was clinically trained, appeared to have most authority in the team. The patients remained untreated, psychotic and disturbed. They spent much of the day and night banging on the doors and windows of the papered-up nurses' station. Finally, a patient set fire to a rubbish bin. No serious damage was done but this triggered an alarm and an investigation by senior management who were appalled that the situation had become this bad. They believed that they had neglected the ward and felt guilty themselves. The ward was closed for a period of time to allow for a full assessment. During this time the staff group were give space to reflect and process previous trauma. The ward reopened three months later in a healthier place, with new leadership, senior support for a weekly reflective practice group, regular senior management input and supervision for all the team members.

In this case the ward team had become paranoid and terrified. There was a loss of structure and healthy authority. It was only with time to think and process that the situation could be resolved.

The Care Organisation

The powerful countertransference effect of the work with patients can permeate health organisation, affecting the systemic processes. Menzies Lyth, a psychoanalyst who had an analysis with Bion, first described these 'Organisational Systems of Defence' in her seminal study: 'A case-study in the functioning of social systems as a defence against anxiety' [7]. This work developed from her observation of nurses in a general medical hospital where she noticed how organisation systems and processes were developed to defend against the life and death anxieties faced by the staff on a daily basis. These social defences allowed the staff to 'avoid anxiety, guilt, doubt and uncertainty' and the organisation to protect staff from mental pain, at the expense of carrying out their real task. She identified the following defences.

- Splitting up the nurse–patient relationship
- Depersonalisation, categorisation, and denial of the significance of the individual
- Detachment and denial of feelings
- The attempt to eliminate decisions by ritual task performance
- Reducing the weight of responsibility in decision-making by checks and counterchecks
- Collusive social redistribution of responsibility and irresponsibility
- Purposeful obscurity in the formal distribution of responsibility
- The reduction of the impact of responsibility by delegation to superiors
- Idealisation and underestimation of personal development possibilities
- Avoidance of change

There are so many examples of how these Organisational Systems of Defence manifest in Mental Health Organisation that it is only possible to list some brief examples. Two case illustrations of relatively common scenarios follow.

1. Idealisation of care possibilities. Collusion with the phantasy that omnipotent care can be provided irrespective of resource and clinical realities
2. Ritualisation of form-filling without any evidence of clinical effectiveness, e.g. Risk Assessment [8]
3. Organisational collusion with the 'psychotic' side of the personality through scapegoating, suspensions and the complaints processes
4. Concretisation of boundaries and projections of badness into other teams
5. Destructive use of email. Projection through the email system of split off aggressive and psychotic aspects of staff functioning
6. Idealisation of new service initiatives and service change processes that become the 'messiah' – coming to rescue the organisation and solve all the problems
7. Collusion with concrete thinking and the belief that reflecting is less important than action or 'doing' activities
8. Idealisation of patient-led care. The staff and patient needs are considered to be in opposition to each other. In this situation it is considered that it is only the patients who need care, which has to be unlimited and unconditional. Patient responsibility is minimised, and the care needs of staff are denied and denigrated
9. Staff 'sickness' covering up and denying mental breakdown
10. Structural enshrining of unhealthy functioning, for example 'the patient is unable to attend the therapy group this morning because it is timetabled at the time of their smoking break'.
11. Use of language to confuse and deny difficulties. 'Cost improvement' for cost cutting, 'pursuit of excellence' denying all developmental struggles etc.

Example 1

In this case, the psychotic parts of patients were activated by the possibility of enlisting the Patient Advice and Complaints (PAC) service and the organisation to amplify the attack on sanity represented by the team and the consultant.

The PAC service decided that they could save time responding to patient complaints by 'nipping them in the bud'. They decided to come every week to the acute inpatient ward and ask the patients if they had any complaints about their treatment. Some of the patients said they were delighted to be asked about this and took up this offer with enthusiasm. After their visits, the consultant regularly received emails from the PAC team with various complaints to be resolved many of which had delusional content. For example, in one the consultant was asked to stop injecting one of the patients at night with hormones transforming him from a man to a woman.

Example 2

The following is a common scenario where the organisation colludes with the psychotic attacks on staff through Human Resource processes.

The mental health trust had a serious nursing crisis. The lack of employed nurses contributed to the lack of containment on the inpatient wards. Each night there were different locum or bank nurses who did not know the patients, the systems or the processes of the wards. The disturbance on the ward increased, as did the financial burden on the Trust.

On one of the acute inpatient wards, a young woman suffering severely with a manic illness took all her clothes off and ran around the ward in a disturbed and vulnerable state. She was finally restrained by the four remaining employed nurses on the ward, two of whom were men. The woman then reported the two male nurses saying that they had sexually assaulted her. They were immediately suspended so as the accusation of sexual assault could be investigated. It took six months before the investigation was completed and they could return to work. They were found to have no case to answer, but their morale and well-being had been profoundly affected and they decided to leave the mental health organisation, further reducing the number of permanent nurses.

How Staff Can Recognise They Are Overwhelmed and at Risk

When clinicians and ward teams are penetrated and controlled by psychotic functioning, they behave in strange and unusual ways without recognition that this is happening. This effect can be subtle or profound, transient or long-lasting resulting in 'burn out'. Some phenomena that can indicate that this has occurred include:

- Acting out of character, or at odds with a previously understood management plan or their usual method of working
- Feeling overwhelmed, fearful and/or angry. They might find themselves sending aggressive emails, losing their temper and/or not sleeping well
- Working late into the evening and find it difficult to separate from the workplace to go home
- Dread of going into the workplace and lack of pleasure in the job
- Feelings of detachment from personal or patient distress

Supportive Reflective Interventions That Increase Staff Resilience

In this environment, the importance of having space to think and reflect on the work cannot be emphasised enough. Reflection is fundamental to ensuring a therapeutic milieu on a ward or in the community. If there is no room to reflect the team becomes overwhelmed and enacts the psychotic disturbance of the patients.

To be effective, alleviating interventions need to be built into the structures and process of the organisational functioning. Broadly these interventions consist of:

1. Regular and reliable spaces to think, reflect and process the work, examples include:

   • Reflective practice groups
   • Supervision
   • Team meetings of different types
   • Risk Forums or Panels

2. Interventions to encourage, nurture and value staff, team and organisational development, examples include:

   • Stable and regularly reviewed ward and team structures, clear timetables that are regularly reviewed
   • Support and work on personal, professional and clinical boundaries
   • The fostering of individual team members' development
   • Organisational staff well-being initiatives
   • Team awaydays

Reflective Practice Groups

Establishing reflective groups in mental health environments can be challenging. The profound attack on thinking that occurs in psychosis can permeate the environment so that any spaces for thinking come under attack. These reflective spaces can then be difficult to launch and retain. To establish these groups often needs some perseverance. They need to be concretely maintained, at the same time and same place, with the same regularity. Having two or more people facilitate the group is very helpful so that if one facilitator cannot attend the group can still continue at the same time (see Chapter 23).

Complex Case/Risk Panels

Many Mental Health Organisations now have Risk Panels that support the thinking of the clinicians in the management of their patients. These are multidisciplinary panels of senior members of the organisation; often including a clinician with psychoanalytically trained perspective can be key in identifying unconscious psychotic processes in the clinical presentation. When clinicians experience a patient as posing a high level of threat or risk to themselves or others it can become very difficult to develop a management plan. The overwhelmed clinicians can bring such patients to the panel where there is space to think with others who are not directly involved and are free of the countertransference effects. The clinicians can also get senior support for their management.

Summary

Working with patients with psychotic illness can be challenging, frightening and disturbing. It is strenuous and demanding work exacerbated by the current climate in health services.

It is important to have space to process the powerful unconscious forces and digest the psychotic material projected. When this does occur this work provides an interesting and a privileged view into the fascinating processes of the unconscious mind. When overwhelmed the deadly pull towards hopelessness can lead staff to lose contact with the reality of how much they are able to help many of their patients. The numerous that have improved, often with almost miraculous transformations occurring over a short period of time, can be forgotten. This chapter concludes with an excerpt from an article published by a psychotherapy trainee about her thoughts on an acute psychiatric ward where she had a placement [9].

The reality is that, for many patients on the ward, being sectioned turns out to be a solace. It is the only way out of a state of mind that has become unbearable: the last resort. . . . When I started observing ward rounds I was shocked by the extremity of suffering . . . I had never seen seriously mentally ill patients close up. . . . There was a broken and silent 20-year-old who seemed almost catatonic following a suicide attempt. . . . Yet within a month he had made an astonishing recovery. He was smiling and chatting, . . . This is an experience repeated with patient after patient. . . . I often see incredible transformations . . . It is clearly so important for patients truly to be thought about, often for the first time.

References

1. Bion WR. Differentiation of the psychotic from the non-psychotic personalities. *Int J Psychoanal* 1957; 38: 266–75.

2. Money-Kyrle R. On the fear of insanity. In D Meltzer, ed., *The Collected Papers of Roger Money-Kyrle*. Strathtay: Clunie Press, 1978.

3. Lucas R. *The Psychotic Wavelength: A Psychoanalytic Perspective for Psychiatry*. Hove: Routledge, 2013.

4. Klein M. Notes on some schizoid mechanisms. In *The Writings of Melanie Klein*. Vol. 3. *Envy and Gratitude and Other Works*. London: Hogarth Press. 1946; pp. 1–24.

5. Rosenfeld H. A clinical approach to the psychoanalytic theory of the life and death instincts: an investigation into the aggressive aspects of narcissism. *Int J Psychoanal* 1971; 52: 169–78.

6. Dartington T. Brilliant stupidity: madness in organizational life—a perspective from organizational consultancy. In D Bell, A Novakovic, eds., *Living on the Border*. Abingdon: Routledge. 2018; pp. 208–25.

7. Menzies Lyth I. A case-study in the functioning of social systems as a defence against anxiety: a report on a study of the nursing service of a general hospital. *Hum Relat* 1960; 13(2): 95–121.

8. Quinlivan L, Cooper J, Meehan D et al. Predictive accuracy of risk scales following self-harm: multicentre, prospective cohort study. *Br J Psychiatry* 2017; 210(6): 429–36.

9. Blundy A. The drugs do work. *Prospect*, Issue 184, 22nd June 2011.

Further Reading

Evans M. *Making Room for Madness in Mental Health: The Psychoanalytic Understanding of Psychotic Communication*. London: Karnac Books, 2016.

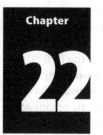

Introduction to Organisational Dynamics

Phil Stokoe

This chapter introduces an approach used by the author, an experienced organisational consultant and senior manager in caring organisations, to organisational dysfunction. The author describes how combining his training experience as a psychoanalyst and in organisational consultancy allows key ideas from psychoanalytic and open systems theories to be combined as the bedrock of his approach.

The chapter will define some of the psychoanalytic terms and concepts that are essential to the model as well as describing what organisational consultancy is and how it is requested. A model is described of what a 'healthy' organisation looks like as a template against which to map the features of any organisation under study [1–3]. A brief description of a consultation to an organisation will further illustrate the work.

Organisational Consultancy

Organisations, like groups, are simply collections of people gathered to perform functions that are designed to achieve a task. Collections of people, like individuals, can lose their way. In the same way that we go to a medical expert when our bodies or minds seem broken, so organisations often seek advice when aspects of their functioning become dysfunctional. This is not surprising; by and large organisations are set up and run by people who have a particular interest and expertise in the tasks and subtasks required to achieve the particular aim of the organisation; they do not necessarily have any expertise in how organisations work or don't work. The organisational consultant is that expert and he/she provides an understanding of the mechanics of the system rather than the nature of the tasks the organisation undertakes. In fact it is actually quite helpful for the consultant not to have any experience of the work of the organisation because it can be a distraction from the mechanics.

It is rare to be invited to look at the overall functioning of an organisation. It is much more often the case that the consultant is asked to help sort out one part of the larger system that seems to be uniquely problematic: for instance, a particular ward in a hospital or a team in a social service department. The not-so-subtle implication is that the rest of the business is functioning perfectly well. A ubiquitous symptom of organisational dysfunction is that there is a preoccupation with people, personalities and personality conflicts. This is very often part of the referral, 'team A is in a mess, there's a clear personality conflict and nobody can do anything about it'.

Another way in which an organisational consultation may be sought is for 'executive coaching' for specific individuals who work there. Once again the error is to believe the propaganda that the problem lies at a personal level, either with the person referred for consultation or with some colleague who is making the identified client feel bad.

It is important to approach such requests on the assumption that what appears to be bad or unprofessional behaviour on the part of an individual or individuals will be an expression of underlying (i.e. below the surface or unconscious) dynamics. It is illogical to start with the individual because there will always be some reflection of the individual's own personality in the problematic behaviour, so you will never move on from that. If you start by searching for an organisational dynamic that is expressed in this behaviour, either you will find one and then you are focussed on your expertise as an organisation mechanic, or you won't, in which case you have proved, beyond doubt, that it really is about the individual.

Drives or Instincts: The Pleasure Principle and the Reality Principle

Freud's theory of the mind begins with drives (also referred to as instincts). He describes drives as essentially biological and that they stimulate *feelings* in the psyche. A drive has a source, the place where the stimulation develops; pressure, which means the sense of urgency; an aim, which is to reduce that pressure and an object, which will be the site of satisfaction [4].

At first, he identified two groups of instincts, the ego, or self-preserving, instincts and the sexual instincts. The sexual urges can be in conflict with society's expectations for acceptable behaviour and the self-preserving instincts act to inhibit those urges. The consequences of this conflict can be symptoms of 'neurosis'. From the observation that the aim of the instinct is satisfaction or the reduction of the level of stimulation, Freud deduced that the basic psychic principle, the governing organisation of the mind, was the 'pleasure principle', by which he meant the reduction of discomfort.

By 1915, he was already indicating that this theory might not be accurate. This hint led to his radically new suggestion [5], that the real instinctual conflict lay between 'life instincts' and 'death instincts'.

At this point, his theory might be re-expressed in the terminology offered by Wilfred Bion [6] in which he described drives as emotional links between the self and another. The life instincts, Eros, is 'love' represented by 'L' and the death instinct is 'hate', represented by 'H'.

To summarise by using the classic example of hunger; this is experienced as a level of excitation which increases its urgency as time goes by. The evoked feelings are unpleasant, and we are thus 'driven' to reduce the unpleasant sensations by seeking something that will make us feel better, this is the aim. The object, traditionally the nipple, provides 'satisfaction' which is experienced as pleasure.

Freud describes this main, unconscious, biologically driven mental process as the *pleasure principle*: an urge to replace unpleasure with pleasure or, at the very least, the absence of unpleasure. As the baby develops, he understands that the reduction of unpleasure (in terms of hunger) is represented by the breast; so, he is able to tolerate the frustration of waiting for the breast by 'hallucinating' it. However, this only lasts a little while and, in the face of the return of frustration, Freud says,

> It was only the non-occurrence of the expected satisfaction, the disappointment experienced, that led to the abandonment of this attempt at satisfaction by means of hallucination. Instead . . . A new principle of mental functioning was thus introduced; what was presented in

the mind was no longer what was agreeable but what was real, even if it happened to be disagreeable. This setting-up of the reality principle proved to be a momentous step [7, p. 219].

As indicated by Bion [6], L & H alone, the drives that link to the pleasure principle, cannot account for this move to looking at reality. Why would a baby, driven only by the need to reduce 'excitement', suddenly decide, 'oh, the hell with that, let's have a look at what's really going on?' Only the assumption of a third drive, curiosity (K for Bion), which operates like a computer programme, requiring us continually to explain to ourselves what is happening to us [8], would result in an impulse to see what's really going on. This is why curiosity is a vital element in healthy functioning of the individual and, therefore, for the group and the organisation.

It is the K-drive (curiosity) that generates the collection of 'explanations' for what is happening to us that gradually accumulate and become our conscious mind. These explanations have been known to psychoanalysts for a long time as 'unconscious phantasy' (a tautological expression because phantasy spelt with a 'ph' *means* unconscious fantasy!). We know that these explanations are always in the form of pictures or images of ourselves in relation to others or parts of others.

Thinking

Freud [7] and Bion [9] took the view that thinking was the consequence of development. In other words, it is an 'achievement', not a given. Bion's theory of thinking begins with the idea of an 'expectation'; for instance, the baby, confronted with the arousal of hunger, is 'programmed' to expect a source of satisfaction. It is easy to see this in animals; a baby lamb, the moment it is born, starts seeking the nipple. Bion described this expectation as a preconception and said that there are two outcomes that will occur in the face of the excitation that seeks satisfaction. One is that the preconception will 'mate' with the actual nipple and this will result in a 'conception'. In other words, there will be an internal 'image' of the nipple, the preconception is no longer an expectation but a discovered entity. The other outcome is the preconception mating with absence of the nipple; this stimulates a 'thought'. This is identical to Freud's idea of an hallucination, the image of the nipple is now a psychic element available for rudimentary processing. It follows from this that thinking is the processing of feelings by turning them into symbols that can be used instead of the thing they represent. Over time and with experience, the baby will develop greater skills with this process, so that thinking becomes a central means to manage the data from the outside and the inside that is received as raw feelings. This capacity will finally become a conscious skill although the original form of thinking will always go on unconsciously as well. In our conscious experience, thinking provides us with the mechanism to manage 'not knowing', by transforming the competing feelings into symbols that can be manipulated in the mind. This is an essential process for healthy function and, therefore, groups and organisations will have to create an apparatus for carrying out the same process.

State of Mind: Paranoid-Schizoid and Depressive Positions

The last psychoanalytic concepts that we need to know about before reflecting on what goes on in organisations are the two states of mind that the baby develops in his earliest development. These were first observed and described by Melanie Klein [10] and this is a necessarily brief summary. Babies are born without any internal defences, meaning that there are no internal psychic systems to protect the baby from the full impact of his raw emotions. Without such internal defences, we would not be able to function, we wouldn't be able to think, we'd remain stuck in a state in which we are motivated by the stimulation of drives and seek only a state of low stimulation. The development of the primary or primitive defences occurs in the first weeks of life. Initially experiences are quite simply divided into wonderful and horrible. One of the earliest defences against the horrible feelings is based on one of the few things a baby can choose to do, close his eyes – denial. In other words, the baby's universe is simply divided between ideal and its opposite, we might say, 'hell'. Clearly the yearning is to be merged with the ideal, usually experienced as the carer. The loss of that position is so terrifying that we are justified in describing it as a life and death level of anxiety; in other words, any anxiety feels like a threat to survival. This view of the universe is the 'default' state of mind and we are plunged into it in the face of any significant anxiety. When we do move into this state (which Melanie Klein called the paranoid-schizoid position – P/S), we are in a world characterised by the following qualities.

Paranoid-Schizoid Position

- RULED by the Ideal
- GOVERNING PRINCIPLE: Pleasure
- ANXIETY one's own Survival
- LANGUAGE is that of Blame
- MENTAL STATE of choice is certainty
- SOLUTIONS are all omnipotent
- THREAT is difference, e.g.
  - Help
  - Valuing
- RELATIONSHIPS are either mergers or sado/masochistic

Hell is the experience of the activation of a drive, typically represented in the literature by hunger and the baby's explanation to himself of what is happening is, 'something is attacking me'. When the carer appears and manages to work out what's wrong and then apply the necessary solution, the baby is overwhelmed with pleasure and experiences this object, the carer, as magical; able to turn something horrible into something marvellous. This is why the only language available in this state of mind is blame (if I'm not with the ideal, who is to blame?). And the only available relationships are either mergers or attack and submission. Clearly, this is the world of the pleasure principle. However, if the baby is able to absorb the carer's capacity to transform the bad into the good, that capacity allows the creation of that hallucination that Freud talked about. When this is strong enough, the baby, applying the 'reality principle', discovers that he isn't being attacked by a hunger monster, nobody is there. This shocking realisation stimulates the next stage of development in which the baby forms a new view of the universe. One in which the major sort of anxiety is the loss of the loved one. This is the state of mind that is often referred to as the 'adult' state. This is an error. True adults move between this and the P/S position all the time. Klein called it the *depressive* position because it requires the baby to mourn the loss of the ideal (the baby has realised that what is absent, when there is no hunger monster, is his carer, being absent means she isn't ideal). The loss of ideal and hell allows a more nuanced view of the world because objects can be seen to be a mixture of good and bad. These are its features:

Depressive Position

- RULED by the ordinary (there are shades of grey)
- GOVERNING PRINCIPLE: reality
- ANXIETY is about the loss of the OBJECT (concern)
- LANGUAGE of achievement (small steps can be valued)
- MENTAL STATE: thinking (predicated on uncertainty)
- SOLUTIONS are based on doing the best you can
- THREATS take the form of losses. This is because:
    - We understand the Facts of Life.
    - We can face Psychic Reality
    - We can acknowledge that we are Needy
- Difference is tolerated and recognised as a source of Creativity and of Hope
- RELATIONSHIPS are reciprocal (creative intercourse)

Although this state of mind is the one in which healthy and effective work can be done, it is the P/S state that will be most significant in our study of groups and organisations.

Initial Observations about Groups and Organisations

Groups, and that collection of groups that we call an organisation, ought to be the most effective way to address most complex human tasks. This raises the question, 'why is it that groups and organisations seem so often not to function well?' The same answer that would be offered about an individual who presents with a problem provides the model for problems in groups and organisations. Namely, individuals are designed rather well, which is why we are the dominant species on the planet, enabling us to contribute so powerfully to its demise. Essentially, we are designed to survive well, form relationships and create new life, thus preserving our DNA [11]. If there is a problem and the individual with that problem seems unable to solve it, it seems reasonable to assume that this must be because that individual cannot see what is causing the problem. In other words, the source of difficulty lies below the surface; it is unconscious. The same is true with organisations; if there is a problem, and the individuals within the organisation cannot solve that problem, the obvious starting hypothesis must be that it is because they cannot see the source of it. What follows are the necessary components for a healthy organisation, which will enable us to deduce the sorts of things that can happen to undermine healthy functioning, all of which might be described as unconscious dynamics.

Among the features that *always* occur in the context of dysfunction in a group or an organisation is what might be described as personalisation. The individuals within the organisation move their attention from the task inwards onto each other. Organisational events feel personal and the explanations for things going wrong will be about the behaviour of *people*. The entire system appears to agree that any solution will involve identifying individuals who are causing the problem and either changing their behaviour or sacking them. One of the many distressing things about the way that organisations attempt to address their problems is that they employ firms who manifestly agree that this belief is true and that they are experts in identifying the problem individuals and either training them or managing them out of the organisation. These firms make an enormous amount of money from this activity partly because, sometime later, similar problems occur again and so they are called back in. This is like a doctor seeing a patient complaining of a pain in his guts and agreeing with that patient that the solution is to remove his colon.

Healthy Organisation Model

This model begins with the rather obvious assumption that, because organisations are created by human beings to achieve things that human beings want to achieve, the best functioning ones will be those that have been able to reflect in their design the features that make individuals function best. In order to do this successfully, we should begin by identifying those processes that seem essential to healthy individual functioning, so that they can be watched for in the group or organisation. Finally, it may seem obvious that, whereas the processes that make individuals function well are an intrinsic part of the design, these things must be consciously, thoughtfully and clearly built into the structure of the organisation; they don't just pop up!

So, what makes for a 'healthy human being'? On an individual basis this requires the mind to have achieved by and large the following abilities summarised below:

1. to face reality
2. to make relationships
3. to absorb information
4. to transform this information into symbols
5. so that it can be thought about
6. all of which leads to the ability to make decisions, and finally
7. to reflect on our own performance

Since these achievements are the result of the development of the mind, through the activities of the three drives, L, H and K, I suggest that any organisation that wants to operate well must also encourage these emotional states and the most important for the organisation, is curiosity. In other words, a central concept for the 'personality' of the organisation is *human values*.

What threatens this constellation of healthy capacities? Fear, or, in its other manifestation, anxiety. As individuals, we begin to operate inefficiently when our psychic energy is diverted to defend us against something that we believe threatens us. This is often something that we don't want to see or be seen by others, either within ourselves or outside us. The same is true of organisations.

There are four governing structures that enable these capacities to be replicated within an organisation, they are:

1. The Primary Task (or Mission Statement)
2. Basic Shared Principles for work
3. A Culture of Benign Enquiry
4. A Hierarchy of Decision-Making

The Primary Task is essentially the *identity* of the organisation, its raison d'être and, as such, it describes the system's relationship to the outside world. All activity within the organisation must be in the service of the Primary Task but this must also be written down, so that it can be under review. This is because things change, and a healthy organisation will operate successfully only as long as it remains relevant.

Shared Principles for Work are also known as the elements of 'governance'; they include Financial, Ethical, Behavioural and Professional standards. These provide the parameters within which work is carried out. Like the Primary Task, they should be written down so that they can be monitored for relevance; they provide essential reference points for decision-making and activity within the organisation.

The Culture of Benign Enquiry might be thought of as the personality of the organisation. Proper maintenance of the work, of the Primary Task and shared principles and of feedback of information will be natural to an organisation that is interested in its own workforce, its own performance and the attitude of the outside world towards it. Benign enquiry, as a feature of management, provides both a flow of information and a sense of containment.

Finally, the structure that enables work to be done is one in which activities are initiated and monitored. This is the **Hierarchy of Decision-Making**. It is the organisational equivalent of the circulation of the blood. Its purpose is to enable activity on behalf of the mission statement and to absorb information about how it is functioning and about the interface with the external world. In other words, it provides the opportunity to link to reality.

This hierarchical framework often starts with the boss who delegates a decision-making function to the next level down, for this example called a manager, who delegates a decision-making function to a level that, for the purposes of simplicity, can be called an operative, see Figure 22.1.

Delegation of decision-making only works if it is accompanied by clear authorisation. The principle is that decision-making authority should be passed to the *lowest sensible level*. This is the beginning of that equivalent to the circulation of the blood. Authority to make decisions gets passed down the line but it must be accompanied, at each level, by a requirement for the subordinate to give a regular account for his/her work to his/her manager. The process of account is the mechanism through which information is passed up the line in two forms, conscious, or formal account, and unconscious communication. The latter is the most important. It is usually communicated as an emotion and, very often, this is anxiety. This completes the circulation system. Put simply, authority is passed down and anxiety is passed up. From the point of view of healthy function, it is any interference with

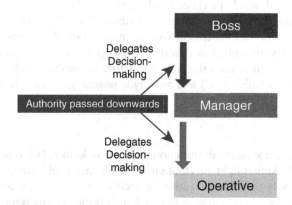

Figure 22.1 The Hierarchy of Decision-Making.

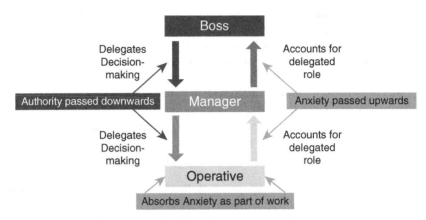

Figure 22.2 The Core Circulatory System of Authority/Anxiety.

the core circulatory system (authority/anxiety) that causes, or is an expression of, dysfunction (Figure 22.2).

On the shop floor, the operative engages with the work and, while doing that, absorbs anxiety. Next, the operative accounts for his/her work to his/her manager and the manager accounts to his/her boss. It is through the accounting system that the healthy organisation encourages anxiety to be passed up the line. The reason for this is that anxiety is so often the emotional experience that accompanies unconscious information and, particularly at work, the accompaniment to the most important connection to reality. In the same way that good decisions require best information, a healthy organisation requires constant feedback about both its internal processes and also its encounter with the outside world. This very often occurs through its most junior staff.

The most important parts of the structure of the circulatory system are the encounters where the 'account' takes place. These are usually meetings between a manager and one or more of his 'direct reports'. Where the approach of the manager is a genuine interest in the others, especially in how they feel about their work, the exchange of anxiety can take place and much of it can be unpacked and turned into information to enable the system to maintain or improve its practice. In my estimation, this is the organisational equivalent of what, in the individual, would be called thinking (Figure 22.3).

When an organisation is clear about the Primary Task (Mission Statement) and the Shared Basic Principles (or elements of Governance), all of which provide the containing parameters; when it is committed to a Culture of Benign Enquiry and when the Hierarchy of Decision-Making is built around the core circulatory system in which authority is passed down (to the lowest sensible level) and anxiety is passed up, then this conforms with the Healthy Organisation Model.

Dysfunction

It is often helpful to see what the dysfunctional system looks like. This is one example among many (Figure 22.4). At first sight, this looks just like the managed hierarchy described above. The difference is only that the delegation of decision-making is *not* accompanied by the provision of authority. This is a system in which only responsibility is designated, authority

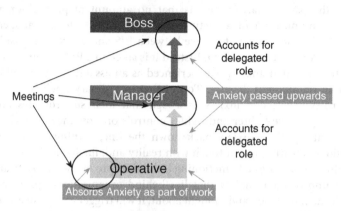

Figure 22.3 Encounters where 'account' takes place.

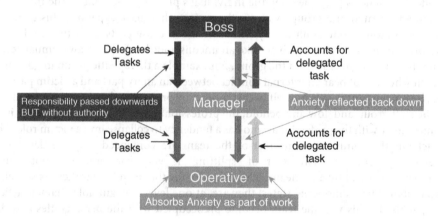

Figure 22.4 A dysfunctional system.

has to be created by the individual. Very often the unconscious reason such a system is set up is that the organisation does not actually want to face reality. This will become apparent in the process of account. In this sort of organisation, there is an absence of curiosity, the culture of benign enquiry is replaced with a culture of blame. Thus, the subordinate reporting to the manager will be rewarded for achieving whatever tasks he/she has been given responsibility to achieve but any expression of anxiety will be treated as a sign of failure either of self or of resolve and the manager will make it clear that such behaviour puts his/her job at risk. This is an organisation in which the management system is essentially bullying. The process of thinking has been replaced by a simplistic system of tasks or outcomes to be ticked. Failure to tick all the boxes is not 'interesting' to the organisation, it is merely a sign of the failure of the individual. In this way the individual is made anxious and is forced to carry out his/her responsibilities from his/her own personal authority. Anxiety is passed down the line and only reassurance is allowed to pass up the line.

Of course, the psychoanalytic view is that no amount of prohibition will stop the unconscious communication of anxiety from a subordinate to a manager. This is an organisation that has no capacity to move between P/S and depressive positions which is an important sign of adult functioning. Instead it is stuck in a P/S (or fundamentalist) state of mind which means that anxiety is experienced as an assault at a survival level and will only result in an omnipotent defence. To put that in ordinary English, the people in the management roles experience anxiety as a sign that their subordinates aren't working properly, so they produce tighter and tighter controls on how they should function. This 'tick-box mentality' pushes anxiety back down the line, turning the organisation into something rigid, uncreative, out of touch with reality and, finally, toxic.

Key to healthy organisational functioning is the ability to manage anxiety and it is always some form of unprocessed anxiety that lies behind organisational problems. If anxiety cannot be noticed, understood and thought about, it will trigger a defensive structure within the organisation with the purpose of avoiding it. A ubiquitous symptom of a problem in an organisation is a preoccupation with specific personalities. People will be drawn into playing out *roles* on behalf of the defensive system within the organisation. This happens through individuals' valencies [12], meaning the individual's preference for one of the three defensive systems created in a group. Many authors since then have expanded this concept to mean our personal vulnerabilities, by which we mean those parts of us that we have not really worked through, and which act like an unconscious hook that draws similar feelings in from the unconscious swirl of the group. For example a therapeutic group might contain a patient who cannot bear an internal conflict between an angry part and a victim part of his mind; he unconsciously rids himself of this conflict by projecting these two emotional states into the staff group and, low and behold, the professional who struggles with 'anger issues' becomes angry with the professional who has a tendency to collapse into a victim role. These two act out the conflict and the rest of the team are convinced they are damaged by a 'personality conflict'. This sort of 'splitting' is very common and not only in a therapeutic context by any means. The difficulty for the team is that there is something familiar about these emotional states, they are, at one level, recognisable characteristics of those people. In this way the team become preoccupied with the personalities and don't realise that the source is in the work and not the team.

As a rule of thumb, the first test for whether an organisation is functioning satisfactorily will be whether everyone in it knows the overall task, understands their specific task and how it serves the overall task. This is enabled by the principle of delegation of decision-making to the lowest sensible level because this will engender the expression of one of those human values, trust. The manager trusts his/her subordinate to get on with the task; the manager who micromanages undoes that instantly and the result is persecutory. When this process works well, the manager discovers that his/her primary concern is looking after his/her staff (not getting the shop-floor work done, because that is the responsibility that has been delegated). When you look after your staff, you are *interested* in how they are, another of the basic human values. That interest will result in information from the interface of organisation and client. This is vital to the process of thinking described above.

This system is constantly under pressure, like the tyres of a car; emotional activity wears down the structure that processes it, so a sensible organisation expects things to go wrong and maintains an overview that picks up indicators so that repairs can be made. For instance, a regular meeting on a ward, like the changeover meeting, might begin on task by being interested in the experiences of those who are just ending their shift, but over time degenerates into the passing on of tasks. In other words, it is exactly like the dysfunction in Figure 22.4, the anxiety exchange (one shift talking about their emotional experience in the work to the oncoming shift) has been shut down and replaced by a task. Coming from the outside, one can see straight away that the unconscious explanation for this is fear of the exposure of anxiety. It might be actually spoken of as a belief that it would be detrimental for the oncoming shift to be made anxious by the passing on of anxiety from the outgoing shift. It's easy to see how compelling this thought is. But it is a thought that has 'forgotten' that talking about these anxieties will always generate useful insight into the work.

To summarise, individuals, groups and organisations have an antipathy towards anxiety. The understanding that anxiety is the same as the 'excitation' that Freud described as the stimulation of a drive and that it is normal and can be turned into information (e.g. I am hungry) once a system to do that is in place (thinking), disappears and is replaced by the language of certainty. Enquiry is turned into certainty and certainty is expressed in rigid structures such as tick boxes and restrictive regulations. It is also expressed in compulsive rumination about people and their personalities, with the same sense of seeking the certain and absolute explanation for why everything feels bad. The job of any of us who would address such problems is to come from a third position, in other words try to remove ourselves from the turbulence of the system and have a look from above, or outside in our imagination. This can only be done by noticing first what has been stirred up in you and adding it to the various narratives coming from the organisation. Even if your own experience feels familiar and, therefore, makes you think it is about you, the principle of valency means that it is also something about the system you are treating. Then you find the story that includes everyone's views because everyone's view will be a truth but not necessarily a truth at the level they believe it to be. If someone feels persecuted by someone else, then 'persecution' is a thing, all you have to do is discover where it really comes from. This sort of intervention, which is really only a form of active, attentive listening and feedback, can actually change everything.

Case Example

A consultant was invited to an inner-city practice by a new, but experienced, practice manager. On joining the practice she felt 'something was wrong'. Newly employed reception staff left frequently and there had been lots of complaints, by patients, about delays for appointment, abruptness of the receptionists and poor communication from the practice as a whole.

The initial meeting was attended by 20 people. The consultant opened the discussion by asking the group what issues they would like to talk about?

A GP who had been there longest started by summarising the current situation, which was a combination of a growing practice, a population of socially deprived patients and major financial pressures.

Eventually a nurse that worked part time with the practice spoke. What struck her about this practice was the work ethic. On the face of it, everyone was committed to working hard and did so. She said that she didn't really know what she was trying to say other than that other practices that she worked in felt more friendly.

This provoked an interesting response, the reception staff spoke about how they felt that they were able to feel friendly towards each other and they knew that they could go to their line manager to get support if things were difficult.

At this point, the consultant intervened by asking what sort of difficulties might happen in reception. They described exactly the sorts of problems that the consultant was used to hearing about in general practice; patients who were angry or very demanding and wanted to be seen straight away. Patients who became threatening. Patients who turned up without an appointment and demanded to be seen.

The consultant asked if an alternative to talking to their line manager would be to talk to the doctors. This created a stir in the reception staff and gradually a sense of frustration emerged. They said that most of the difficulties with the patients had been caused by decisions made by GPs who were then 'too busy' to deal with them. It was left to them to manage the challenging situations that arose. The GPs began to join in with thoughts about whether or not they'd be available to be called if necessary. The discussion was becoming more emotional.

The consultant wondered whether there was a blockage in communication between the different professional groups, illustrated by the GPs being 'too busy'. The consultant put it to them that the encounter between patient and reception was the beginning of the clinical meeting, therefore, whatever happened in that encounter must be important information for the GP in their work with the patient. The current situation actually deprived the GP of vital information about the emotional and psychological state of the patient. The reception staff were also left without important information that would help them to understand what the doctor wanted for the patient.

The meeting ended with a much more creative feel; reception, nurses and doctors began thinking together about how they might ensure that there was a proper exchange of information. For the first time a doctor said that she was really concerned to hear about how difficult it had been for their receptionists.

This illustrates a common example of what can happen in teams and organisations. The Primary Task, which in this case was 'to provide care to the patients' had been lost. The team had become dysfunctional and overwhelmed by growing demand and reduction in resources. There were realistic fears that the practice would not survive. This survival anxiety triggered a move to P/S functioning and all possibility of thinking together was lost. Doing was prioritised over thinking, and the GPs higher up the hierarchy projected their anxiety down. The reception staff had no place to take this anxiety and could only act it out with the patients, or leave.

The consultation provided the thinking space, where emotions could safely be expressed and heard by staff at all levels of the system. Although not a demanding process in terms of time or resource this consultation led to a significant shift in the relationships within the practice and improvement in organisation as a whole was able to function.

References

1. Stokoe P. The healthy and the unhealthy organisation: how can we help teams to remain effective. In A Rubitel, D Reiss, eds., *Containment in the Community: Supportive* *Frameworks for Thinking about Antisocial Behaviour and Mental Health.* London: Karnac Books. 2011; pp. 237–60.

2. Stokoe P. Loss in organisations. In S Akhtar, ed., *Loss: Developmental, Cultural, and*

Clinical Realms. Abingdon: Routledge. 2019; pp. 67–84.

3. Stokoe, P; 2020; The Curiosity Drive: Our Need for Inquisitive Thinking, Bicester, Phoenix Publishing House.

4. Freud S. Instincts and their vicissitudes. In J Strachey, ed., *The Standard Edition of the Complete Psychological Works of Sigmund Freud, Volume XIV (1914-1916): On the History of the Psycho-Analytic Movement, Papers on Metapsychology and Other Works*. London: Hogarth Press. 1957; pp. 109–40. (Original work published 1915)

5. Freud S. Beyond the pleasure principle. In J Strachey, ed., *The Standard Edition of the Complete Psychological Works of Sigmund Freud, Volume XVIII (1920-1922): Beyond the Pleasure Principle, Group Psychology and Other Works*. London: Hogarth Press. 1955; pp. 1–64. (Original work published 1920)

6. Bion WR. *Learning from Experience*. London: William Heinemann,1962. [Reprinted London: Karnac Books]

7. Freud S. Formulation on the two principles of mental functioning. In J Strachey, ed., *The Standard Edition of the Complete Psychological Works of Sigmund Freud, Volume XII (1911-1913): Case History of Schreber, Papers on Technique and Other Works*. London: Hogarth Press. 1958; pp. 213–26. (Original work published 1911)

8. Morgan M, Stokoe P. Curiosity. *Cpl Fam Psychoanal* 2014; 4(1): 42–55.

9. Bion WR. A theory of thinking. *Int J Psychoanal* 1962; 43: 306–10.

10. Klein M. Notes on Some Schizoid Mechanisms. *Int J Psychoanal* 1946; 27: 99–110. (Updated 1952 in Klein M. *Envy and Gratitude and Other Works 1946-1963*. London: Hogarth Press, 1975.)

11. Dawkins R. *The Selfish Gene*. Oxford: Oxford University Press, 1976.

12. Bion WR. *Experiences in Groups*. London: Tavistock, 1961. Reprinted Hove: Routledge. 1989; pp. 116–17.

Further Reading

Stokoe P. The healthy and the unhealthy organisation: how can we help teams to remain effective. In A Rubitel, D Reiss, eds., *Containment in the Community: Supportive Frameworks for Thinking about Antisocial Behaviour and Mental Health*. London: Karnac Books. 2011; pp. 237–60.

Stokoe P. Loss in organisations. In S Akhtar, ed., *Loss: Developmental, Cultural, and Clinical Realms*. Abingdon: Routledge. 2019; pp. 67–84.

Stokoe P. *The Curiosity Drive: How Inquisitive Thinking Develops the Mind and Protects Society*. Quezon City: Phoenix Publishing House; 2020.

Reflective Practice and Its Central Place in Mental Health Care

Maria Eyres

Introduction

It is of primary importance for organisations in the field of mental health to provide opportunities for clinicians of all backgrounds to reflect on their work. This enhances their ability to provide high quality care, supports staff in their work and can prevent burnout.

The General Medical Council recognises and supports this in their guidance for the reflective practioner, stating 'Medicine is a lifelong journey, scientifically complex and constantly developing. It is characterized by positive, fulfilling experiences and feedback but also involves uncertainty and the emotional intensity of supporting colleagues and patients. Reflecting on these experiences is vital to personal well-being and development, and to improving the quality of patients care.' [1]. There has been a real grassroots movement to create a variety of additional reflective spaces in the shadow of the COVID-19 pandemic, not only in mental health but also in physical health settings. This powerfully demonstrates their usefulness to staff when facing emotional distress.

There are many definitions of reflection and reflective practice; for the purpose of this chapter it is understood as a way of making contact with the emotional aspects of clinical work and finding the meaning of this experience in the context of the team. Reflective practice is often carried out in a group setting. It provides the participants with a safe space that is managed by a facilitator to explore the feelings stirred up by encounters with both patients and colleagues in work situations. Models of reflective practice vary, from psychoanalytic approaches, underpinned by the concept of the unconscious mind, to more cognitively informed paradigms.

Reflective practice can be provided in many settings including:

- Supervision
- Case-based discussion groups
- Staff support groups
- Reflective practice groups
- Case discussion groups, including Balint groups

Balint groups have a special place in medical training, starting in medical schools and being the first mandatory component of psychotherapy training for all new psychiatric trainees. Recognising and attempting to understand and process the emotional complexities at work has been recognised to foster the developing doctor's empathy and resilience [2].

This chapter is specifically focussed on psychoanalytically informed reflective practice including case discussion and Balint groups. It will consider the ways these models can be applied to psychiatric practice and illustrate their value using clinical examples.

The Theoretical Underpinning of Reflective Practice in Groups

Psychoanalysts have put forward a model of the mind which emphasises the importance of moving from the initially dyadic relationship between the baby and the mother towards recognising the painful reality of exclusion in psychological development [3]. This realisation is key to establishing the ability to be separate and to think for oneself. As the dyadic relationship is challenged by the presence of a third, usually a father and the baby experiences being outside in terms of the mother's preoccupations, a triangular space becomes opened up in the mind where thinking can take place. The concept of reflective spaces is rooted in this idea of finding a 'third position' from which both oneself and others can be observed and thought about.

It is a very remarkable thing that the unconscious of one human being can react upon that of another, without passing through the conscious [4].

This observation by Freud speaks helpfully to the unconscious processes that occur between staff and patients within mental health organisations. These processes can powerfully increase anxiety and disturbance if they are not recognised and digested. Capturing and reflecting on the emotions engendered by contact with patients can become a lens through which the unconscious can be glimpsed.

Psychiatric breakdown can be a very painful and frightening experience, giving rise to unbearable feelings such as helplessness, dependence, avoidance of responsibility and shame. Defences against awareness of these feelings include projection and projective identification into the staff that work with them. Those processes are particularly potent with psychotic patients whose projections can threaten to overwhelm the clinicians' mind. Due to the intensity of those experiences, recognising and understanding the countertransference often needs the presence of another, which can relieve the dyadic relationship between clinician and patient and create space to think. As patients are likely to see a number of professionals from the same team, discussing the effect of this phenomenon in the group allows for more thorough examination and multiple perspectives can emerge. This is then a valuable tool helping us to understand the experiences of our patients.

Without opportunities to reflect on those processes, the mind of the clinician can become controlled and trapped by powerful projections and may also react against the projective pressures. Responses from staff to such powerful communication may include:

- Over-involvement or emotional detachment, driven by a disowning of one's own emotional response
- Identification with the patient as if they are of one mind
- Taking action in a reactive way which can become a doing-to the patient rather than a being-with
- Fragmentation of patients' care which is seen as a sum of tasks rather than holistically considering all aspects of the presentation
- Inability to maintain a perspective about risk, leading to risk avoidance or under-recognition of any threats to patient safety in treatment plans

We all have our own blind spots, likely to be linked to our reasons for choosing mental health as a profession. These are deeply personal and we are drawn to particular responses when facing powerful conscious and unconscious communication from patients as a result. Working in teams amplifies those phenomena potentially leading to conflicts and difficult team dynamics. To prevent possibly destructive enactments it is vital to develop an understanding and awareness of our own limits, vulnerability and tendency towards taking up a particular role within a team and towards patients.

Bion's concept of containment [5] is particularly helpful while thinking about the impact of projections on staff. Containment describes the capacity of the mother to recognise that frightening and disturbing projections from her infant are attempts to communicate with her. She receives and thinks about them. In the process they are detoxified and rendered understandable and communicable. These can then eventually be returned to the infant who feels understood, held in mind and becomes calm. Bion postulated that with time the process of feeling contained leads to the infant internalising this capacity and becoming able to think about his emotional states and to manage them himself. There are clear parallels here to be drawn in terms of how patients project unbearable states of mind in mental health settings. The motivation is similar to the infants in that they are searching for a container which will accept the projections and think about them, transforming 'raw bits of experience' into thinkable form.

To be able to act as such a container, staff need thinking space to safely unpick the disturbing threads of their emotional response to patients, making use of their counter-transference in a way that frees them up to support and to understand their patients more deeply. Thinking under the fire of powerful projections is hard work. There are times that both individuals and the team resist engaging with such a painstaking task.

Why Teams May Resist Reflection

Anyone that has tried to set up a reflective practice group in a mental health setting will be aware that it can be difficult. On occasion teams express their desire for the space but then find it difficult to attend or fully engage. Bion's concept of basic assumptions [6] is helpful in terms of the theoretical underpinning of the team dynamics that help explain this. He proposed that groups of people continually engage in a cycle of working towards the primary task, and then disengaging with it due to the emotional challenges the work demands. This disengagement is marked by the group resorting to unconscious 'basic assumption' functioning. This is evidenced through three main 'positions' or dynamic patterns taken up by the group as a whole, dependence, fight/flight and pairing.

- Dependence: if the unconscious assumption is that the group's primary task is to fulfil the dependency needs, the group is passive and relies on authority to solve all problems
- Flight/fight: if the unconscious assumption is it is only fight/flight that can preserve autonomy, the conflict with authority is prevalent, expressed through avoiding the challenges of the task
- Pairing: if the basic assumption is a phantasy that pairing of powerful individuals will resolve the group's problems, the group sits back and waits for the magic solution, avoiding engagement

While basic assumptions are more visible in therapy groups, less pronounced versions might be also observed in reflective practice groups and at times, can be accessible for discussion.

Winnicott's concept of maternal holding and the holding environment [7] can be extrapolated to wider social environments, including those of psychiatric wards. For the mother to be able to provide a holding function which includes the ability to contain the baby's primitive anxieties projected onto her, she needs her own containment as described by Bion. This function is usually provided by the father, extended family and the wider social environment around her. To enhance the ability of staff to contain their patients, they too need support from the wider organisation, rather like the paternal function described by Winnicott, and reflective groups is one of the ways in which this can take place.

Mental health teams are constantly under pressure from the patients, the organisation and their own members which can make it difficult to think and to create and maintain its reflective capacity. The team's diversity (including ethnicity, age, gender, sexuality, religion, status, academic achievement and personality) creates a powerful mix which can become negatively amplified when the team is under pressure, leading to splits. Klein described splitting as unconscious mental phenomena in the infant's mind of separating good and bad parts of the object driven by the fear of good ones becoming destroyed by the bad, toxic ones [8]. In this process experiences and people can be experienced as polarised, only good or bad. The potential to split can continue throughout life and can be seen in mental health care teams, for example; with good nurses and junior doctors but a bad consultant, a good female therapist and a potentially harmful male one. Yet, providing patients with a safe and containing environment demands cooperation and interdependence; it is a combined effort of admin staff, nurses, doctors, occupational therapists, therapists, psychologists and others which makes key contributions to the patients' experience of health care. Reflective practice provides a setting where such splits can be noticed, thought about, understood and worked through in the best interest of patients' care.

Organisations also play their role in staff's attitude towards reflective practice taking a range of positions towards it, from actively promoting, scepticism or a degree of resistance seeing it as not a productive time. The latter might be for a variety of reasons and is likely to be linked to high levels of unprocessed anxiety within the organisation. Organisations might need support in understanding this link and in changing the organisational culture to embed reflective spaces so that staff feel supported to engage with them.

Setting Up a Reflective Practice Group: The Process

Authority

Reflective practice groups can be requested by the staff themselves, either as a team or individual (usually a consultant or a manager), or be suggested as part of an organisational strategy; both approaches can lead to development of a space which is valuable and supportive and/or dreaded and anxiety provoking. Sometimes they are requested in the aftermath of a particularly traumatic event the team has been exposed to. The overt and covert reasons behind the request need to be thought about. It is important that the wish for reflective practice is held within the leadership of the team.

Facilitator: External/Internal

The facilitator can come from the organisation where the team is working or be contracted from the outside. There are advantages and disadvantages of both. The internal facilitator is familiar with the culture and workings of the organisation and aware of the issues it is facing. There is a concomitant risk that an internal facilitator might be perceived as colluding with the organisation and as not being neutral, especially in times of heightened anxiety.

A facilitator from outside the organisation might have knowledge of external factors the team might be unaware of that may be contributing to the issues they are struggling with. These might be difficult not to divulge. The external facilitator might also have unrealistic ideas about the task of the team and come across as disconnected from the real world challenges the team is facing.

The Facilitator: Expertise Required

- The organisation needs to authorize and support the setting up and maintenance of the group. The facilitator needs to show her/his authority to provide a consistent and boundaried setting and to hold a clear view of the task of the group and manage the setting and the process
- The capacity not to be disillusioned by poor attendance, anxiety or even hostility
- The ability to maintain a neutral and reflective stance under pressure
- Genuine interest in the experiences of the staff
- A theoretical model of the development and workings of the mind and thorough understanding of organisational dynamics

The Facilitator: Key Tasks of the Role

The facilitator provides an overall containment through the following activities:

- Reducing initial anxiety by preparing the physical space and maintaining a safe environment
- Making a regular commitment to the group and to prioritise this
- Boundary maintenance; there may be challenges to this thinking space from within the group and from the outside
- Language needs to be accessible, for example projective identification described as gut feeling or splitting as seeing things in black and white
- Helping the group to agree and meet its aims; making sure that the group is on target
- Monitoring the pace; silences; slowing down and accelerating; helping members to talk
- Ensuring that the level of the distress and anxiety at the end of the group is acknowledged and addressed as far as possible

Practical Issues: The Setting

- The frequency of the meetings should be discussed with the team and a balance between what is realistic and what is required to develop the culture of the group; monthly sessions are recommended as a minimum to create a containing and safe space. Some teams can be authorised to initially meet more frequently to help with the process of team development
- A regular time and place for the meeting is important
- The meeting needs to be held in an undisturbed and private space
- The length of the meetings should be discussed and set. The usual parameters are between 60 and 90 minutes
- The duration of the group needs to be agreed. Is it for a set time period or open-ended? An agreement to review at some point may be useful

- It is important to discuss how staff can be released from their usual duties for the duration of the group
- Attendance (voluntary or mandatory) needs to be agreed at the management level; there are advantages and disadvantage of both. This needs to be discussed further with the team at the preliminary meeting

Preliminary Meeting with the Team

The first meeting with the team includes finding out how involved the team feels in planning the group, clarifying the ownership of the proposed group as belonging to the team and listening to the concerns or doubts. If there is a large gap between the expectations of the authorising manager and the team, this needs to be discussed with the management before the regular meetings start.

The Beginning

During the first session time needs to be spent negotiating the framework for the reflective practice group in a particular team. This discussion is key to setting the parameters and exploring the expectations of the group. It includes arriving at a shared understanding of the purpose and the task of the group, the way that the group functions, its boundaries, time, place, frequency, group membership, including the position of temporary staff, attendance and of course, confidentiality. The staff need to recognise that the group is a confidential space with the specific task to encourage reflection towards enhancing clinical understanding separate from the usual organisational processes. While the learning from the session might be taken to a different forum for further discussion such as supervision or team meeting, this is not a decision-making meeting. The facilitator might summarise this discussion in a written contract to be discussed and agreed on in the following session. It can then be distributed to all staff, including new group members.

The Middle

Well established, engaged staff, attendance fluctuating within reason. The length of this phase varies, depending on initial agreement.

The End

Planned – optimum of six months if the group meets monthly.

Reviews/Evaluation

Regular reviews can be agreed upon in the preliminary meeting or proposed later by the group or facilitator. They can take the form of a review session, anonymous feedback forms which can be fed back to the manager who proposed the group through discussion or a written report if requested. If attempting a written survey, it is helpful to ask the contributors how many sessions they attended over the last 6 or 12 months, followed by a series of questions with responses in the format of a Likert visual rating scale with five available responses to each questions ranging from *Strongly disagree* to *Strongly agree*. The questions may include asking about helpfulness of the session, how easy it was to bring an issue for discussion, if the participants felt listened to, how they rate the discussions in terms of moving things forward and how they rate the facilitator. The last part of the survey may offer an opportunity to give examples of something helpful, something unhelpful and any suggestions for improvement. Engaging the team in evaluation might lead to a decision to continue the group as it is, to change something about it or to decide that it has achieved its task and it is time to finish.

Overall Task of Reflective Practice Group

The aim of reflective practice groups is to enhance team functioning through containing and working through the emotional impact and anxiety related to the work. This primary task can then be broken down to a number of overlapping elements:

- To provide the experiential and safe space to bring one's vulnerable parts, to open up emotionally without being too defended in order to talk about feelings evoked by the work. This leads to understanding better the anxiety and provides the opportunity for staff to support and learn from each other and to improve communication
- To enable the staff to express, discuss and manage difficult or painful emotional responses to clinical situations, such as guilt, hostility, envy, states of persecution and anxiety
- To regain the capacity to think; to move from basic assumptions to working group
- To enhance the group's capacity to act as its own container
- To hold in mind the pressures of the work and how it impinges on the capacity to function as a group or team
- To enhance the creativity and deepen clinical understanding towards optimising clinical care
- To become more aware of the realities of scarce resources, including time to promote more egalitarian and cooperative state of mind
- To enable the team to discuss the obstacles to the work
- To repair splits in the team and to understand better their origins
- To improve staff well-being due to more cohesive team functioning and to optimise clinical care

Common Themes in Reflective Practice Groups

While each group is different, there are some recurring themes and issues that tend to emerge in reflective practice groups in mental health settings.

- Attendance, especially of a manager and/or consultant can become a preoccupation. All members of the team are generally encouraged to attend
- Being at the receiving end of the expression of patients' disturbance, in a conscious and unconscious way as staff may vary in their awareness of this and stand to learn from each other in this group setting
- Risk of physical violence from patients towards staff and various ways of coping with it ranging from accepting it as a part of the job, taking sick leave or even leaving the team
- Impact of the witnessing physical violence between patients, towards staff and towards patients during restraints
- Persecutory anxiety relating to patients' risk of suicide and self-harm (see Chapter 19)
- Frustration with having to manage very distressing and disturbing situations with continuously shrinking resources and perceptions of not being heard by the management

- Disagreements about formulation and clinical care, as different members of the team have sensitivities to different aspects of the patient's presentation

Clinical Vignette 1: A Patient Impossible to Nurse

At the first session of a newly established fortnightly reflective practice group on the ward a nurse spoke about her patient, The patient, whom she found impossible to nurse. The patient was admitted under Section of the Mental Health Act. She refused to cooperate with any activities on the ward, including self-care. As a result, the smell from her room started to permeate the whole ward. The cleaning staff refused to enter it and were threatening to abandon cleaning the ward if something wasn't done. Many discussions were held in the multidisciplinary team with no avail.

In the reflective practice group, the staff initially saw her refusal to wash or change her clothes as a passive resistance against the intrusion of being sectioned, moved to an unknown ward and her flat being blitz cleaned. The staff spoke of feeling hopeless and unable to create a therapeutic relationship with the patient which in turn made them feel bad about themselves. The discussion about the roles and duties across the team followed. The nurses felt that their job was seen as inferior to other professionals, doctors, psychologists and occupational therapists. The perceived lack of appreciation of nursing as a discrete and valuable contribution to the working of the ward was explored. The nurses spoke about being taken for granted and most frequently physically attacked by the patients and how this diminished their pride in the job as well as their confidence in doing it well. The link with patient's race was made and how her complaints of racism somehow paralysed the team.

Towards the end of the session other professionals expressed their gratitude to the nurses, with the psychologist describing them as a backbone of the team. The patient's refusal to engage with the ward was discussed in the context of her being uprooted from her home and brought to the hospital without her consent or agreement, unable to function in her usual way, feeling stuck and wanting to exercise control and also to express her rage in the only way she could, by refusing to do what the staff wanted her to do. The initial anxiety about not knowing what to do and a sense of hopelessness shifted. At the next reflective group session the nurse who brought this case for discussion spoke of how the discussion allowed her to reconnect with her own professionalism, which lead to her approaching the patient differently, leading to establishing a more helpful connection and successful encouragement enabling her to attend to her personal hygiene.

Clinical Vignette 2: Suicide and Persecutory Anxiety

A junior doctor who thought that he had the last contact with the patient in the community before his suicide a month later spoke about his hopelessness, despair and fear of repercussions on learning what has happened. The patient had a long-standing chronic depression and a progressive physical illness. He had many different treatments, including being hospitalised and an unsuccessful attempt at therapy. The discussion in the reflective practice group revealed that the patient had been in touch by phone with other professionals since seeing the doctor and memories of the patient were shared in the team, including his early history of growing up in a violent household. The doctor's despair was linked to the patient's experience. This helped the doctor recover some capacity to think and he remembered that he presented the patient to his consultant and they reviewed his treatment together and agreed that it was a good plan. The discussion led to the conclusion that the patient was a complex individual who presented in various states of mind over many years. The fact that the team could not control everything or be responsible for everything was discussed, with recognition the team wanted to help but was not omnipotent.

Clinical Vignette 3: Personal Links

A young pharmacist whose training didn't include exposure to clinical environments spoke about the task of going to the wards and being left alone with patients, with various difficulties from depression to psychotic illness, to discuss medication the medical team prescribed. She spoke of those encounters making her feel at times very lonely, misunderstood, hopeless, frustrated and angry. The group wondered if the presenter's feelings of exposure and isolation might be linked to the ways patients can feel, especially if they are detained on a section of the Mental Health Act or on a locked ward. The presenter then spoke of how one of the patients reminded her of a friend who struggled with mental ill health while another aroused very intense feelings which seemed familiar. The other group members, all of them pharmacists, spoke about having similar experiences. They felt that the expectation was for them to manage without any supervision that addressed this aspect of the job. A new manager became aware of those conversations and suggested reflective practice group for the team; she was aware of them being run for clinical teams which found them helpful. This could be thought of as an example of a paternal, supportive function of the organisation, supporting the staff in their task.

Specific Examples of Reflective Practice Groups

Staff Support Groups

Staff support groups provide a particular forum with the explicit task of supporting staff in their everyday work. They share some similarities with reflective practice groups and the boundaries between them are not rigid, with some significant overlap. Staff support groups tend to have a more explicit focus on the emotional impact of the work on staff, including the relationships between team members and with the organisation itself, whereas reflective practice groups tend to examine relationships staff have with patients, the management and at times with the wider organisation. Staff support groups in psychological therapy services are sometimes facilitated by a group analyst, which can lead to unconscious dynamics within the staff group explored more robustly. They are sometimes called sensitivity groups.

Balint Groups

Balint groups are another form of reflective practice groups. They were initially set up in London by the Hungarian psychoanalyst Michael Balint and his wife Enid as seminars for General Practitioners [9]. Balint groups offer a semi-structured form of psychodynamic reflective practice, which allows members with little psychotherapy or group experience, using everyday language, to explore the emotional aspects of the patient–clinician relationship in a contained manner. Balint groups place the relationship between the clinician and the patient at its heart and examine the clinician's countertransference as an important source of information about the patient's state of mind.

Balint Group Structure

- One or two facilitators who ask who would like to bring the case
- The presenter takes about 10–15 minutes to present the encounter with the patient with the emphasis on the feelings stirred up by it. This is an informal oral presentation, without notes, focussing on the interaction between the patient and the clinician
- A few clarifying questions might follow, with the curiosity about what might be behind the question rather than seeking clarification alone
- The presenter is then asked to sit back and restrain from further discussions until invited back; in traditional Balint groups this might be marked by moving the presenter's chair a few inches back, therefore symbolically removing themselves from the circle and focussing on listening
- The group reflects on the presentation, relating to the experiences of the presenter and bringing in their own emotional responses to the material, including free associations. In newly created Balint groups the participants might be tempted to focus on actions rather than stay with the feelings, wanting to discuss the management plan or come up with solutions and it is the task of the facilitator to gently remind the group of the primary task. This part of the group might include periods of silence which might initially be difficult for the group to manage and need to be thought about
- Once the discussion is over, the presenter is invited back to the circle and given 5 minutes or so to describe their experience of listening to the discussion
- The whole group discussion takes the remaining 5 minutes, with the facilitator keeping an eye on the time and inviting the presenter to have the last word at the end of the session

Balint Group Principles and Process

- Members of the group collectively explore the emotions towards the patient revealing unconscious processes that may be present. This allows new perspectives to emerge regarding the patient's presentation and impact upon the team as reflected in the Balint group
- Negative emotions such as frustration, guilt, shame, lack of empathy or even anger towards the patient can be voiced safely and accepted allowing release of repressed feelings that may otherwise negatively influence clinical care
- Sharing those experiences in a safe and contained space and listening to multiple perspectives of colleagues, some of them similar to the presenter's, creates new insights and a more complete and realistic view of the clinical encounter
- Through examining the relationship between staff and patients Balint groups can also bring the clinician's own struggles closer to the surface and by doing that, helping them to get to know themselves as individuals
- Discussion can lead to increased understanding of the impact of mental illness on patients as human beings, with their own specific history, circumstances and relationships
- The Debate can help to recognise how aspects of early formative relationships can be reflected in patients' relationships with staff members and in team dynamics

- Balint groups can also help to understand various ways in which teams and organisations might defend themselves against powerful emotional experiences that threaten to disturb their own equilibrium

A number of studies show that Balint and Balint-type case discussion groups enhance psychological skills, empathy, attitudes towards patients and colleagues and job satisfaction, and reduce burnout [10–13].

The Balint Society organises a number of events including study and training days and weekends across the country. In the UK Balint groups are being rolled out nationally with the aim of each medical school offering them to medicals students. The model has been adopted by psychiatrists around the world, with the International Balint Society coordinating Balint thinking, development and research among member countries.

Clinical Vignette 4: An Uninteresting Patient

The presenter spoke about a patient she came in touch with on the ward and found difficult to relate to. The patient was initially admitted to the hospital under Section of Mental Health Act, subsequently discharged from the Section and was staying on the ward informally. The patient discharged himself after a few days and his admission was thought about by the ward staff as unhelpful. The staff felt the patient caused problems on the ward, was difficult to contain and unlikable. In the discussion that followed the group members spoke about the ward itself being uncontained at the time, struggling with drugs and alcohol finding their way to patients and the problems this caused. The link between the level of disturbance on the ward and in the patient's early life was made, which made self-discharge more understandable. The presenter was surprised by the feelings of helplessness, loss and trauma of being on such an unsettled ward evoked by her presentation in other group members. While the patient couldn't escape the family home as a child, his self-discharge was seen as something potentially developmental, a movement towards a more active position of taking responsibility for his predicament. At the end of the group the presenter thanked the group for helping her to relate to the patient more fully and concluded that her patient became unexpectedly interesting.

Clinical Vignette 5: An Ungrateful Patient

A first-year male trainee introduced the group to a mixed-race female patient from a working class background in her 30s who presented in crisis. He has been trying very hard to help her and yet ended feeling frustrated and angry with her. This feeling stayed with him and he found it difficult to shake it off. The patient had a long history of presenting to and then disengaging from services, of self-harm and was homeless. The presenter went out of his way to help, found temporary accommodation for her and recommended various organisations and services that could support her. The presenter learned the patient didn't take up the place he arranged for her in the refuge and the following week she presented to mental health services in a very similar way. The presenter didn't say anything about the patient's past. The group seemed impressed by the amount of time and effort the presenter put into helping the patient. Some questions were posed about her history and lifestyle. With help from the presenter and a couple of other attendees who knew the patient it transpired she had an early history of emotional, physical and sexual abuse and of neglect. She was working in the sex industry and used drugs. Her two young children were taken into care as she wasn't able to look after them. An observation was made about the patient's history, how painful it seemed and how the patient had many reasons to be angry. Some questions were raised about the meaning of the patient's encounter with a white middle-class male doctor who could have been perceived as an authority figure, someone who wanted to take advantage of her and possibly an object of envy. This was discussed in the context of the patient's history and possible mistrust of authority. The group wondered about the meaning of accepting help for this patient, including coming into contact with potentially very painful feelings of hopelessness, uselessness, loss and despair rather than the oblivion drugs offered. The group thought about the presenter's wish to save the patient in the way he thought was right and about the external and internal pressure doctors often feel under to save or to heal completely. Group members spoke about their own encounters with patients with similar presentations and how they shared some of the emotions described by the presenter. At the end of the session the presenter reported a sense of relief linked to feeling understood, of having a range of emotions in response to the patient after the discussion and how realising there are limits to his interventions was helpful.

Case Discussion Groups

A wide variety of case discussion groups are routinely run in mental health teams which may have a differently structured approach and aim, such as a meeting between a team and a panel to discuss clinically complex or risky cases. Although these may not be explicitly set up as reflective practice groups, they also provide opportunities to address the emotions evoked in the team by the patient, which may considerably help to shift the thinking and to develop the clinical understanding.

Clinical Vignette 6: The Risk Panel and Reflective Practice

A mental health trust set up a monthly risk panel in order to support staff with the anxieties elicited when working with high risk patients, and to further the clinical understanding of the presentation. A community team presented a young man who had grown up in a violent and chaotic household, with a terrifying alcoholic father and a mother who had been helpless to intervene. He frequently presented to mental health services intoxicated, severely self-neglected and threatening violence to the terrified staff. His provocative behaviour in public meant he frequently got into fights and would be injured as a result. The team felt stuck and were highly anxious about him, and when asked directly how she felt about the patient the consultant psychiatrist said she felt like his mother must have felt, a helpless witness to violence and self-destruction she was unable to change. This helpful insight meant the team were able to recognise the role they had been unconsciously allocated in repeating the patient's past relationships in the present. Able to recognise and consider the projected feelings of fear and helplessness enabled them to develop ideas, feel more in control of his management and to consider alternative ways to intervene.

Other Examples of Reflective Practice

- Complex cases meetings: these are discussions about the management of challenging clinical cases. An attempt to understand the patient's early history and the dynamics stirred up in the professionals can become a helpful part of the management plan and free the team to make their decisions from a more holistic perspective
- Psychosis workshops: first described by Richard Lucas [14], these were built on Bion's understanding of psychosis as dismantling patients' ability to manage reality as a defence against unbearable psychic pain. Lucas' psychosis workshops utilised clinicians'

countertransference as a valuable insight into patients' internal world helping them to bring psychotic and non-psychotic parts of the patient's mind together (see Chapter 21)

- Reflective consultations to teams (see Chapter 22)
- Schwarz Rounds: these have become increasingly used across a range of health care settings in the USA and have become increasingly popular in the UK. There are many similarities with Balint groups and they maintain a focus upon caregiver–patient relationships and the emotional impact of the work. They provide containment and space to reflect and are usually also run with a clear structure. A key difference is that Schwartz Rounds are open to all staff in an organisation, may become a very large group and the membership tends to vary. Themes also vary and are preselected – examples include working with aggression, impact of suicide, and so on and some brief vignettes presented to illustrate some of the issues for consideration by the group. There is an increasing evidence base of the benefits for both staff and patients when there is space to focus upon relational aspects of care and their emotional experiences at work [15].

Conclusion

Reflective practice in mental health setting encourages staff to notice and address the emotional impact of the work through shared examination of their feelings towards the patients, the work the organisation and each other in a safe space. This process aims to deepen the understanding of the clinical presentation and team interactions, making the team feel more supported and therefore able to contain their patients and find fulfilment in the workplace. It also contributes to improving staff's mental health and well-being by preventing stress, burnout and ill health, and therefore increasing the sustainability of the workforce. The COVID 19 pandemic highlighted those points poignantly, with the strong movement to establish reflective spaces to support front line workers in mental and physical health services. Reflective organisations encourage staff to establish a range of reflective spaces as described in this chapter valuing their contribution to creating a thinking and containing environment where staff feel safe and are able to flourish. This in turn leads to a well-functioning, caring and sustainable organisation offering patients high quality of care and cherishing its staff.

References

1. General Medical Council. The reflective practitioner – a guide for medical students. 2019. www.gmc-uk.org/education/stand ards-guidance-and-curricula/guidance/refle ctive-practice/the-reflective-practitioner—a -guide-for-medical-students [Accessed 18/ 11/2020]

2. Yakeley J, Johnston J, Adshead G, Allison L (eds.). *Oxford Specialist Handbooks in Psychiatry: Medical Psychotherapy*. Oxford: Oxford University Press, 2016.

3. Freud S, Cronin AJ. *The Interpretation of Dreams*. Redditch: Read Books Ltd, 2013.

4. Freud S. The unconscious. In *The Standard Edition of the Complete Psychological Works of Sigmund Freud, Volume XIV (1914–1916): On the History of the Psycho-Analytic Movement, Papers on Metapsychology and Other Works*. London: Hogarth Press. 1957; pp. 159–215. (Original work published 1915)

5. Bion WR. *Learning from Experience*. London: Karnac Books, 1962.

6. Bion WR. *Experiences in Groups and Other Papers*. First published in 1961 by Tavistock Publications Limited, Reprinted in 2001 by Brunner-Rutledge.

7. Winnicott D. The theory of the parent-child relationship. *Int J Psychoanal* 1960; 41: 585–95.

8. Klein M. Notes on some schizoid mechanisms. *Int J Psychoanal* 1946; 27: 99–110.

9. Balint M. *The Doctor, His Patient and The Illness*. London: Tavistock Publication, 1957.

10. Turner AL, Malm RL. A preliminary investigation of balint and non-balint behavioral medicine training. *Fam Med* 2004; 36(2): 114–17.

11. Kjeldmand D, Holmström I. Balint groups as a means to increase job satisfaction and prevent burnout among general practitioners. *Ann Fam Med* 2008; 6(2): 138–45.

12. Ghetti C, Chang J, Gosman G. Burnout, psychological skills, and empathy: Baliant training in obstetrics and gynecology residents. *J Grad Med Educ* 2009; 1(2): 231–35.

13. Santos G, Alves M, Moreira A. Baliant group training and physician empathy – systematic review [Abstract]. *Eur Psychiatry* 2018; 48S: S141–358.

14. Lucas R. *The Psychotic Wavelength: A Psychoanalytic Perspective for Psychiatry*. Hove: Routledge, 2009.

15. The Point of Care Foundation. Impact Report 2019: How the Point of Care Foundation's programmes support healthcare staff and patients. 2019. www.pointofcarefoundation.org.uk/resource/impact-report-2019/ [Accessed 18/11/2020]

Further Reading

Armstrong D, edited by French R. *Organizations in the Mind, Psychoanalysis, Group Relations and Organization in The Mind*. London: Karnac Books, 2005.

Balint Society. https://balint.co.uk/ [Accessed 18/11/2020]

Evans M. *Making Room for Madness in Mental Health: The Psychoanalytic Understanding of Psychotic Communication*. London: Karnac Books, 2016.

Hartley P, Kennard D (eds.). *Staff Support Groups in the Healing Professions: Principles, Practice and Pitfalls*. Hove: Routledge, 2009.

Obholzer A, Roberts VZ (eds.). *The Unconscious at Work, Individual and Organizational Stress in Human Services*, 2nd ed. Abingdon: Routledge, 2019.

Omer S, McCarthy G. Reflective practice in psychiatric training: Balint groups. *Ir J Psych Mod* 2010; 27(3): 115–16.

Wilke K. Beyond Balint: a group-analytic support model for traumatized doctors. *Group Analysis* 2005; 38(2): 265–80.

Working Psychotherapeutically with Children

Margot Waddell

Introduction

The essential goals of the child and adolescent psychotherapist are not dissimilar to those of the adult therapist: to understand and render meaningful troubled aspects of the personality. The process brings insight to bear on the nature of the internal world and its mixed population of figures, benign and persecutory. Mental development occurs not so much through 'ironing out' the difficulties, but rather through 'an increase in the capacity to bear reality and a decrease in the obstructive force of illusions' [1, p. 51]. Bearing reality lies in being able to reintegrate aspects of the personality that have been disowned, or disavowed as too threatening to psychic equilibrium. The process of integration involves taking back projections and bearing the discomfort of being brought into relation with the less manageable aspects of the self. The method is based on the observation and interpretation of the transference and countertransference relationship, the elucidation of dreams and, in the case of children and adolescents, the underlying meaning of play and enactments of whatever kind that take place both in and outside the consulting room.

Some years ago, I listened to a child psychoanalyst vividly recollecting her first training case, seen in the early fifties. The little boy in question, I'll call him Simon, was two-and-a-half when he was referred to the Clinic. His father had died soon after the birth of Simon's younger sibling. For most of the session, we were told, Simon stood anxious and uncommunicative. Then, towards the end of the time, he turned to his toy box, hitherto unopened. He set out a street scene with cars and buses and people crossing the road. Finally he spoke, 'There was an accident and a man was killed, and then a policeman came.' Simon looked very anxious. With few words, he was managing to communicate a great deal about the state of his inner world: there *had*, in reality, been an accident there, a mortal accident – his father had died. Perhaps he also regarded the birth of his younger sibling as a terrible accident. But of particular interest is his reaction to the presence of the policeman. His stated upset may have been a way of registering relief at an authority figure being at hand who might help out – as with a child's tears when the testing time is over. But the policeman's approach seemed to bring not so much reassurance as further anxiety – a possible indication, one might infer, of some kind of guilt. Since this was a first session and Simon did not yet know his therapist, his response might also have indicated his worry as to what kind of policeman/person he was about to encounter; fear too, perhaps, about punishment for what, in his mind, he may have felt that he *had* somehow done. Maybe he had an unconscious fear that he was implicated in the accident – had he, quite naturally, hated his father as well as loved him? Beyond the everyday feelings of ambivalence towards a parent, he may have felt a special antipathy towards his father at this particular time – for somehow giving his mother another baby, for example, and then for having abandoned them by dying. Had his ordinarily angry impulses been experienced, now, to be death-dealing?

This little episode is full of possible meanings and it also seems a very hopeful beginning to therapy. For Simon, young as he is, and despite inevitable anxiety about being with a strange lady in such an unusual situation, was able to find symbolic expression for his internal predicament – one which his therapist could, in turn, emotionally register, explore over time and find ways to talk to him about.

This description stayed in my mind because it contrasted so starkly with the first session of another boy whose case I was supervising at the time. 'Peter' came into therapy when he was 11. He, too, had experienced an 'accident' – his parents had separated when he was four and his mother had moved away with Peter to another country, with the result that son and father seldom saw one another. As a little boy, living alone with his mother, Peter had, according to her, seemed to manage this total and sudden upheaval 'surprisingly well'. In particular, as she recounted, he had excelled at school and, in reading and writing, was well ahead of his peers. By 11, however, a different picture presented itself and he was referred for treatment by a child psychiatrist who was alarmed by the intensity of his withdrawn and depressed state: friendless, earnest and obsessional, by turn clinging to and icily rejecting of his mother, Peter would, not infrequently, talk about suicide. His first session was in stark contrast to little Simon's. He, too, remained silent and withdrawn for most of the time, but towards the very end of the session he commented, rather sourly, that he didn't feel there was any point talking, and anyway, he was too clever for any professional, or anyone come to that, to understand him. With his insistently negativistic responses to whatever his therapist ventured, he effectively 'killed off' any possible link with her, leaving her feeling guilty, inadequate and anxious about ever being able to reach this rather cold and seemingly arrogant youngster who was so clearly in terrible pain. It might be assumed that 'guilty, inadequate and anxious' was a fair description of Peter's own feelings, if he could have allowed himself any contact with them.

At the very end of the session Peter precociously asserted that it was pointless talking about his feelings because he didn't have any. Or, he added, with a touch of uncertainty, if he did, he 'strangled' them as soon as possible. Asked what he meant, he said: 'It's like crying. When I want to cry in a film or watching TV, I tell myself it's just a mass of pixel points. Then I feel better. It's the same with books – if they're upsetting I tell myself that they are only a lexical arrangement.' This strangling of emotions by cognition was very chilling. And it was a long time before Peter even opened his toy box or showed any capacity for creative or symbolic thought.

The impact of this first session was enormous. His therapist felt quite overwhelmed by the intensity of the feelings that Peter was seeking to deny by the impenetrability of his defensive, precociously intellectual carapace. It would seem that, early on, Peter had adopted 'cleverness' as a defence against feeling and against fears about the risks attached to establishing any meaningful emotional link with somebody else who might then betray him, and/or disappear. Was *he* the reason his parents had separated? Was it *his* wish to have his mother all to himself that had brought about that very situation – so dreaded and so desired? Child therapists are particularly aware of how cognitive abilities, quite as much as apparent cognitive deficits, can act as defensive procedures, as bastions against the turbulence of emotional experience, especially when that experience involves unmanageable degrees of anxiety and guilt. Had Peter also been in therapy when the 'accident' first occurred, perhaps he could have been spared the isolating, obsessional, aloof, frozen self that he had developed in order to protect himself from the pain within.

Historical Development of the Theory and Practice of Child Psychotherapy

It was interest in these kinds of anxieties and guilts in young children and the way in which they affected later emotional growth and development – in particular their natural curiosity and ability to learn – that first stirred the compassion and involvement of the pioneers of child therapy and characterised their earliest cases.

An early quote about work with children can, perhaps surprisingly, be found in the writing of Elizabeth Craig in her 1948 encyclopaedia of housekeeping tips, among entries about baking and laundry (1948 edition of Elizabeth Craig's Compendium of Lively and Up-to-Date Information on Every Household Subject):

> *Nervous Children: If in spite of all your care and patience, a child continues to show signs of nervousness, never neglect them. The happiness of his whole life may depend on your seeking expert advice now. Psychoanalysis, which uncovers the core of the fears, examines it in the light of day and so minimises it and removes it, is a form of treatment that is becoming more and more widely used and successful. Your doctor may be able to help you set about obtaining this treatment or you can get into touch with the Institute of Child Psychology, 26 Warwick Avenue, London W9.*

Awareness of the plight of children was particularly acute during and after the two World Wars. Trauma, bereavement and massive displacement of children characterised both periods. The early child practitioners were all too aware of the relationship between external experiences of separation and loss and that between these events and internal, not consciously known, impulses. They also recognised how these experiences might be engaged with and mitigated through their symbolic representation in play. It was during and after the First World War that work directly with children first began and the end of the Second World War saw the founding of three training schools for the psychoanalytic treatment of children, funded both privately and by the NHS, now under the umbrella of a joint registering body – the Association of Child Psychotherapists.

Turning first to an historical overview: strictly Freud's 'Analysis of a Phobia in a Five-Year-Old Boy' [2] (Little Hans, 1909) was the first recorded case of intensive psychotherapy with children. But this 'treatment' was a sort of analysis by proxy – that is, it was based on Freud's comments on a series of detailed observations of Hans as noted by his psychoanalytically well-informed father. Freud himself met Little Hans only once. The outcome of the father's discussions about this delightful, intelligent and articulate little boy who, in anticipation of his next sibling's birth had developed a fear of horses, did much to reassure Freud about the nature of his early theoretical reconstructions of the Oedipal period and the idea that the so-called 'infantile neurosis' was a precursor of later adult neuroses. Although the treatment was largely successful, Freud was, apparently, perturbed by the response to the paper's publication [2]: ' ... a most evil future had been foretold for the poor little boy because he had been robbed of his innocence at such a tender age and had been made the victim of psychoanalysis' [2, p. 148]. Although implicitly repudiating such a response, there was, nonetheless, a sense that the psychoanalysis of children might be dangerous lest the 'soul is disturbed instead of freed', as one of the first to work directly with children, Hermine von Hug-Hellmuth [3, p. 289], put it.

Freud himself was sceptical about whether the deeper strata of a child's unconscious was therapeutically penetrable and was also concerned about the limited range of expression (by which he meant words and thoughts) available to the child [4]. It was three redoubtable women who, though working in rather different ways, effectively pioneered the treatment of children in person: Hermine von Hug-Hellmuth, Anna Freud and Melanie Klein. I shall briefly sketch these early approaches before concentrating, primarily, on the Kleinian development, which is the one most rooted in the child's earliest and later development.

In these early days Anna Freud thought of the child therapist's role as that of a kind of educator – a view largely shared by von Hug-Hellmuth – and advised that attempts to address the transference relationship with the therapist should focus on the positive aspects rather than on the negative. 'It is in their positive relationship to the therapist that truly valuable work will be done' [5, p. 41]. It was considered important to gain the child's affection and cooperation the better to support his or her weak ego functioning.

In general, Anna Freud tended to resist, even disapprove of, embarking on intensive (three or more sessions a week) work with a child until he or she was at least seven or eight years old. She also tended to favour one aspect of her father's thinking – his scientific concern with the organic energy that propelled the individual from within. She formulated an impressive model detailing the emotional growth of children and meticulously worked out the various stages of normal and pathological development with their specific anxieties and defences. In her emphasis on the ego's complex tasks in its moves towards an adaptation to reality, her focus tended to be more on the id-ego model of internal drives and impulses than on that of internal object relations [6].

While Anna Freud's position remained close to her father's, Klein's ideas, by contrast, resulted in what amounted to a fundamental reframing of psychoanalytic thought. Certain pivotal concepts (example penis envy or castration anxiety) lost their centrality, to be replaced by an extraordinarily rich and complex picture of the inner life of the young child, and even of the baby. In this account it was the nature and quality of emotional relationships that took precedence rather than a picture based on the quantitative intensity of impulses and drives. The language of instinct and impulse remained but its significance was much altered.

Klein and others, notably Fairbairn and Winnicott, traced a crucial developmental shift from anxiety about self-survival to concern for others, emotional responsibility and a desire to repair. With the linking of development to ethical concerns and matters of value, psychodynamic work with young children and adolescents gradually became less instinct-bound and more interested in emotional life and in meaning. This interest in the formative effect of early relationships became known as an 'object relations' approach, a term which, albeit clumsy, stresses the primary significance of the nature and quality of relationships between self and other, from the very first, as being central to a person's continuing psychological development.

It was with these ideas about the role of infantile anxiety and the impact of environmental failure on young people's lives, later detectable in the symbolic arena of speech and play, that the ground was laid for the psychoanalytic understanding and treatment of psychotic processes (on the whole regarded by Freud as not amenable to psychoanalytic treatment) and, more recently and extensively, of autistic and borderline states. Clinical experience, especially with children, continued to yield new insights. The origins of severe learning and developmental difficulties began to be located in disturbances of thought, of which the emotional determinants were sought in the earliest unconscious exchanges, and in the quality of care in the infant's primary relationship with mother or caretaker.

Wilfred Bion's work in the 1950s, 1960s and 1970s concentrated attention on the relationship between the way in which a person uses his or her mind and that person's capacity for emotional development. Bion did not, himself, work with children, but some of his theories had a fundamental, indeed, transformative effect on how child analytic thinking has developed. Despite their radical and innovative ideas, both Bion and Klein always considered their work as adhering to Freud's earlier psychoanalytic principles:

> I was also guided throughout by two other tenets of psychoanalysis established by Freud, which I have, from the beginning, regarded as fundamental; that the exploration of the unconscious is the main task of the psychoanalytic procedure and that the analysis of the transference is the means of achieving that aim. [7, p. 5]

Kleins own first paper, 'The Development of a Child' [8] was, like Little Hans, based on the analysis, at home, of a boy of five-and-a-quarter, Fritz – later revealed to be her own son, Erich. Her observations from this work led her to conclude that in-depth analysis of very young children was possible but incompatible with the therapist taking up an educative role [8].

It was Klein's view that it was precisely those areas of the child's emotional experience that were not consonant with what he had been taught that gave access to the internal world of psychic reality – thus to the nature and character of the various figures (primarily, at first, parental) who populated that world. These were figures who, as she soon noted, usually bore little resemblance to the external people whom they appeared to represent and seemed more based upon strongly held intuitions. Her own analysis in Budapest with Sandor Ferenczi, allowing intense examination of her own past relationships and also her passionate interest in the inner lives of her own children, further confirmed these ideas to Klein and many of Ferenczi's own ways of thinking about children's development were reflected in her later theories.

The Role of Play

It was in order to facilitate and intensify the transference to the therapist, Klein concluded, that the psychoanalysis of children should occur not in their own homes and playrooms but in a distinct and separate setting, as little influenced by known and familiar relationships as possible. Into this setting Klein introduced toys – not the child's own toys, as previously, but ones chosen to invite and encourage both as much symbolic representation as possible, un-interfered with by day-to-day or conventional meanings, and also to offer a potentially creative function – that of playing, building or dismantling, separating and joining, bouncing, tying, gluing or pouring. There would be small doll figures of different genders, generations and, these days, colour. Some wild and tame animals would be included, possibly some pieces of fencing, usually a few small vehicles, perhaps including an ambulance, a police car, a truck of some kind and a couple of cars. As child psychotherapist Shirley Hoxter put it, these toys

> ... are not provided to reassure the child or to give him a joyous time or to provide a creative or an abreactive outlet – although they may function for him in all these ways. Primarily they are there to provide the child with a vocabulary, as it were. They are a means of facilitating the

expression of his thoughts and feelings and clarifying their exploration. Klein considered that the child's play could be understood and interpreted in very much the same way as the psychotherapist interprets adults' dreams. [9, p. 208]

This notion of play as providing 'a vocabulary' for the inner world of the child is precisely what is demonstrated in my description of Simon's first session. Klein stressed the need to consider the child's play in the context of his total behaviour in the session, but also recognised that many children, for example Peter, are too traumatised or inhibited, indeed overwhelmed by anxiety, to be able to establish the degree of symbolic capacity that underlies the ability to play in the first place. As Shirley Hoxter suggests, these children's communications are 'not only non-verbal, they are even of a "pre-play" nature' [9, p. 208]. The potential shift in very disturbed or developmentally arrested children from non-symbolic to symbolic registers of emotion and feeling has increasingly become central to the work of the child therapist and of those engaging psychoanalytically with severe psychotic and borderline conditions.

To go back to the history, each child's play materials would be kept for their exclusive use in an individual box or drawer. Klein's premise in introducing the toys was that children's play, like adults' dreams, constituted the royal road to the unconscious. Her extraordinary capacities for observation and attention enabled her to engage with the underlying meaning of the child's world as enacted in play, in their associations to the play, in behaviour and activities around the play, and, especially, in relation to how she, the therapist, was variously related to in the course of these tremendously complex activities. It could be said that the most important part of the whole setting lies in this capacity for receptivity on the part of the therapist – what Bion was later to call 'reverie'.

There were two underlying intuitions in these Kleinian developments, ones that were to have a very significant impact on the future of psychoanalysis generally. The first was the observation that the transference is not so much, or not only, the projection of past relationships onto present ones, but is, rather, an ongoing, here-and-now re-experiencing in the room of infantile states. 'By re-experiencing early emotions and fantasies, and understanding them in relation to primal objects, the patient can revive these relations at their root, and thus, effectively diminish his anxieties' [10, p. 431]. Thus, for Simon, the policeman may have represented not only a version of his internal or external father, but also of his present experience of his new therapist. The second 'intuition' related to what Klein perceived, and her colleague, Susan Isaacs, theorised, as being the constant underlying operation of a kind of primary mental activity – not split off from present experience (in a conscious/unconscious layered model of the mind) but rather informing and shaping the meaning of that experience in an active way, all the time. Apparently conscious mental activity is thus constantly affected, shaped, and even determined, by this kind of unconscious phantasy, as external reality becomes informed or infused with internal meaning. All such suggestions reached far into very early states of mind, into what Freud had referred to as the 'dim and shadowy area of the mind', one which he himself did not feel confident about exploring.

The capacity or incapacity to play, that is the ability or inability to represent mental states in symbolic form, was at the heart of these new analytic developments and remains central to child analytic practice today.

Play, wrote Klein in 1932 [11],

is the child's most important medium of expression. If we make use of this play technique, we soon find that the child brings as many associations to the separate elements of its play as adults do to the separate elements of their dreams. These separate elements are indications to the trained observer: and as it plays, the child talks as well, and says all sorts of things which have the value of free association. [11, p. 30]

Countertransference

By 'trained observer' Klein was referring to the child therapist and an ability to engage with the total situation of the analytic session, including the impact of the contact with the child and his or her activities upon the therapist. This latter development, loosely called the countertransference emerged as a central psychoanalytic concept, highlighting the importance of the therapist's self-reflective responses in the work.

In a paper given at the first symposium on child analysis at an International Congress in 1961 [12], child therapist Esther Bick placed particular emphasis on what she describes as the specific countertransference problems that affect the child therapist, and suggested that 'the countertransference stresses on the child therapist are more severe than those on the therapist of adults, at any rate of non-psychotic adults'. She rightly noted the constant problem for the child therapist with his or her unconscious identifications – both with the child against the parents, the parents against the child or with a protective, reassuring and parental attitude towards the child. As Bick described, 'these conflicts often lead to a persecutory and guilty attitude towards the parents, making the therapist over-critical of them and over-dependent on their approval.' Added to this is the tremendous strain on the child therapist imposed both by the contents of the child's material and often by its mode of expression. As Bick described:

The intensity of the child's dependence, of his positive and negative transference, the primitive nature of his phantasies, tend to arouse the therapist's own unconscious anxieties. The violent and concrete projections of the child into the therapist may be difficult to contain. Also the child's suffering tends to evoke the therapist's parental feelings, which have to be controlled so that the proper analytic role can be maintained . . . Moreover the child's material may be more difficult to understand than the adult's, since it is more primitive in its sources as well as in its mode of expression, and requires a deeper knowledge of the primitive levels of the unconscious . . . It imposes on the child therapist a greater dependence on his unconscious to provide him with clues to the meaning of the child's play and non-verbal communication. [12, p. 171]

To these somewhat dark thoughts should, perhaps, be added something of the enormous pleasure and gratification the child therapist derives from the work. Right from the beginning of the training, which involves a two-year observation of an infant in the context of family life, there is a tremendous sense of the privilege of being entrusted with such intimate knowledge of a young individual's psychic development, especially one who has the rest of life to benefit from what help he or she receives for his or her growing potentialities, who, as one so often sees, can responsively achieve a better relationship with his or her internal objects and be encouraged to maintain that relationship despite the incursions of more savage and destructive impulses.

Container/Contained

Wilfred Bion's theories [13] have made a fundamental contribution to the enormously complex area of the nature of the internal setting of the therapist's mind. In elaborating

Freud's 'Two Principles of Mental Functioning' and Klein's theory of projective identification, Bion posited, as models of mental functioning, a notion of emotional linkage, and of the process by virtue of which one individual's (initially the baby's) inner experience can not only be mentally received and accommodated by a mother/therapist, but can also be transformed into a version which is understandable and therefore meaningful. This process was conceptualised as container/contained.

Bion extended Klein's concept of projective identification to include ordinary communications of feeling and emotion, and not just toxic ones of which the infant is seeking to rid him or herself. These communicative, as opposed to evacuatory, projections formed the basis of the crucial capacity to establish and sustain links of relatedness with the other, the emotional ties which lie at the root of the developmental process. Essential to the establishing of such links is the availability of a mind – a kind of 'thinking breast' – which is able to register and receive those projections for what they are, one that can, in Bion's terms, contain and mentally digest them. Not surprisingly, the concept of container/contained has become central to psychotherapeutic thinking, for it so exquisitely encompasses the many-faceted process that renders unmanageable states of mind bearable and enables learning from experience to take place. It also encompasses the possible consequences when, lacking such a container, the infant/young child, or, indeed, adolescent, has to fall back on his own defensive devices, ones which, as we saw at the beginning with Peter, may distort or deform the growing personality or, at worst, put a stop to the thinking and learning capacities altogether.

In work with children and adolescents, being able to contain and to go on thinking, to be able to 'think under fire', as Bion once put it, is often tested to its uttermost. In a quite physical way, any kind of unexpected change or absence can be felt as a breach in the containing function of the setting itself. It is for this reason that the closest attention has to be paid to consistencies of time, of self-presentation, of arrangement of furniture, of personal attitude, etc. It is likely that the more disturbed or deprived the child, the more absolute will be the importance of reliable boundaries and limits and the more threatening any slight alteration.

> Gary had been seen regularly by a therapist at school where the 'time out' provided relief from the tumult and stress of his classroom and had come to be valued by him inordinately. Usually disorganised and chaotic, he never missed his session-time and was never late. On the occasion described, the therapist was one minute late. Gary thrust a broken milk bottle in her face in the opening moments of the session. 'If you do that again I'll kill you', he hissed.

In this case the experience of being let down, even by a minute, had aroused unbearable feelings of betrayal and abandonment. The attacking force of his infantile fear had to be projected violently because it was literally uncontainable. The therapist was to experience the impact, on Gary himself. In this situation it can be very difficult to respond therapeutically rather than parentally. This point is made particularly clearly by child and adolescent psychoanalyst Donald Meltzer [14]:

> It is Bion's theory that the mother can understand her baby through her unconscious receptiveness to the baby's projective identification and that the therapist who is sufficiently in touch with his own unconscious can be aware of a similar receptivity and responsiveness in himself. Notice that he must first of all be sufficiently receptive and then secondly be sufficiently in touch with the unconscious processes in himself which result from this receptivity. By this second step he is able to respond analytically rather than parentally. [14, p. 9]

This attitude of receptiveness and thoughtfulness and the desire to understand cannot be counterfeited. It may *in itself* be felt as therapeutic, for much can be introjected before it is possible to verbalise things accurately. Indeed the very capacity to hold mental states and to bear not knowing – not prematurely interpreting and reaching for explanation – that capacity for what Keats termed 'negative capability' lies at the heart of analytic practice, especially in relation to work with children and young people.

In this early work of Klein and her colleagues, there were three very significant modifications of the early images of children's mental life. These were the revelation of very early psychotic anxieties; the nature and significance of psychic reality; and the elaboration of the paranoid-schizoid and depressive positions.

Case Example

Sammy had a very difficult beginning. He had been born prematurely and had several quite serious physical problems which resulted in his being kept in hospital for two months after his mother and twin sister had gone home. His mother had been very depressed following the twins' birth and had been convinced for a long time that Sammy would die. He spent his first three weeks in an incubator and suffered many brief stays in hospital thereafter. He was eventually referred for psychotherapeutic treatment because of his parents' distress over the nightmares which had begun around the time when his mother had started to wean him from bottle to cup. Scarcely a night passed without his mother having to spend long periods attempting to calm Sammy down, to stop him bashing his head against the wall or against the side of his cot, and to try to render more manageable the persecutory world in which he seemed to exist. She described how, when he awoke, he would often seem to experience her as a frightening, rather than as a comforting figure. This increased her own distress – making her feel, by turn, angry and inadequate.

There seemed to be a complete split between the happy, chatty, day-time Sammy and the terrified and tyrannical night-time Sammy. Now that he was three, he could demand his mother's reassuring presence, unlike before when, as a tiny infant, he was not only helpless, but physically separated from her as well (in the incubator). He may also have had a sense of her lack of an emotional capacity to contain his own fear of dying, since she, herself, was so frightened of death.

As time went on and Sammy began to experience his therapist as someone who could bear the naughty, messy and destructive 'boy' (as he referred to himself when in this mode) as well as the charming 'Sammy', the terrifying nature of his inner world, hitherto confined to his nightmare life, started to appear explicitly in the sessions. Violent fantasies began to be played out, usually attributed to the 'nasty, biting crocodile' or to 'Jenny', his twin, or to 'Spencer', one of his soft toys and, at the same time, a lively representative figure in his internal world. At first, the play was only very occasionally preceded by the pronoun, 'I', for Sammy, at this stage, found it almost impossible to take any responsibility for his rage and aggression.

As a consequence of experiencing his therapist's ability to tolerate his own unbearable feelings of anger, jealousy and distress, and realising that she could take in and hold these feelings without being dominated by them, nor driven into action herself, Sammy was able to re-engage with his 'thinking' self. In being receptive and understanding to all he expressed in the sessions through his words and his play, including scenes of intense fear, jealousy, murderousness and hatred, his therapist was able to divest his feelings of excessive anxiety and to return to him a 'thought-about' and therefore meaningful version of his pain. The session provided a safe place and time for thinking about Sammy's feelings and actions.

Sammy gradually became brighter and his nightmares reduced eventually disappearing altogether.

Conclusion

The work of a child psychotherapist provides a necessary setting for the extraordinarily passionate, destructive and persecutory experiences that the baby/child needs to have modified externally and internally in order to be able to proceed with his development. These experiences in the internal world of the child may be expressed in a variety of ways – through words, behaviour, play and the countertransference responses of the therapist. The early discoveries of pioneering child psychotherapists have elucidated and refined the understanding of early, primitive states of anxiety, unconscious phantasy and the development of thought and the ability to learn. The process whereby some of the ways that development may be distorted and arrested, and how these can be modified before they are again played out in adolescence and so-called, 'adulthood', is the task of the child therapist.

References

1. Bion WR. *Elements*. London: Heinemann, 1963. Reprint, London: Karnac Books, 1984.

2. Freud S. Analysis of a phobia in a five-year-old boy. In J Strachey, ed., *The Standard Edition of the Complete Psychological Works of Sigmund Freud, Volume X (1909): Two Case Histories ('Little Hans' and the 'Rat Man'*. London: Hogarth Press. 1955; pp. 3–152. (Original work published 1909)

3. Hug-Helmuth H von. On the technique of child analysis. *Int J Psychoanal* 1921; 2: 287–305.

4. Freud S. From the history of an infantile neurosis. In J Strachey, ed., *The Standard Edition of the Complete Psychological Works of Sigmund Freud, Volume XVII (1917–1919): An Infantile Neurosis and Other Works*. London: Hogarth Press. 1955; pp. 7–122. (Original work published 1918)

5. Freud A. The role of transference in the analysis of children. In *Introduction to Psycho-Analysis*. London: Hogarth Press, 1974.

6. Likierman M, Urban E. The roots of child and adolescent psychotherapy in

psychoanalysis. In A Home, M Lanyado, eds., *The Handbook of Child and Adolescent Psychotherapy: Psychoanalytic Approaches*. London and New York: Routledge, 1999.

7. Klein M. The psycho-analytic play technique: its history and significance. In *New Directions*, op. cit. 1955.

8. Klein M. The development of a child. In *The Writings of Melanie Klein*. Vol. 1. *Love, Guilt and Reparation and Other Works, 1921–1945*. London: Hogarth Press. 1975; pp. 1–53.

9. Hoxter S. Play and communication. In M Boston, D Daws, eds., *The Child Psychotherapist and Problems of Young People*. London: Wildwood House. 1977; pp. 202–31.

10. Pick I, Segal H. Melanie Klein's contribution to child analysis. In J Glenn, ed., *Child Analysis and Therapy*. London and New York: Jason Aronson. 1978; pp. 427–50.

11. Klein M. *The Psycho-analysis of Children*. London: Hogarth Press, 1975.

12. Bick E. Child analysis today. *Int J Psychoanal* 1962; 43: 328–32.

13. Bion WR. *Learning from Experience*. London: Heinemann, 1962. Reprint, London: Karnac Books, 1984.

14. Meltzer D. *Sexual States of Mind.* Strathtay: Clunie Press, 1973.

Further Reading

Abraham K. A short study of the development of the libido, viewed in the light of mental disorders. In E Jones, ed., *Selected Papers on Psycho-Analysis.* London: Hogarth. 1927; pp. 418–501. Reprint, EB Spillius, ed., *Melanie Klein Today: Developments in Theory and Practice.* Vol. 2. *Mainly Practice.* London: Routledge, 1988.

Edgcombe R. *Anna Freud: A View of Development, Disturbance and Therapeutic Techniques.* London: Routledge, 2000.

Geissman C & P. *A History of Child Psychoanalysis.* London: Routledge, 1992.

Harris Williams M (ed.). *Collected Papers of Martha Harris and Esther Bick.* Strathtay: Clunie Press, 1987.

Hoxter S. Play and communication. In M Boston, D Daws, eds., *The Child Psychotherapist and Problems of Young People.* London: Wildwood House. 1977; pp. 202–31.

Hurry A. *Psychoanalysis and Developmental Therapy.* London: Karnac Books, 1998.

Isaacs S. The nature and function of phantasy. *Int J Psychoanal* 1948; 29: 73–97. Reprint, M Klein, P Heinarm, S Isaacs, J Riviere, eds., *Developments in Psycho-Analysis.* London: Hogarth Press, 1952.

King P. Steiner R (eds.). *The Freud-Klein Controversies, 1941–1945.* London: Tavistock/Routledge, 1991.

Klein M. Symposium on child analysis. In *Love, Guilt and Reparation and Other Works, 1921–1945,* op. cit. 1927

O'Shaughnessy E. A 3½-year-old boy's melancholic identification with an original object. *Int J Psychoanal* 1986; 67: 173–9.

O'Shaughnessy E. A commerative essay on W. R. Bion's theory of thinking. *J Child Psychother* 1981; 7 (2): 181–9. Reprinted as W.R. Bion's theory of thinking and new techniques in child analysis. In EB Spillius, ed., *Melanie Klein Today: Developments in Theory and Practice.* Vol. 2. *Mainly Practice.* London: Routledge. 1988; pp. 177–90.

O'Shaughnessy E. *Melanie Klein Today: Developments in Theory and Practice.* Vol. 2. *Mainly Practice.* London: Routledge, 1988.

Rustin M, Rhode M, Dubinsky A, Dubinsky H (eds.). *Psychotic States in Children.* London: Karnac Books, 1998.

Szur R, Miller S (eds.). *Extending Horizons: Psychoanalytic Psychotherapy with Children, Adolescents and their Families.* London: Karnac Books, 1991.

Waddell M. *Inside Lives: Psychoanalysis and the Growth of the Personality.* London: Karnac Books, 1998.

Waddell M. *On Adolescence.* London: Routledge, 2018.

Therapeutic Communities

Steve Pearce and Adam Dierckx

Introduction

Therapeutic communities (TCs) have a long history in mental health care, and the approach is now used in the areas of personality disorder, intellectual disability, forensic services, addictions, education and psychosis. They form the basis for tier 3 personality disorder services when delivered as day services. TC principles have had an enormous impact on current psychiatric practice and were influential in the foundation of social psychiatry. This chapter outlines the history, principles and practice of democratic TCs (DTCs) and traces their impact on service development more broadly. It describes DTCs as a treatment method. It does not treat the use of TC approaches in education, intellectual disability services, addictions, or TC as a philosophy of care in any detail.

Note: vignettes are given to illustrate aspects of DTC practice. They are taken from a DTC in the UK, and reflect some procedures and nomenclature specific to that TC.

TCs have been used as a leading treatment model in health care going back to the Second World War. DTC principles are used in education and with disturbed children and young people, to create mutually respectful communities in intellectual disability, and in prisons [1]. Hierarchical TCs, which emphasise mentoring and seniority, have been used in the treatment of addictions since the 1950s [2]. DTCs, emphasising democratisation and a flattened hierarchy, have been used to promote change and recovery in patients we would now recognise as suffering from medically unexplained symptoms, post-traumatic stress disorder, psychosis, personality disorders (PDs) and affective disorders. In the 1940s pioneers such as Wilfred Bion, SH Foulkes and Tom Main used these principles with soldiers invalided out of the war, and informed later work by Maxwell Jones at the Belmont Clinic/Henderson Hospital and later Dingleton Hospital in the Scottish Borders, and Tom Main at the Cassel Hospital in London, among many others. In the 1960s DTCs became associated with the anti-psychiatry movement, partly through the influence of RD Laing, and in the 1970s and 1980s experienced an enormous expansion across the UK and the USA, with large numbers of psychiatric hospitals and wards adopting DTC principles [3]. In 1978 the TC movement was instrumental in a major reform of psychiatric services in Italy (Law 180) in which the 'democratic psychiatry' movement resulted in the closure of the asylums, replacing many of them with TCs [4]. In the UK, interest in DTCs coincided with the discovery of phenothiazines, and was instrumental in the unlocking of mental hospital wards [5]. DTC pioneers such as Maxwell Jones and Tom Main, and the TC model, were instrumental in the establishment of social psychiatry [6].

Over the 1990s and 2000s DTC approaches in health care gradually focussed on the treatment of PDs, and all but a few residential services closed or became day services [7]. Government policies designed to improve PD provision led to an increase in outpatient and day DTC services for PD in the early 2000s [8].

At the time of going to press (2020), the number of DTCs in the UK National Health Service (NHS) probably number about 30 but are unevenly distributed geographically. There are in addition 15 DTCs operating in HM Prisons, including 3 for prisoners with intellectual disability and PD [9]. The need to adopt therapeutic approaches in psychiatric practice was highlighted in 1953 by the World Health Organization Expert Committee on Mental Health, which noted that the correct role of a psychiatric hospital was 'that of a therapeutic community' [10], while in 2019 the NHS Long Term Plan noted that 'for people admitted to an acute mental health unit, a therapeutic environment provides the best opportunity for recovery' [11, s3.102, p. 71]. The Enabling Environments initiative, part of the Royal College of Psychiatrists, provides a quality mark for services aiming to create or bolster their therapeutic and relational aspects, and grew out of the DTC approach. DTC approaches have given rise to innovative relational models outside psychiatry, including in homeless hostels (psychologically informed environments, PIEs), and probation hostels and prison wings (psychologically informed planned environments, PIPEs) [12]. DTC principles have been incorporated into quality assurance networks, often founded on peer review processes. The Royal College of Psychiatrists Accreditation for Inpatient Mental Health Services (AIMS) process, for example, recommends that staff should be trained in group methods, and that a patient community meeting be held regularly, with shared decision-making and spontaneous staff–patient activities, principles taken from DTC practice.

Theoretical Foundations of DTC Practice

Rapoport: An Anthropologist's Observations of an Early DTC

In 1959 an American anthropologist and his team visited the Belmont (later Henderson) Hospital, a residential DTC, for a number of months in order to study and describe the interactions and social environment. He published *Community as Doctor* [13] the following year, which set out what he regarded as the four most prominent characteristics of the TC. These were observations rather than instructions, and were restricted to a single residential DTC in the late 1950s, but the four elements described below have come to be regarded as central features of DTC functioning.

Democratisation

Decision-making was devolved to the community, consisting of all patients and staff, with all participants having an equal influence over outcome. Decisions are taken in community meetings with all members present, and if necessary, can be voted upon. The process of reaching a decision is itself therapeutic, promoting empowerment, encouraging prosocial skills in a shared endeavour and giving each community member a stake in the common life. DTCs vary in the extent to which reaching decisions is prioritised over discussion.

Before acting on behalf of the group, a group member must seek a 'vote of confidence' and must not act without majority agreement. Tom was a timid man who had decided to chair another group member's review after lots of group encouragement. When it came to time to start, he got cold feet. The group reminded him that they had all expressed, through the vote, that they were confident he could do it. The group stopped him backing out and he chaired successfully, later saying he felt this represented a breakthrough.

Permissiveness

Delinquent behaviour was not proscribed, but was tolerated with a view to understanding the underlying drivers and meaning.

Barry was a socially awkward character who expressed critical views about mental health problems (including denying his own), the value of groups generally and the TC in particular. He launched into tirades about authority and 'young people'. Nevertheless, he did not offend individual group members. The group tolerated his rants, seeing them as a distancing strategy. Several months later he remarked this was the first group of people who had tolerated him long enough to get to know him properly. Other group members said they had learned patience with 'off-putting' people and felt pride in being welcoming.

Reality Confrontation

Delinquent behaviour, while tolerated, was also confronted by other TC members, both patients and staff. The impact of the behaviour on the community was regularly fed back to the patient.

Eva talked in group about her relationships with a series of men who inevitably treated her badly. Another group member wondered if such relationships might be another form of self-harm. Initially Eva seemed offended, misinterpreting him as blaming her. As they talked, she was able to consider his points and subsequently questioned her own part in maintaining her problems.

Communalism

The members of the community regarded themselves as mutually accountable, and spent formal (in-group) and informal time together.

Susie repeatedly missed group meetings, especially the morning community meeting. She said that was OK as she was the one missing therapy, ignoring the effects on others. She missed volunteering for tasks to help the group, and hearing other members' problems. When she arrived, she expected help. Once this was explained she began to see the effects of her lateness on others, and to attend earlier.

Haigh's Quintessence: A Developmental Model of Progression in DTC Treatment

In 1999 Rex Haigh, a British psychiatrist, developed a model to describe the stages of development that a member of a DTC typically goes through, mirroring the stages of development undergone in normal infancy [14].

Attachment

In the early stages of membership, members attach to the group as a whole, as well as the group members individually. The sense of belongingness this engenders becomes one of the motivators for change.

> Laura was new to the community but volunteered to chair the morning meeting, despite her anxiety. Jim talked about his anxiety when he first chaired, helped by support from senior group members and practice. Next week, Laura sat next to Jim when chairing and on several occasions looked across to him as she faltered. Staff noticed him giving her a quiet nod at times and she chaired the meeting successfully.

Containment

This element stems from ideas about containment developed by Bion [15] (see Chapter . . .). TC structure, in particular mutual care and predictability, produces the safety and security necessary for therapeutic change, and minimises acting out.

> Alice, a woman who often got into unsafe situations during crises, arrived in group highly distressed. The group helped her to fight the urge to constantly talk about what had gone on over the weekend and to focus on the planned structure of the day. Later she said this structure helped by giving time for her distress to settle, having protected but limited space to talk, and the encouragement to refocus on others.

Communication

Freedom of communication (see below), treating behaviour as a communication, and the Culture of Enquiry (see below) start to play an increasingly important role in the TC members' journey by its mid-point.

> In the morning community meeting group members are expected to give an update on any risk-related behaviour since last group. All are expected to participate in turn, and to be honest about risks. In large group one afternoon, Paul wanted to discuss his self-harm. While the group wanted to hear about this, they also highlighted him choosing not to disclose it earlier in the morning meeting.

Inclusion

All community members are included in the life of the community, the Living Learning Experience.

> Sheila had a long history of rejection by services either due to mental health problems, the wrong diagnosis or her risk profile. In selection she discussed this rejection, along with other aspects of her problems that left group members wondering if the TC was right for her. She was offered a place, given the 'benefit of the doubt' and became a valued group member, benefitting greatly from the community. Several months later, during a period of depressed mood, she

doubted whether anyone wanted her around. Several group members challenged this perception, reminding her that the community as a whole voted for her to join, just as it had for each member there.

Agency

As the TC member becomes more senior, democratisation and reality confrontation gradually mobilise his or her sense of agency. Members come to recognise their own ability to effect change and take responsibility for doing so.

John was open about his problems asserting himself with powerful authority figures, tending to become submissive. Encouraged by others, he volunteered to chair meetings and started to lead meetings without either dominating or deferring to staff and more experienced members. Later he was also able to help the group keep ownership of a problem, demarcating the limits of his authority by reminding the group that the decision was theirs not his.

The Four Principles of DTC Treatment: How TCs Work

More recently, the principles by which DTCs have their effect have been described in more detail [16, 17].

Belongingness

People who feel they belong, who have the sense that they are important to others and care about those others themselves are better able to regulate their mental state, learn and retain prosocial behaviours and are less prone to aggression and suicidal feelings [18]. Many people referred to DTCs are isolated, and the feeling of belongingness that they find in the community becomes a key factor in their willingness and ability to adopt new coping strategies.

Cathy had always felt alienated from society and been rejected by various institutions over time. Initially she saw herself as different from others and that the TC wasn't really for her. During a meeting for people who had applied to join the TC, Cathy described life in 'our group'. Afterwards the group remarked on this. She bashfully admitted she had started to think of the TC as her group and perhaps the first place she felt she belonged and felt accepted.

Social Learning

Higher animals, including humans, learn socially as well as through direct behavioural mechanisms such as operant conditioning. This process is central to the therapeutic effect of DTC treatment, and was described in detail by Clark [19]. TC members imitate more senior members, respond to praise and critical feedback and are sensitive to the actions of the staff.

Don had severe agoraphobia, avoided going to the shops and minimised time spent outside. An early goal was to volunteer as a group shopper. Reviewing this, he stated it was only possible if accompanied. The other shoppers observed that he went to another aisle of the store to fetch bread alone. He replied he had seen one of them do the same two weeks earlier and thought he'd try this. This small change presaged greater changes in behaviour and attitude later.

Narrative Development

Psychologically traumatic events can be difficult to incorporate into a person's life narrative, or be incorporated in an unhelpful way, leading to maladaptive beliefs and behaviours. In talking and thinking about past events in the presence of non-judgemental others, their meaning changes, and can be incorporated into a self-concept that is more adaptive. For example, a woman who was raped as a child may think of herself as complicit and therefore guilty; it can take many retellings before this changes [20].

The Promotion of Agency, and Responsibility without Blame

Many patients, particularly those with PD, may feel powerless and that any change needs to originate outside themselves. This can be related to a history of childhood abuse and victimisation. Changes to maladaptive behaviours such as self-harm and abnormal eating patterns may get easier with insight and improvements in mood, but will still require the exercise of the patient's will, and a sense of agency. In DTC, responsible agency is encouraged through the devolved and democratised structures of the community [17], but, crucially, is separated from the attribution of blame [21]. Blame is the normal accompaniment to responsibility when behaviour is harmful, in particular when it harms others, but blame is countertherapeutic and likely to lead to early loss from treatment. This leaves a dilemma: how not to blame someone, while retaining their sense of being responsible for their actions and therefore empowered to change. DTC practitioners practice responsibility without blame, in which members are treated as responsible for their actions and decisions, but are not blamed for them. An online course in this way of working is available at www.responsibilitywithoutblame.org/.

Justine often spoke angrily and condescendingly to other group members, leaving them feeling hurt or angry. Sometimes they would try to challenge her, but the conversation would get derailed by her distress at 'all of you attacking me'. Eventually the group proposed to use the community's 'participation' process – a contract to change behaviour that is obstructing good participation. Although she initially disagreed, by working on this specific behaviour she came to see that others telling her how they experienced her differed from criticising or attacking her. She realised that the only one who could change the way she spoke to others was herself.

Other Principles of DTC Treatment

Over the course of the last 60 years, a number of additional essentials of DTC practice have been described. These are described as essentials as their absence is likely to seriously disrupt DTC functioning.

Culture of Enquiry

Tom Main coined the phrase culture of enquiry to describe a situation in which all decision-making is open to question [22]. Each member is responsible for their communications, and can expect to have them challenged, albeit compassionately. The principle encourages assertiveness and responsible agency.

On Sally's first day things seemed to go wrong from the start. The normally smooth running of the day became haphazard; many group members were fractious and irritable; a review was undertaken hastily; and shoppers bought insufficient food for lunch. Later in large group, members struggled to identify what they wanted to talk about, but complained there was inadequate time. Staff expressed curiosity about all this, also that the group had been uncharacteristically unwelcoming to the new group member, for example forgetting to show her around and not taking her with them at break time. Group members asked each other about this and made amends to the new group member. The community identified a general feeling that 'there isn't enough space for all of us here to get looked after'. An experienced group member suggested that 'in not looking after Sally we stopped looking after ourselves'.

Freeing of Communications

Closely related to the culture of enquiry, freeing of communications is a term coined by Clark [19] to describe the principle that any topics can, and potentially should, be discussed in the TC. Difficulties with staff communication also used to be dealt with in TC meetings, a habit less common in modern DTCs. This facet of DTC practice reveals the close relationship between the development of the approach and that of Group Analysis, many of the pioneers having worked together (or indeed being the same people). In Group Analysis, freeing of communications is a central concern, serving the same function as free association in psychoanalysis.

In an 'Information Meeting' for prospective group members, the group candidly answered questions from a sceptical visitor, giving positive experiences while not hiding their experiences of frustration and disappointment. When he came to a selection meeting a few weeks later, he said that something that had convinced him to proceed with his application was the group's honesty about therapy's imperfections. He said he was used to staff being over-optimistic about therapy and it then being disappointing and useless.

Analysis of All Events

Another of Clark's terms, all events in a DTC potentially have meaning. Behaviour is neither dismissed, proscribed nor merely tolerated, but is understood as a communication, to be analysed and understood in the group by the TC members. This is a fundamentally psychoanalytic approach, undertaken by the TC.

In the example above given for 'Communalism', this technique enabled consideration of the effects each member had on others without blaming. Imagining others' perspectives and hearing robust feedback from peers helped Susie to see why others were annoyed and what needed to change.

No Secrets

Many TC members have been subject to abuse and exploitation, and may continue to be vulnerable to this, while others may have been exploitative. All interactions between members, whether in informal group time (milieu time), meetings of subgroups such as work groups and small groups, or outside of TC time, are brought back to the community. This prevents abuse or unhealthy relationships developing between members (including between members and staff), and avoids recreating situations reminiscent of the secrecy that accompanies abuse.

> The group elects three shoppers as a safeguard against private conversations. Perhaps because Tony was a quiet person, Jody and Ruth had been talking together when Ruth told Jody she had cut herself that morning, though she had withheld this from the group. She swore Jody to secrecy. Tony, whom they had forgotten, objected. To Ruth's chagrin he told the group on their return. The group discussed Ruth's attempts at secrecy and her concealment of self-harm. They realised they had underestimated Ruth's self-harm and asked about it each week thereafter, thus supporting her efforts to stop.

Being Alongside

'Being alongside' is related to the flattened (or fluid) hierarchy that typifies DTCs [19]. Rather than an expert-driven model, in which a patient is advised and treated by an expert, the main interactions are between patient members. When staff contribute they are guided by the principle of authenticity; rather than providing a detached expert view, they bring their own feelings and experiences to bear as members of the TC themselves.

> In the example for 'Culture of Enquiry' above, staff tried to imagine Sally's feelings on her first day, to be curious why other members were behaving differently and to comment on how they felt being in this TC now without criticism or guidance.

Living and Learning

The members of the TC engage in the normal activities of life, cooking, cleaning, shopping and being together. It is through their experience of this, the living learning experience, that they learn about themselves and acquire the skills to form and sustain healthy relationships elsewhere.

> Asha struggled to join the group for lunch. When she ate her own sandwiches elsewhere the group gently but firmly restated that everyone was expected to share lunch. Subsequently, Asha stayed in the room with other group members at lunchtime, eventually joining them at the table, though not eating anything. Group members included her in conversations. One day they offered her some fruit they were enthusing about. Asha timidly accepted, looking quietly pleased to be asked. The following week she started to take a little more food and after several months she was eating a full meal with the group.

DTC Practice

DTCs can be residential or run as day programmes. The latter normally have a support system for when the TC is not meeting, either by telephone or electronic communication, or in person. Day programmes can run for any number of days per week, at the time of writing the most common frequency is one day per week. In general, intensity decreases through the day and (for those that run on more than one day per week) through the week, so the most psychologically strenuous interventions, such as psychodrama and analytic small groups, would normally occur near the start of the day/week, and more relaxed activities, such as work groups and social groups, would be more frequent towards the end. The communities vary in size from 6 in some of the children's TCs to 40 in some prison TCs. Although most commonly attended by individuals, some TCs cater for families.

TC structure generally follows a sandwich pattern, each day starting and normally ending with a community meeting, which is the main forum for business, and it is here that any tensions or important events from the life of the community are discussed, votes taken when necessary and decisions made. Specialist groups may include art therapy, psychodrama, analytic small groups, work groups (in which TC members take care of their environment, including for example cooking, gardening and cleaning) and other specialist psychotherapeutic approaches such as mentalising, coping skills, mindfulness and transactional analysis.

Typical daily structure	
Opening community meeting	Opening and closing community meetings involve all TC members, and are the main decision-making body of the TC. Community processes are investigated, plans made, admissions and discharges planned and when necessary votes taken. At the beginning of the day members sometimes check in, particularly if the TC did not meet the day before, so that the community knows if any members are struggling or if new problems have arisen
Break	
Specialist group	
Lunch	
Business meeting	A meeting which staff members may not attend, in which menus and rotas are often decided upon
Specialist group	
Closing community meeting	Similar to opening community meeting. Includes plans for the evening, and review of any issues that have arisen during the day

Diagnosis

DTCs have traditionally taken an idiographic (treating each individual as a unique case) rather than nomothetic (attempting to derive broad types into which individuals fit) approach to classification, reflecting shared roots with the group analytic and psychoanalytic traditions. Diagnoses are commonly used when helpful for research, for deciding whom the intervention is likely to benefit, for identifying areas of difficulty and to help members feel their problems are not unique to them.

Medication

Some DTCs have in the past required members to reduce and stop psychotropic medications on the basis that they might interfere with the effective development of healthy coping strategies by numbing the experience of distress, and remove incentives to change. More recently most DTCs have taken a flexible approach, recognising that the more disabled members might require the support of medication in the early stages as the containment and attachment to the TC develops, but encourage members to reduce their reliance on medication where evidence of long-term prescribing being necessary is lacking.

Boundary Maintenance

Many people who join TCs have experienced inconsistent care, and so the consistent maintenance of boundaries, and dynamic administration in general, is central to successful treatment. Boundaries are set by the community democratically, and are maintained by the community, with staff being more or less active according to circumstances. The principal governing staff action is that the community are encouraged to be self-governing, which has a therapeutic impact in encouraging empowerment and the development of responsible agency, stepping in when necessary to ensure consistent and safe boundary maintenance. A TC that is working well will require minimal staff intervention. Care is taken that boundary maintenance does not become harsh or punitive. TCs use specific structures and instruments to maintain boundaries.

Structures and interventions used in DTC	*Note, different DTCs tend to evolve their own approaches and names for interventions, but will commonly have approaches that mirror those below*
Special or Crisis meeting	Called anytime a formal group is not meeting (i.e. during milieu time), when a community member feels in need of support, or an urgent issue has arisen that cannot wait until the next group. May be called by ringing a bell
Contracts	An agreement made by members with the community. Usually used to support and encourage new coping strategies or prosocial approaches to replace maladaptive and harmful behaviours
Mini case conferences	A brief (typically 10 minute) slot in a community meeting in which a particular issue is brought by a community member for dedicated consideration

(cont.)

Rejoining case conferences	After a severe boundary break, or if a member's commitment to the community becomes a concern, they may be invited to present their reasons for being a community member in a similar way to when they first joined. There may also be a vote as to whether they remain a member of the community
Suspension	A serious boundary break, often comprising very harmful behaviour, may result in temporary suspension of the member's place in the community. This approach is used with careful attention to the principles of permissiveness and belongingness (see above)
Discharge	Only in the most serious cases, for example if the behaviour of a member is deemed to be damaging the community or its members, or if the member is themselves in danger of harm through the treatment, might a therapeutic discharge from a community be considered

Research

DTCs have in the past had difficulties carrying out experimental research, but for different reasons to those that have affected psychoanalytic approaches. TCs have attracted a rowdy crowd, often allied to countercultural philosophies, and suspicious of positivism (in this context, the idea that firm conclusions can be drawn from experimental or observational evidence and applied generally). At various points in its development the movement has also had a political element, which has been hostile to systematisation and dispassionate investigation. People who have experienced life in a TC also have a tendency to become identified with the method, and to resist the idea that it should be subject to the same proofs of effectiveness as less immersive approaches. In short, people often find their exposure to DTC life-changing, and consequently can be reluctant to interrogate its effectiveness.

In the early years research mostly centred around the big residential units and inpatient TCs, which were the main expressions of the method in the 1970s, 80s and 90s. In 1999 a large systematic review was published of TC research to date, which concluded that evidence for effectiveness was strong, particularly in addictions TCs, but that there was a lack of high quality randomised controlled trials (RCTs) [23]. There were a number of subsequent case-controlled studies and case series in healthcare settings, but the barriers to running an RCT seemed high.

Difficulties running an RCT of DTC treatment (adapted from [24])

Ethical objections
1. TC practitioners' concerns over subjects being denied TC treatment. Many TC practitioners regard the approach as 'fundamentally human' and obviously beneficial
2. Concern that running an RCT would damage the culture of the TCs taking part
3. Current TC members should be given the choice of whether their TC should participate, and may decline

Feasibility

4. Difficulties measuring and ensuring adherence to the treatment model
5. Uncertainty over the active constituents of TC treatment
6. Selection of candidates for the TC by current TC members leading to a proportion of subjects randomised to TC treatment being turned down for treatment
7. Effect on participating TCs of a reduction in members joining due to randomisation
8. Problems stemming from referrer attitudes to the possibility of patients not receiving an otherwise available specialist resource
9. Problems obtaining consent to randomisation: due to the emphasis in DTC practice on transparency and shared decision-making, candidates for DTC treatment are often committed to the treatment and unlikely to agree to an alternative (or no) treatment
10. Effects of TC 'health': TCs can go through cycles of disturbance and effectiveness

Problems shared with other group therapeutic models

11. Non-independence of observations: a technical statistical problem, often ignored in the analysis of group-based interventions.

In 2017 the first RCT of DTC treatment for PD reported positive outcomes [25]. The research group have described the way they overcame the anticipated difficulties [24].

Research in prison DTCs has tended to focus on recidivism, with a separate and growing literature on addictions TC interventions in prisons. There is good evidence of effectiveness in reducing recidivism in prisoners in DTC programmes, with ancillary findings of reductions in adjudications [26]. RCTs have not been carried out, and are rare in prison populations for any intervention.

Training

Training in TC theory and practice has, for most of the twentieth and early twenty-first centuries, been based on an apprenticeship model. Since the 1980s a twice yearly workshop, the Living Learning Experience, has provided an opportunity for experiential learning, through the creation of a temporary TC in which attendees participate for three days (http://growingbetterlives.org/living-and-learning/). More recently a year-long course, the Therapeutic Environments Practitioner Course, has been available for students who want to progress to practitioner level (http://tcept.org/). The course is based on the Democratic Therapeutic Community Handbook, published in 2017 [16], provides training in therapeutic community and related approaches such as milieu therapy and the operation of therapeutic and enabling environments, and incorporates the Living Learning Experience weekend. Developments in DTC training are covered in more detail elsewhere [27].

TC Influence on Current Service Development, and the Future

Several of the currently fashionable ideas in psychiatry owe their core ideas to the widespread influence of therapeutic community ideas in the 1970s and 80s. Social psychiatry arose substantially out of the work of the TC pioneers in the 1950s. The Recovery movement, with its emphasis on learning rather than treatment, and patient empowerment as a route to recovery, itself arose from social psychiatry and incorporates elements of DTC philosophy. Co-production, the planning and delivery of services and research as a partnership between clinicians/researchers and patients or ex-patients has its origins in the use of experts-by-experience by TCs, and the valuing of peer support and expertise in TCs.

References

1. Kennard D. The therapeutic community as an adaptable treatment modality across different settings. *Psychiatr Q* 2004; 75(3): 295–307.

2. De Leon G. *The Therapeutic Community: Theory, Model, and Method.* New York: Springer Publishing Company, 2000.

3. Pearce S, Haigh R. Milieu approaches and other adaptations of therapeutic community method: past and future. *Ther Communities* 2017; 38(3): 136–46.

4. Foot J. *The Man Who Closed the Asylums: Franco Basaglia and the Revolution in Mental Health Care.* London: Verso Books, 2015.

5. Adams J. Nursing in a therapeutic community: the Fulbourn experience, 1955–1985. *J Clin Nurs* 2009; 18(19): 2747–53.

6. Leff J. The historical development of social psychiatry. In C Morgan, D Bhugra, eds., *Principles of Social Psychiatry*, 2nd ed. Wiley Online Library. 2010; pp. 3–11.

7. Pearce S, Haigh R. Mini therapeutic communities: a new development in the United Kingdom. *Ther Communities* 2008; 29(2): 111–24.

8. Crawford M, Rutter D, Price K et al. *Learning the Lessons: A Multi-method Evaluation of Dedicated Community-Based Services for People with Personality Disorder.* London: National Co-ordinating Centre for NHS Service Delivery & Organisation, 2007.

9. Community of Communities. Community of Communities Member Directory 2019–2020. 2019.

10. World Health Organization. *Expert Committee on Mental Health: 3rd Report.* Geneva: WHO, 1953.

11. NHS. The NHS Long Term Plan. 2019. www.longtermplan.nhs.co.uk/ [Accessed 27/11/2020]

12. Johnson R, Haigh R. Social psychiatry and social policy for the 21st century: new concepts for new needs-the 'Enabling Environments' initiative. *Ment Health Soc Incl* 2011; 15(1): 17–23.

13. Rapoport R. *Community as Doctor.* London: Tavistock, 1960.

14. Haigh R. The quintessence of a therapeutic environment. *Ther Communities* 2013; 34 (1): 6–15.

15. Bion WR. *Learning from Experience.* Sterling, VA: Stylus Publishing, LLC, 1984.

16. Pearce S, Haigh R. *A Handbook of Democratic Therapeutic Community Theory and Practice.* London: Jessica Kingsley Publishers, 2017.

17. Pearce S, Pickard H. How therapeutic communities work: specific factors related to positive outcome. *Int J Soc Psychiatry* 2013; 59(7): 636–45.

18. Baumeister RF, Leary MR. The need to belong: desire for interpersonal attachments as a fundamental human motivation. *Psychol Bull* 1995; 117(3): 497–529.

19. Clark DH. *Administrative Therapy: The Role of the Doctor in the Therapeutic Community.* London: Routledge; 2013.

20. Pickard H. Stories of recovery: the role of narrative and hope in overcoming PTSD and PD. In JZ Sadler, CW Van Staden, KWM Fullford, eds., *The Oxford Handbook of Psychiatric Ethics*, Oxford: Oxford University Press. 2015; pp. 1315–27.

21. Pickard H. Responsibility without blame: empathy and the effective treatment of personality disorder. *Philos Psychiatr Psychol* 2011; 18(3): 209–23.

22. Main T. The concept of the therapeutic community: variations and vicissitudes. *Group Anal* 1977; 10(2): S2–16.

23. Lees J, Manning N, Rawlings B. Therapeutic community effectiveness: a systematic international review of therapeutic community treatment for people with personality disorders and mentally disordered offenders. York: University of York, 1999.

24. Pearce S, Autrique A. On the need for randomised trials of therapeutic community approaches. *Ther Communities* 2010; 31(4): 338–55.

25. Pearce S, Scott L, Attwood G et al. Democratic therapeutic community treatment for personality disorder: randomised controlled trial. *Br J Psychiatry* 2017; 210(2): 149–56.

26. National Offender Management Service. Do Democratic Therapeutic Communities Reduce Reoffending? 2010.

27. Pearce S, Dale O. Training for democratic therapeutic community practitioners, and workers in therapeutic and enabling environments. *Ther Communities* 2018; 39(2): 93–7.

Further Reading

The approach and theoretical background to DTC practice described in this chapter are treated in more detail in:

Pearce S, Haigh R. The Theory and Practice of Democratic Therapeutic Community Treatment. London: Jessica Kingsley Publishers, 2017.

Chapter 26

The Open Dialogue Approach

Miomir Milovanovic

Introduction

The Open Dialogue Approach (ODA) has introduced radical changes in the approach to treatment of psychiatric disorders, particularly for those with psychosis. The model recognises the key value of family and social relationships and places specific emphasis on these aspects of the patient's life, both in understanding the psychiatric breakdown and providing the tools for recovery. This is actively translated into practice where patients are seen together with members of their family and significant others by the treating team, from their first presentation and throughout their treatment. With open and active involvement of all present, including the patient, an understanding of the presenting symptoms is jointly sought, formulations are co-created with relationships seen as playing a central role. Within this social group all decisions about management are made.

Open dialogue takes a primarily psychotherapeutic and relationship-based approach but is also open to pragmatic use of other therapeutic approaches in an integrated way to find meaning and to support recovery in psychiatric breakdown.

What Is Meant by an Open Dialogue Approach?

ODA refers to both:

a. A **treatment approach**, applicable to any psychiatric disorder where relationships within families and social networks are prioritised as the key to understanding the breakdown

b. An **organisational model** applicable to all mental health care and services for all patients within a defined catchment area

It involves:

1. **Integration with the local services and institutions**, who are involved in the patient's life, for example schools, police, employers and social services

2. **Early referral of new patients**, which leads to a significant reduction in the duration of untreated psychiatric disorders

3. **A creative integration of psychoanalytic and systemic treatment models**, providing a base which is also open to the pragmatic use of other different therapeutic modalities (individual psychoanalytic therapy, pharmacological, cognitive behavioural therapy (CBT), couples therapy . . .). These are provided in response to the changing needs of the patient, his/her family and other members of the group in a seamless, synchronous and comprehensive manner

4. **A treatment model appropriate for all patients** regardless of their diagnoses, presentation or level of complexity. This includes, and is particularly relevant for, patients whose presentation is complex and considered treatment resistant

5. **The addressing of issues at different levels**, from the depths of the individual unconscious to interpersonal relationships and the broader social context within which the breakdown has occurred

6. **Flexibility and adaption** according to the nature of the service. ODA as a treatment modality can be used within mental health services that are primarily organised along ODA principles, or in a more conventional manner, in which the ODA teams work within teams in Mental Health Trusts

Brief History

ODA is a modification of the Need Adapted Treatment (NAT) model, a psychotherapeutically oriented approach to psychosis that was originally developed in the 1960s by Yrjo Alanen and his team in Turku, Finland. It was initially called the Schizophrenia Project, created for the treatment of schizophrenia and psychosis and was renamed and modified into the ODA in the 1990s. In the province of Länsi-Pohja, Western Lapland, the entire mental health service has been organised according to these principles.

Alanen worked in close collaboration with a dedicated group of psychiatrists and psychoanalysts, who were also trained in systemic family therapy. The main principles of the NAT model drew upon psychoanalytic ideas regarding treatment approaches with individual schizophrenic and psychotic patients that started with Freud and Abraham, and continued in the USA with Theodor and Ruth Lidz [1]. For this work Professor Alanen was awarded the World Psychiatric Association's Pinel prize in 2008 in recognition of his contribution to psychiatry.

Professor Alanen and his colleagues stated aim was 'to develop our psychosis ward into a psychotherapeutic community, which would be characterized by a shared empathic attitude towards patients, open communication, frequent group activities and meetings, and close relationships between all staff and patients'. They were of the opinion 'that specialized psychiatric nurses, who work on the ward and become profoundly familiar with patients' problems, constitute a therapeutic resource that is far too seldom made use of' [2]. More than 40 per cent of therapies at that time were conducted by nurses who had 'on-the-job training and supervision' [3]. Successive cohort studies undertaken by Alanen and his team found that when they introduced family therapy meetings, the already impressive outcomes from individual therapy were significantly enhanced. A further step was therefore taken to introduce engagement of family members in regular meetings from admission onward. These family meetings had informative, diagnostic and therapeutic functions. Eventually they used the same meetings for outpatient appointments immediately after referral.

The results were impressive with rapid elimination or alleviation of psychotic symptoms, and a 50 per cent reduction in readmission rate within the next five years. The approach was welcomed by participants with 87 per cent of families in the early cohorts agreeing to participate in the family meetings [4]. The importance of family therapy was recognised, and multi-professional family therapy training was initiated in Finland, with the first training seminars started in 1979. The majority of the members of the first training team were psychoanalysts and 'combination of psychoanalytic and systemic expertise was a great asset both in the training and in the subsequent development of family therapy' [3, p. 148].

The early promise of the ODA led to widespread adoption of the model in other areas of Finland, Sweden and in psychiatric units around the world including the USA, Germany, Greece and the UK [5]. It remains to be seen how the treatment approach and research findings can be replicated within more urban environments where there may be a high volume of referrals and patients may be socially isolated and not in close contact with family members. Particularly important are questions concerning fidelity to the original model and whether the level of training of clinicians achieved in the new environment is adequate in comparison with original model, which may affect subsequent outcome data and research [6, 7].

The Seven and Other Principles and Clinical Practice of ODA

For clinicians working in the NHS mental health services today the principles and description of ODA may sound difficult to achieve and removed from the everyday reality of their clinical practice. On this point it is important to emphasise that at the time of its development levels of resources within services operating on ODA principles were generally comparable with services that have not previously used it.

There is a difference in emphasis, with resources allocated early on in the treatment pathway. The aim is to contain the crisis and to reduce the risk of the patient developing chronic and entrenched disorders with potential to escalate into continuous and repeated crises. When successful this reduces the financial impact in the longer term. ODA therefore has the potential to change the clinical pathway for the patient and enable them to experience recovery, supported by a network of relationships around them, in a positive way.

In Lapland ODA is practised in its purest form and the services are available to patients with any presentation across the spectrum of complexity and urgency, with or without psychotic symptoms. A referral can be made by the patient, a family member, someone from their social network, or from any involved professional, such as the GP.

Responsibility

The team member who takes the referral has the responsibility of arranging the first meeting. He/she will organise the time and the place, which is often the patient's home. In discussion with the patient he/she will identify who will be invited and how they will receive this invitation. The meeting can include anyone in the immediate social and family network. This team member also recruits another clinician/s into the case-specific team.

- The case-specific team (usually consisting of two members) takes all the responsibility for identifying and understanding the current problem, and planning and conducting the treatment and management from then on

Immediate Response

- The first meeting is arranged within 24 hours of referral and the crisis service operates over 24 hours
- This immediate response provides important containment for the patient and his/her family who may have become overwhelmed with intense fear, feelings of confusion and

helplessness. Being listened to in an open manner, with all their thoughts and feelings taken seriously by experienced clinicians who are prepared to see them again very soon (the next day if necessary), provides reassurance and allows key information to freely emerge. This leads to a recovery of a sense of agency and confidence for the patient and those closely involved in their lives. It also lays the foundation for a trusting collaborative relationship with the patient and their social network

- All participants from the outset are invited to engage in an open forum. All those present in the meetings speak for themselves and hold responsibility for what they say
- The team member who has taken the referral takes charge of leading the dialogue only in the initial meeting. There usually is no prior planning or agenda. The pathway for therapeutic intervention and treatment is derived from the discussion in the group meeting

Social Networks Involvement

- From the outset, the patient, family members, important people from the social network and all relevant professionals are all included in all meetings for as long as it is required. At the first meeting the issue of other key people who have not so far been invited is discussed. The presence of those with important past and present relationships with the patient means that some very difficult experiences can be shared and processed. In cases of violence and abuse within these relationships an ODA is not ruled out but may raise specific issues particularly around the needs for boundaries and privacy
- A conversation is created in these meetings using questioning in as open-ended a manner as possible to create an inquiry into the patient's struggles and what they may be expressing through their symptoms. All those present are invited to share what they feel is important, their thoughts about the crisis and what should be done. The aim is to try to open and facilitate dialogue/s. Everybody has the right to comment whenever he/she is willing to do so but comments should not interrupt an ongoing dialogue

Dialogism

- One of the main aims of the team is to develop and maintain a dialogue where all the different 'voices' – which includes thoughts, feelings, memories, fantasies, hallucinatory or delusional experiences – can be expressed and heard from all present. A 'voice' is also considered to be expressed not only through verbal utterances, but also through different non-verbal means; for example, through a sigh or a particular look during the meetings
- An emphasis is placed on resisting any urges to promote positive change in the patient and family at the expense of listening and facilitating dialogues. These insights and emerging issues may never have been talked about before and addressing them can lead to important changes in the patient and the family. It can help them acquire a sense of agency and confidence in their ability to make changes in the way they communicate, understand and relate to each other

Tolerance of Uncertainty

- The attitude and availability of the team provides the necessary containment for the patient and family from the outset when little may be known about the situation. The team needs to have the capacity to tolerate uncertainty, and to prioritise development of therapeutic relationship during this early stage. It is important not to rush and 'do something', or 'fix' the problem prematurely – such as early use of medication which may increase sedation, decrease the ability to think and to communicate, and potentially increase the likelihood of inpatient admission

- If the patient presents with psychosis, he/she is understood to be experiencing something that has been unappreciated or unacknowledged within their close relationships. Although the patient's comments may sound incomprehensible in the first meetings, after a while it may become apparent that the patient is speaking of real incidents in their lives. These incidents may include some terrifying issue or threat that they have not been able to articulate before the crisis. This is also the case with other forms of difficult behaviour. In extreme anger, depression or anxiety, the patient is seen as speaking about previously unspoken themes. The group works towards a shared language, to make sense and start to understand the meanings of these experiences [8]

Case Example 1

Mark, a 22-year-old man living with his parents, presents with a third episode of what has been diagnosed as schizophrenia. In the first meeting, attended by his close family and two of his friends, he talks in a way that is not easy to follow or to understand. Eventually one of the team members says that it seems to him that Mark is trying to tell the group about a communication difficulty with someone where he puts in an enormous effort, hope builds up and then somehow everything collapses. In the ensuing silence it is clear Mark cannot say more. Then his sister suddenly says what Mark has said makes complete sense to her. That is exactly how she feels with their mother – you put in a lot of effort and you start to hope you can make some connection with her but then everything collapses. At that point it is clear she is very angry. She adds: 'That is why I was staying at home as little as possible!'. This was in contrast to Mark who had remained living at home and continued to experience difficulties in his relationship with his parents. He had not been able to find a way to establish more independence from them. It was immediately clear that what she has said made sense to all members of the family and a discussion developed about the strains in the relationships within the family, which included the mother's depression which the family had not been able to talk about before.

Flexibility and Mobility

- The treatment is continually adapted to the specific and changing needs of each patient and his/her family using pragmatically therapeutic methods best suited to each family (individual psychoanalytic therapy, pharmacological, CBT, couples therapy etc.)
- During the most acute phase where anxieties may be at their most intense, it is advisable to hold a meeting every day (usually during the first 10–12 days). This will no longer be necessary once the situation has stabilised
- The place for the meeting is jointly decided (homes, working places, schools, clinics etc.) as well as the frequency and the length of meetings
- The meetings are usually held for 90 minutes. This may vary as the treatment progresses. The length of the overall intervention is decided at a later point
- The team tries to avoid prescribing antipsychotic medication at least for the first two weeks to allow symptoms not to be suppressed, as they are an important source of information. If sedation is necessary benzodiazepines are considered

- If the patient does not want to join the meeting or leaves during it, a discussion ensues about whether to continue the meeting. If the family wants to continue, a staff member informs the patient that she or he can return if they want. During this discussion, no other decisions concerning the patient are made

Psychological Continuity
- The same case-specific team that meet with the patient, family and others in their first therapeutic meeting will continue to work with them for as long as needed in both outpatient and inpatient settings
- According to the developing understanding of the issues, new clinicians can be co-opted into the team. For example, if there is a need for medication a psychiatrist could be included, if they haven't been part of the team from the outset. So, all the necessary resources are present in the team and there is no need for referrals outside of the team
- If the patient presents again to services after discharge, an effort is made for him to be seen by the same team or at least some members of the original team

Other Principles
- All discussions, treatment decisions and management plans should be made openly and reflectively in the presence of the patient and the whole network so everybody has a chance to take part in them
- If a key person is not present at the meeting this may be acknowledged, but this person would not usually be discussed in their absence
- At the end of each meeting the main themes of the meeting are summarised, including whether or not decisions have been made, and if so, what they were [9]
- Family members are not seen as the cause of the difficulties, or the focus of treatment, but as competent partners in a therapeutic recovery process. It is important to promote a 'No blame' culture
- Staff should have flexibility to intervene in an emergency, for example if risk escalates

Theoretical Models
Although the ODA can be used with patients with any presentation, NAT and ODA have been mainly developed to treat patients with schizophrenia and other psychotic disorders and a large body of research has been accrued working with these patients. ODA represents a very different treatment approach to traditional Western psychiatric practice which tends to rest mainly upon the premise that psychosis represents an illness of the brain, has an organic cause and needs primarily biological, that is pharmacological, treatment. Other approaches towards understanding and treating psychosis are regarded as much less important and may be ignored. An example of this is illustrated by the limited availability of family therapy as a treatment modality, despite the clear research evidence of its positive impact in reducing relapse rates for patients with schizophrenia [10].

Psychiatry aims to be a biopsychosocial discipline; however, it is the biological model of mental disorder that dominates in everyday clinical practice, teaching curricula and research. Current diagnostic systems, DSM and ICD focus on description and gathering of signs and symptoms without consideration of inner experience or psychological processes [11]. This often results in difficulties in understanding, appreciating and applying different theoretical models, for example those based on psychological, psychodynamic or social paradigms, theoretically but even more importantly in everyday management and treatment of psychotic patients. Working with psychotic patients is rarely included in formal psychotherapy training and practitioners themselves may lack confidence and experience in this field. Alanen also draws attention to how socio-political ideologies have tended to reduce the availability of social support and public care which are essential for the comprehensive treatment of psychotic patients. To change to a true biopsychosocial model of psychiatry, Alanen suggests there will need to be a fundamental change in the paradigm of mental illness and in how the brain and mind are understood [3].

Alanen's work is based upon his experience and conviction that schizophrenia is not a single nosological entity and that the pathogenesis and development of this group of psychoses is a multifaceted and multilevel process in which both biological and psychosocial factors interact and contribute [4].

In the early days of the development of NAT Alanen and his team drew heavily upon psychoanalytic ideas. They subsequently recognised the importance of the involvement of the patient's family and underwent further training in systemic family therapy, which led to initiation and widespread presence of family therapy training across Finland.

The psychoanalytic roots of the model are evident in many of the ideas and clinical practice. As an example, 'Voices' is the term used in the ODA to point out that every member of the group should be supported to freely express anything that he/she wants, and thinks is relevant. This can be through both verbal and non-verbal means and is taken seriously by others as something that is manifestly or potentially meaningful even if it does not immediately appear to be. The same term is applied to multiple points of view/different feelings or beliefs, sometimes within the same person, that could be discordant or even contradictory. This accords with psychoanalytic ideas in which the term 'voices' can refer to expressions of internal and external objects, that is, these are representations of people in external reality or of past experiences, stored internally in the mind such as an internal mother, father, colleague, with whom we consciously or unconsciously are engaged in continuous internal dialogues.

Case Example 2

John had a very difficult relationship with his father. He knew that his father loved him and was supportive of him; however, at the same time he was deeply convinced that his father expected more of him and considered him to be a failure. This conviction led him to hate himself, which in turn formed the basis of depressive episodes in which he would hear a paternal 'voice' constantly criticising himself and devaluing everything he had done. His hallucinatory voices came to be seen by the team as an expression of the critical voice he heard from his father that he carried with him at all times with no respite. Acknowledgement of this within the family led to an important discussion about his father's childhood that had not been talked about within the family.

Within the ODA the team members assume an 'Open' stance. This means that a non-judgemental attentive and inquiring attitude is maintained to whatever is presented or arises, rather like the evenly suspended attention and non-directional approach in other forms of therapy and particularly in psychoanalysis. This openness and curiosity mean that the material is not taken simply at face value. The emotions elicited within the team, known as the countertransference response, are an important part of the process even if not couched in such terms. A key emphasis is on relationships, both in the external and the internal world of the patient, and early formative templates are seen as informing how we perceive and respond to others in later life. In common with a psychoanalytic approach, the relationship with the treating teams and the key others in the external world are seen as crucial to the resolution of their difficulties and recovery from breakdown.

Table 26.1 Comparative table of two models of psychiatric practice: current dominant model versus ODA model

Current dominant model	ODA model
Mainly a biological, medical approach	A fully biopsychosocial approach
Main treatment pharmacotherapy	Main treatment psychotherapeutic
Fragmentation	Integration
Patient is treated by services organised in fragmented ways and he/she is perceived as consisting of fragmented aspects and relationships	Focus on integration of experiences of the patient, family and others as well as services and institutions and perspectives towards understanding what has happened
Delaying of referral process and interventions increase the risk of development of chronicity	Focussing provision of necessary resources early is the key to success in treatment and better recovery
Patient has a sense of passivity	Emphasis on sense of agency
Patient has a sense of meaninglessness	Searching actively for meaning
Patient has a sense of exclusion	Sense of involvement
Patient experiences as being out of control	Being in control
Treatment resources increase with the duration of symptoms	Resources used early in the presentation

An Open Dialogue Approach to Understanding a Mental Health Crisis

In everyday clinical work a mental health crisis tends to be experienced as something threatening, disturbing and risky. It evokes anxiety in everybody involved. As a consequence, the usual response by most clinicians is to try to quickly extinguish it by any possible means. This usually involves using medication as a very early intervention.

Within an ODA a crisis is seen as a window of opportunity. During the first couple of days/weeks of a crisis, it may be possible to speak of things/experiences that are difficult or impossible to discuss later (or before crisis). Psychiatric breakdown often represents a collapse of the usual defences used by the patient, the family, and/or other social groups that the patient is a member of. It is seen to occur for a reason and to provide a potential opening where underlying and previously unspoken issues can be seen, along with the possibility of questioning previously held beliefs and family, systemic, and cultural 'stories'. This opportunity might quickly fade away as defensive organisations/mechanisms and familiar patterns of relating and behaving become re-entrenched. In such an emotionally charged setting issues of confidentiality are handled in an open way. The patient has a primary role in determining which issues are for open discussion and which are confidential. The confidential issues are addressed in individual sessions that can go in parallel with group meetings. The ODA provides a forum where information from a range or sources is continually shared, debated and used to piece together what underlies the breakdown and allows a comprehensive understanding to be developed.

Research

Since their inception, both NAT and the ODA have been extensively researched and compared with other approaches through multi-centre trials where there has been follow up of patients ranging from 2 to 10 years. The resulting data provide a very robust and extensive evidence base showing that ODA and NAT produce significantly better outcomes to treatment as usual on a number of different measures in the treatment of psychotic patients [12].

Key research findings from a number of studies comparing ODA/NAT to treatment as usual are summarised in Table 26.2 [12–15].

Other points of interest which have emerged from the evidence base include:

- Outcomes in NAT/ODA treatment of first-episode psychosis have remained consistent over a 10-year period thus showing long-term stability
- Families were actively involved in all the cases, having on average 26 meetings over two years
- Only 33 per cent of ODA patients used neuroleptics temporarily during some phase of treatment compared with 100 per cent throughout the treatment in the comparison group.
- Although length of hospitalisations in the ODA services were shorter than elsewhere in Finland this did not lead to more frequent hospitalisations
- As a comparison, in the few long-term follow-up studies of first-time psychotic patients treated by traditional methods, after five years more than half, about 60 per cent, are said to be living on a disability pension [15].

Table 26.2 Summary of the studies comparing ODA/NAT with Treatment as usual

	Treatment as usual	NAT/ODA
Inpatient days/patient	117 (2 y)	14 (2 y)
Relapses 1+	71%	24% (2 y), 29% (5 y)
Symptoms present	50%	17% (2 y), 18% (5 y)
Back to work/study	43%	81% (2 y), 86% (5 y)
On disability allowance	62%	14–16%

In addition to these outcome studies, after the full introduction of the ODA in Western Lapland other important changes also emerged as follows:

- The number of new long-stay schizophrenic hospital patients fell to zero in 1992 and has not emerged since, and the need for this facility has remained very low
- The mean annual incidence of schizophrenia and the proportion of schizophrenia cases diagnosed out of all psychotic patients declined and eventually disappeared while the incidence of schizophreniform psychoses has not changed. A possible explanation is that the ODA arrested progression of psychotic process into a more chronic form of psychotic illness, or that once clinical staff adapted their approach towards seeking meaning in the breakdown, they were less likely to make a diagnosis of schizophrenia

Limitations of Open Dialogue Approach

Alanen pointed to the continuum from patients who are able to benefit from an ODA to those who are too deeply withdrawn into their own worlds and unable to benefit from it. This is very similar to limitations of other psychotherapeutic approaches where patients could benefit from therapy only if they are able to engage in psychotherapeutic process.

In a recent study with very long follow-up (1992–2015) of patients (n = 65) who had first-episode psychosis in 1992–2005 the average length of treatment was 6 ± 2 years, and a significant decrease (p < 0.001) in total use of psychiatric services was observed. The admission rates and duration of treatment were highest with subjects who behaved aggressively (U = 270, p < 0.005), and/or who were hospitalised (U = 157, p < 0.001) and medicated (U = 114, p < 0.001) at onset. Overall, external aggression at onset emerges as a factor that may challenge the application of the ODA treatment principles, being associated with a greater need for hospitalisation and longer treatment duration [16].

Concluding Remarks

ODA offers a creative integration between different strands of practice, theory, research, education and training. This model has been shown through research to be of benefit to most patients with mental disorders and in particular to improve the prognosis of those with schizophrenia and psychosis.

The adoption of the ODA has implications for service planning and organisation of mental health services as a whole. It emphasises continuity of care and changes the basic paradigms of everyday mental health practice.

References

1. Lidz T, Fleck S, Cornelison AR. *Schizophrenia and the Family*. Madison, CT: International Universities Press, 1965.

2. Aaku T, Rasimus R, Alanen YO. Nursing staff as individual therapists in psychotherapeutic community. In *Psychiatria Fennica, Yearbook*. Helsinki: Foundation for Psychiatric Research in Finland. 1980; pp. 9–31.

3. Alanen YO. *Schizophrenia: Its Origins and Need-Adapted Treatment*. London: Karnac Books, 1997.

4. Alanen YO. Towards a more humanistic psychiatry: development of need-adapted treatment of schizophrenia group psychoses *Psychosis* 2009; 1(2): 156–66.

5. Razzaque R, Stockman T. An introduction to peer supported open dialogue in mental health care. *BJPsych Adv* 2016; 22: 348–56.

6. Freeman AM, Tribe RH, Stott JCH, Pilling S. Open dialogue: a review of the evidence. *Psychiatr Serv* 2018; 70(1): 46–59.

7. Tribe RH, Freeman AM, Livingstone S, Stott JCH, Pilling S. Open dialogue in the UK: qualitative study. *BJPsych Open* 2019; \5(4): e49.

8. Seikkula J, Alakare B, Aaltonen J. The comprehensive open-dialogue approach in Western Lapland: II. Long-term stability of acute psychosis outcomes in advanced community care. *Psychosis* 2011; 3(3): 192–204.

9. Seikkula J, Olson ME. The Open Dialogue Approach to acute psychosis: its poetics and macropolitics. *Fam Process* 2003; 42: 403–18.

10. Leff J, Berkowitz R, Shavit N et al. A trial of family therapy v. a relatives group for schizophrenia. *Br J Psychiatry* 1989; 154(1): 58–66.

11. Shedler J, Westen D. Refining personality disorder diagnosis: integrating science and practice. *Am J Psychiatry* 2004; 161(8): 1350–65.

12. Tuori T, Lehtinen V, Hakkarainen A et al. The Finish National Schizophrenia Project 1981–1987: 10-year evaluation of its results. *Acta Psychiatr Scand* 1997; 97: 10–17.

13. Aaltonen J, Seikkula J, Lehtinen K. The comprehensive open dialogue approach in Western Lapland: I. The incidence of non-affective psychosis and prodromal states. *Psychosis* 2011; 3: 179–91.

14. Alanen YO, Lehtinen K, Rakkolainen V, Aaltonen J. Need-adapted treatment of new schizophrenic patients: experiences and results of the Turku Project. *Acta Psychiatr Scand* 1991; 83: 363–72.

15. Seikkula J, Alakare B, Aaltonen J. Open dialogue in psychosis II: a comparison of good and poor outcome cases. *J Constr Psychol* 2001; 14(4): 267–84.

16. Bergström T, Alakare B, Aaltonen J et al. The long-term use of psychiatric services within the open dialogue treatment system after first-episode psychosis. *Psychosis* 2017; 9(4): 310–21.

Neuropsychoanalysis and Relational Neuroscience

C Susan Mizen

Introduction

Opinions vary on the relevance of neuroscience to psychotherapy. Some make the case that there is no relationship between the two disciplines. After all psychotherapists, particularly psychodynamic therapists, work with interpersonally constructed meaning in the present moment. Even if it is the case that this is all transacted in the brain, neuroscience can have little or nothing of relevance to say about that interpersonal dynamic. Others talk about neuroscience as though it offers the hope of biological validation for their models of psychotherapeutic work. This is of particular importance to psychoanalysis, which, being difficult to falsify, has over recent decades lost a degree of credibility in wider scientific debate. Neuroscientists would call the former view a 'dualist perspective' meaning that even if all neural processes associated with an aspect of conscious experience were identified the association between neural events and subjective events can only be correlative not causative. In neuroscientific terms the latter view would be seen as 'materialistic monism', following the assumption that mental life can be seen as the product of, or can be reduced to, innumerable neural interactions. Further to this it could be argued that neuroscience has proceeded well enough without the psychotherapeutic perspective and vice versa so what do these two disciplines have to offer each other?

Another philosophical and neuroscientific position 'dual aspect monism' makes the case that psychoanalytic practice and neuroscience provide two perspectives, namely subjective and objective, on the brain. Psychoanalysis provides perhaps the most detailed and in-depth account of intrapsychic life and the interpersonal mind as it is perceived by the subject, where as neuroscience is the objective study of the structure and function of the brain as a bodily organ. It is this binocular view which offers new metapsychological understanding of clinical phenomena and refines research questions for neuroscientists. For this reason, it is important that psychotherapists and psychotherapeutically interested psychiatrists understand recent developments in neuroscience and are able to think about their implications for clinical work and research. To this end this chapter aims to describe those developments in psychodynamic neuroscience most relevant to psychotherapists and psychiatrists.

The indivisibility of brain and mind and consequent indivisibility of biological and psychotherapeutic psychiatry are well expressed in Kandel's new intellectual framework for psychiatry [1]. Eric Kandel won a Nobel prize for his research on the physiological basis of memory that described the unique domain psychiatry occupied in academic medicine in analysing the interaction between the social and biological. He refers to Freud's own starting point as a neurologist leading to the publication of his Project for a Scientific Psychology [2]

Box 27.1 Kandel's 'New Intellectual Framework for Psychiatry'

Principle 1. All mental processes, even the most complex psychological processes, derive from operations of the brain, even where the causes of the disturbances are clearly environmental.

Principle 2. Genes and their protein products are important determinants of the interconnections between neurons in the brain, their functioning exerting a significant control over behavior.

Principle 3. Genes do not, by themselves, explain all of the variance of a given major mental illness, behaviour and social factors act on the brain by modifying the expression of genes and function of nerve cells. Thus "nurture" is ultimately expressed as "nature."

Principle 4. Alterations in gene expression induced by learning give rise to changes in neuronal connections. These form the basis of individuality as well as initiating and maintaining abnormalities of behavior induced by social contingencies.

Principle 5. If psychotherapy is effective in bringing about long-term changes in behavior, it presumably does so through learning, changing gene expression, altering the strength of synaptic connections and bringing about structural changes.

in which he linked psychological hypotheses with neurophysiological processes. Freud abandoned his project because neuroscience had not progressed to a point that his theories could be tested, not because the endeavour itself was flawed. Kandel argued that during the 1950s and 60s when psychoanalysis dominated academic psychiatry in the USA the discipline was largely unconcerned with the brain as an organ of mental activity. Subsequently biological psychiatry may be in danger of becoming unconcerned with mind as the subject of mental activity. The importance of this extends beyond understanding our patients as people who experience illness which is otherwise defined in biological terms. Kandel makes the case that of greater importance still is maintaining a perspective on both brain and mind with potential to reinvigorate the intellectual life of psychiatry. Box 27.1 sets out the principles of his proposed intellectual framework.

Over the past two decades neuroscience developments have generated renewed clinical and scientific interest in this area. Among other developments a new scientific discipline Neuropsychoanalysis has emerged. This has been led by Professor Mark Solms a psychoanalyst and neuropsychologist promoting interdisciplinary dialogue and research at this interface. Research developments include investigations of the unconscious and memory, the neural mechanisms of drives, dreams, primary and secondary processes and defence mechanisms. What follows is only a small corner of a rapidly evolving field. The areas covered have been chosen on the basis of their relationship with psychoanalytic theory and their relevance to clinicians.

These include:

- Instinct, drive and affect
- Interoception, exteroception and the embodied self
- Self, other and the drive to relate
- Generating an internal model of the world: fantasy and reality
- The role of dreaming in mental life

Instinct, Drive and Affect

Instinct and drive are fundamental concepts in Freud's metapsychology. Instinct in Freud's terminology refers to innate preconceptions about the world linked to uncondi-tioned stereotyped responses such as the rooting reflex. He defined drive, ('Triebe' in the original German text) as 'a measure of the demand made upon the mind for work in consequence of its connection with the body' [3]. When the body deviates from its homeostatic set point this deviation makes demands upon the brain to respond to restore the balance. It may do so by either acting to meet the drive demand or by inhibiting the demand itself. More recent neuroscience findings indicate that these drive demands are associated with qualities of experience or qualia. For example, when blood glucose drops there may be a physical sensation such as feeling faint but there is also a felt mental quality of the experience of hunger and the urgency of the need to find food. These qualities of experience are affects. Affects are defined as distinct from but related to emotional feelings.

The relationship between affect and homeostatic need is a relatively recent neuros-cientific idea. Ideas about the nature, origin and classification of affect have been evolving for over a century. One of the earliest, the James-Lange theory (1884) proposed that emotion did not originate in the brain at all [4]. As an example physiological autonomic arousal on perceiving something frightening such as an oncoming train was thought to give rise to the emotional experience of fear. More recently Silvan Tomkins identified nine primary affects, including shame and disgust, each characterised by particular intensity and physiological expression [5]. This and Eckman's classification were based on the social expression of emotion rather than their neurobiological basis [6]. Joseph LeDoux adopted a neuroscientific approach to the study of emotion. Like many researchers he was interested in the amygdala, thought to process memory and mediate emotional responses. His research on fear conditioning identified two pathways to the amygdala – a fast subcortical pathway transmitting rapid behavioural responses to threats ('Pavlovian threat conditioning') and a slow pathway providing highly processed cortical information responsible for the feeling of fear [7]. His research improved understanding of how the brain responds to threats and how fearful memories are stored which has relevance to exposure therapy. However, LeDoux proposed the brain detects feelings but does not create them. Jaak Panksepp, a professor of veterinary medicine, investigated subcortical networks mediating affect in mammals. He identified subcortical systems with discrete neurochemistries and anatomical distribution each with distinct affective qualities and behavioural correlates. He proposed affects are intrinsic to the brain and stereotypical [8]. The importance of Panksepp's findings cannot be underestimated. Before his research contribution neuroscience research had focussed on cognition and those forms of behaviour which were available to direct observation. Emotion was considered subjective and therefore not amenable to study through empirical methods. As a consequence of Panksepp's findings affect could be studied objectively leading to the development of a new scientific discipline affective neuroscience.

Affective Neuroscience

Jaak Panksepp's primary research in animals identified seven anatomically and functionally distinct subcortical Basic Emotion Command Systems (BECS). These systems are usually described by capitalising their names. They are SEEKING, PANIC, FEAR, RAGE, LUST, CARE and rough and tumble PLAY. These systems, are located between the brainstem and limbic system, parts of the brain which have homologous structures in all mammals, including humans. Their function is to provide information to higher centres in the cerebral cortex about the state of the interior of the body in relation to the external world and to motivate behaviour to meet inner homeostatic and survival needs. In this way the BECS coordinate the multitude of hormonal and neural signals arising from the body into categories with pleasant and unpleasant qualia (affect). The quality of the pleasant/unpleasant affect engendered is particular to each individual affect command system. For example, for the PANIC system the pleasant qualia would be the comfort of closeness with an attachment figure and the unpleasant would be the separation distress. BECS have both a perceptual function in receiving such bodily states and asigning qualia to them but also a function in motivating specific categories of behaviour directed towards meeting basic survival imperatives, the pleasant/unpleasant qualia providing the affective motivation for the behaviour. Table 27.1 illustrates these functions for four of the seven BECS.

SEEKING and PANIC

Examining the SEEKING and PANIC systems in greater detail will clarify the role of BECS and the link between these biological systems and psychotherapeutic concepts such as libido and attachment. The SEEKING system motivates behaviour to locate resources in the environment which will satisfy appetite. It is not itself oriented towards a particular goal but is activated in response to hunger, thirst or sexual desire. If you are thirsty SEEKING provides the motivational drive to look for 'something'. The hypothalamus identifies what you are looking for, that is, water. The SEEKING system is tonically active underpinning the activity of all the other BECS. From Table 27.1 it will be apparent that neuroanatomically it is the dopaminergic mesolimbic, mesocortical pathway which is causally implicated in the major psychiatric disorders. It may become overactive through use of stimulants or as a consequence of mental illness in mania and schizophrenia. It is thought SEEKING may also become active as a consequence of failure of top-down regulation or failure of regulatory mechanisms between the BECS [9]. SEEKING not only motivates behavioural activation but also mental activity. When SEEKING is overactive it is thought to increase the tendency towards making spurious connections between cause and effect and the development of delusional ideas.

Table 27.1 Function, anatomy and neurochemistry of four BECS

BECS	Function	Anatomy	Neurotransmitters
SEEKING	**Behavioural:** energetic exploration locating resources to satisfy appetite, e.g. hunger, thirst and sexual appetite **Psychological:** motivates interest and curiosity cementing the connection between cause and effect giving rise to ideas	**Mesolimbic mesocortical pathway** Periaqueductal grey (PAG)–lateral hypothalamus–nucleus accumbens–ventral tegmental area pathway	**Dopamine** and descending glutaminergic components, opioids, neurotensin, orexin and neuropeptides
PANIC	**Behavioural:** separation distress circuits. Their activity promotes bonding and proximity seeking behaviour in young mammals and social behaviour in adults **Psychological:** mediates the psychological pain and panic/anxiety of separation	PAG–bed nucleus of the stria terminalis (BNST)–pre-optic area–dorsomedial thalamus–**anterior cingulate gyrus**	**Opiates, oxytocin, prolactin** Inhibitory Corticotrophin-releasing factor (CRF), glutamate
FEAR	**Behavioural:** unconditioned fear response to competitors/predators. Fight/**flight** **Psychological:** anxiety from external threat	Dorsal PAG–medial hypothalamus–central and lateral **amygdala**	**GABA** Diazepam binding inhibitor, CRF, cholecystokinin, a melanocyte stimulating hormone, neuropeptide Y
RAGE	**Behavioural:** three distinct aggressive circuits - Affective attack **fight/**flight - Predatory aggression - Inter-male aggression **Psychological:** anger stimulated by threat, restricted freedom of movement, irritation to body surfaces or obstructed access to resources	PAG–BNST–medial and fornical hypothalamic nuclei–medial **amygdala**	**Substance P** (key modulator) GABA and acetylcholine stimulate

The PANIC system motivates proximity seeking behaviour in both infants and adults. As described earlier the qualia associated with the PANIC system are the comfort of emotional and physical closeness and the pain and anxiety associated with separation and loss. It has been suggested that there is an apparent correspondence between the SEEKING system and Freud's concept of a libidinal drive which is blind to its object. In contrast the PANIC system mediates attachment behaviour providing the biological basis for Bowlby's attachment theory [10].

Panksepp identified two systems responsible for different forms of anxiety. The PANIC system being associated with the depressive affect and anxiety associated with social loss and the FEAR system associated with environmental threat. It would seem that the systems underpinning separation anxiety and persecutory anxiety are distinct from one another. The psychopharmacology of these systems appears to correspond with these findings. Benzodiazepines may be effective in moderating the GABA receptors in the FEAR system, tricyclics antidepressants and opiates acting upon the PANIC system. On the basis of Panksepp's findings Yovell undertook a randomised controlled trial which demonstrated the efficacy of short-term low-dose buprenorphine in the treatment of depression and suicidal ideation [11]. For psychotherapists the idea that the therapeutic relationship has its effects at both psychological and neurobiological levels is perhaps surprising and could change our way of thinking about how psychological/biological change happens.

Affective Consciousness and Representations of the Body in the Brain

BECS are also thought to mediate what is described as core affective consciousness. This refers to both the quantitative attribute of wakefulness and the qualitative attributes already described arising from the BECS. Core affective consciousness comprises awareness of the homeostatic status of the interior of the body arising from two systems, the humoral

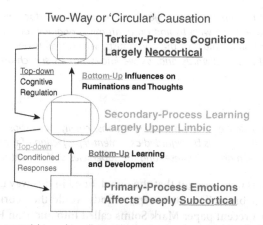

Figure 27.1 Panksepp's nested hierarchies illustrating bottom-up cognisation of affect and top-down affect regulation.

(hormonal) system and the autonomic nervous system. These are the two mechanisms by which the brain perceives the interior of the body (interoception) and this interoceptive mode of perception is core affective consciousness. In this way the body is represented in two ways in the brain. The external surface of the body, perceived objectively through exteroceptive senses and through motor activity, is represented in body maps on the cortical surface. The interior of the body is perceived through interoception and is represented in deep brain regions including the hypothalamus, ventral tegmental area, parabrachial nuclei, nucleus locus coerulus, reticular formation and periaqueductal grey. Somatotopic maps exist in both brain regions. The interior of the body gives rise to both affective consciousness providing the basis for the core quality of subjective being [12]. The two forms of consciousness arising from these two representations of the body differ. Where consciousness of the external world and the objective body is specific to each sensory modality, affective consciousness perceives both the state of the interior of the body and the response of the subject to external events. Antonio Damasio, whose research demonstrated the central role of emotion in social cognition and decision-making, proposed core consciousness is fundamentally dependent on the response of the protoself, which is represented in the brainstem and defined in these bodily terms, and environment [13].

Panksepp's BECS sitting at the interface between brain and body do not mediate emotional feelings in the way we usually experience them. He proposed affects were elaborated in more sophisticated ways at higher levels in the brain through nested hierarchies. Figure 27.1 illustrates the 'bottom-up' relationship between basic affects and 'cognised' affects and top-down affect regulation.

The implications of these findings for psychotherapy and psychiatry are profound. Perhaps one of the most obvious applications to both clinical practice and research is in the area of psychosomatic medicine.

Interoception, Exteroception and the Embodied Self

In his paper 'The Ego and the Id' Freud stated:

> The ego is first and foremost a bodily ego; it is not merely a surface entity, but is itself the projection of a surface. If we wish to find an anatomical analogy for it we can best identify it with the "cortical homunculus" of the anatomists, which stands on its head in the cortex, sticks up its heels, faces backwards and, as we know, has its speech-area on the left-hand side.

He went on:

> The ego is ultimately derived from bodily sensations, chiefly from those springing from the surface of the body. It may thus be regarded as a mental projection of the surface of the body, besides, as we have seen above, representing the superficies of the mental apparatus [14].

As discussed above it is now thought that the Ego defined in this way is just one representation of the body in the brain. The interoceptive body would then correspond with Freud's concept of the Id. In a recent paper Mark Solms called into question Freud's assertion that the Id is unconscious and the Ego conscious [12]. He made the case that the Id is the seat of affective consciousness where those cortical representations of the body are unconscious only becoming conscious when they are attended to. He has written subsequently about the implication of this revision of Freud's theory for clinical practice [15].

Damasio found that interoception plays a central role in self-awareness [13]. More recent findings indicate that interoceptive self-awareness arises in a developmental context [16]. Because infants are dependent upon their parents to maintain homeostasis at the beginning of life the responsiveness of the mother to the baby's physiological needs through bodily interactions is thought to determine the baby's attunedness to their own bodily states. Where these interactions are contingent upon the needs of the baby a dynamic process of embodied mentalisation' takes place. This underpins the constitution of earliest developments of the sense of self upon which more sophisticated distinctions between 'subject and object,' 'self and other' and 'pleasure and pain' are built. The correct identification of the origin of bodily and mental states by the parent is required to establish the self–other distinction, social relatedness and cognition. Conversely the failure of these developmental processes results in the failures of interoceptive awareness and difficulties in regulating endogenous states of arousal which are found in many mental disorders including autistic spectrum disorders (ASDs) and schizophrenia [17].

It seems that the development of the psychosomatic interface is not only relevant to the development of psychosomatic disorders in the context of non-contingent caregiving in early childhood but may participate in symptom maintenance in a wider range of mental disorders.

Self, Other and the Drive to Relate

The Drive to Relate

The PANIC system provides the biological substrate for the drive to relate. Panksepp proposed the PANIC system ensured the survival of young mammals while attachments and survival skills develop. This biological drive to relate along with inborn reflexes such as the rooting reflex, orientation towards faces and to maternal smell comprise the early imprinting process in humans described by Bowlby as preceding the development of maternal attachment at six to eight months [18]. The PANIC system is responsible for the emotional salience of babies' interactions with their parents. Without it there would be no pleasure or pain associated with these interactions, they simply would not matter to the infant. Panksepp proposed an opiate theory of ASD [19]. He suggested 'neurotypical' individuals had a relative deficit of PANIC system opiates. For this reason the absence of social contact is distressing. He proposed that in ASD opiate receptors in the PANIC system were saturated. As a result social engagement was not emotionally salient and isolation was not sufficiently distressing to promote engagement so that from birth infants who would go on to develop ASD did not seek out social engagement. A number of developmental consequences in language, abstract thinking and symbolisation arose from this biological deficit. To test this hypothesis naloxone, an opiate antagonist, was administered to children with ASD in a double-blind study resulting in a degree of clinical improvement in the treated group [20]. While recognising the heterogeneity of ASD this provides some preliminary evidence that the PANIC system may account for one component of the atypical neural apparatus for relating found in these disorders.

Under ordinary circumstances the pain of social exclusion promotes group and social behaviour in adults. The social exclusion of individuals or minorities is associated with separation distress and vulnerability to depression and anxiety. The fear of social exclusion may be a prime motivator towards conforming to conscious and unconscious group behaviour even when doing so opposes an individual's rational beliefs [21].

The Representation of Self and Other in the Brain

Damasio described hierarchical neural structures representing self and other responsible for the generation of consciousness [13]. He proposed the experience of the self to be contingent upon the experience of the other and that consciousness arises from the interaction between self and other. The most basic representation of the 'protoself' is a collection of neurones monitoring the internal state of the body as it responds to the environment in the periaqueductal grey, hypothalamus and insula [22]. More sophisticated representations mediate emotions reaching conscious awareness. At the highest level the autobiographical self moves beyond the here and now and is reliant upon declarative (conscious autobiographical) memory systems.

In the neocortex self and other are represented in two large-scale neural networks, one lateral the other medial [23]. A lateral fronto-parietal network and its associated mirror neurone networks are thought to bridge the gap between the bodily self and others in the here and now. Mirror neurones were first discovered in primate research where they were noted to fire both when an action was performed by the self and when the same action was observed to be performed by another [24]. Mirror neurones respond to prosody in social interactions allowing motor simulations in the subject from which the emotional state of the other is inferred. This lateral self/other network is active during current interactions perceiving their emotional state and intention through body language. The medial network representing self and other is referred to as the Default Mode Network (DMN). This is active when cognition and executive function are 'offline'. The DMN transacts internal thoughts and feelings about social interactions after the event.

The evidence suggests the right lateral fronto-parietal network undergoes a critical period of development during the second year of life [25]. Optimal development is dependent upon the emotional environment including attuned care and contingent emotional interaction with attachment figures. Absence of this interaction may lead to impaired dendritic branching and apoptosis with consequent reduced cortical volume [26]. Feldman and colleagues measured blood oxytocin levels of mothers and infants during cycles of play demonstrating synchrony between their limbic systems [27]. She proposed that mirror neurone systems link maternal and infant limbic systems with significant implications for emotional and neural development.

These findings offer a biological mechanism by which feelings can be evoked between individuals and underline the importance of this evocation of emotion between parents and infants for the neurocircuitry of the developing brain. This evocation of emotion is a commonly observed phenomenon in psychotherapeutic practice being the basis of transference and countertransference. While the identification of this mechanism falls short of directly demonstrating how projection and projective identification occur it does open the possibility of studying these developmental and defensive mechanisms empirically.

Self, Other Perspective Taking and Symbolisation

Studies of infant development confirm that in the first instance babies are egocentric assuming the world is as they see it from their own perspective. When development during the first year of life progresses well, infants engage in dyadic face-to-face and embodied interaction with others. At the end of the first year of life a developmental progression occurs in which the baby realises theirs is not the only perspective on the world, that others have a perspective of their own [28]. From this point on the baby develops a capacity to move back and forth between their own and another's perspective on the world, this being a first step in the development of theory of mind. The ability to triangulate in this way appears to be a nodal step in subsequent development of symbolic play, symbolic use of language and ultimately abstract thinking [29]. Failure of these key developmental stages may impact on future mentalisation and the development of the capacity to express emotions symbolically through language with resultant alexithymia. This is a common finding in many mental disorders including personality disorder, eating disorders and ASD.

Understanding those aspects of psychopathology and therapeutic interaction which contribute to the collapse or development of the capacity for triangulation is likely to facilitate verbal communication of feeling in conditions where body language predominates [30].

Generating an Internal Model of the World: Prediction Error and Free Energy

Contemporary neuroscience started with the work of Hermann von Helmholtz (1821–1894), tutor to Freud's mentor, Ernst Brucke. Helmholtz's ideas contrasted with the prevailing idea that sense organs transmit a 'representation' of 'reality' to a passive receiving brain. He proposed the mind *makes its own model of the world* dynamically, constantly updating its model in the light of experience as a form of internally generated virtual reality. These ideas were the predecessors of Freud's topographical and structural models. Karl Friston, one of the foremost neuroscientists of the past two decades, also draws upon Helmholtz's model. Friston's model of brain function is based upon mathematical principles and the laws of physics, in particular Bayes law and the second law of thermodynamics. He states,

> Considering the whole human organism, the brain perceives external and internal states of the body drawing inferences about the causes of those states in the external world and acts to sustain the internal milieu [31].

Friston's model rests on two principles, The Free Energy Principle and Prediction Error. The term 'Energy' in the Free Energy Principle refers to an explanatory framework for both physiological and mental functioning rather than energy as a physical phenomenon [32]. Friston proposes energy is either free or bound. Free energy arises from the unpredictable nature of the environment and its impact on the organism. He argues that a balance is struck by the organism between the need to explore and sample the environment, which generates free energy in order to build a model of the world so that the organism can sustain itself, and the need to bind energy within the predictive model in order that the sensory apparatus is not overwhelmed with stimuli. Friston's terminology and concepts correspond with Freud's who first put forward his own ideas about the interaction between free and bound energy in his Project for a Scientific Psychology [2].

Regarding prediction error, Friston argues that the purpose of the sensory and motor systems is to maintain homeostasis which the brain does by generating an internal model of the causal order of the world which is constantly updated on the basis of new sensory information. These predictions are then matched with what we actually perceive and the divergence between predicted and actual data yields a prediction error. The better the prediction, the better the fit with perceived reality. Prediction error leads to an adjustment of the internal generative model both immediately and during dreaming sleep so that it is aligned more closely with reality. The internal model applies both to perception and action in that we act upon the world both to update the model and make it conform more closely with our predictions (active inference).

Adjusting the internal generative model takes place through a hierarchical cascade. Lower levels of the hierarchy process simple data, for example sensory stimuli, higher levels process integrated sensory data such as object recognition where the highest levels include mental imagery. Prediction errors move up the hierarchy to adjust the model and predictions move down to influence how the perceptual apparatus samples the external world (Figure 27.2). Each layer in the hierarchy makes predictions about the inputs from the level below. It appears, from a neurological point of view, the brain is intolerant of unfulfilled expectations and so structures its model of the world and motivates action in such a way that more of its predictions are correct.

This cascade applies not only to perceptions of the external world but also those arising from the interior of the body. Low level interoceptive sensations include homeostatic and autonomic status, mid level representations may include those subcortical structures which mediate affect, higher level representations mediating emotional feeling. In this framework emotion is interoceptive prediction and the active inferential process operates by triggering physiological change.

Friston proposes that in mental disorder the generative model is not updated, instead perception of the external world is adjusted so that it conforms to the internal model. In psychotic disorders this results in perceptual disorders such as hallucinations [33].

In Friston's model we do not perceive reality as it is but our internal representation of the world and the inferences we have made about the hidden causes of external events. This applies to interpersonal relationships as well as the physical reality of the world, to the

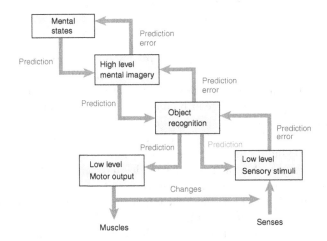

Figure 27.2 Friston's hierarchical prediction error.

external world, and to the interior of our bodies which gives rise to emotion and subjectivity. In short we live in a fantasy about the external world which is updated in our dreams and the correspondence of that internal phantasy with external reality is dependent upon a range of factors both emotional and biological which can interfere with our ability to update the model. While it is easy to overstate the correspondence between Friston's model and Freud's metapsychology, it is apparent that the similarities allow for the ready transfers of ideas between clinical and neurobiological disciplines [34]. This has led to a number of publications outlining models of mental functioning and disorder which can be tested empirically [35, 36].

Dreaming

Freud stated that the interpretation of dreams was the royal road to the unconscious [37]. He was referring to the dynamic unconscious as the location of contents of consciousness which are repressed and rendered unconscious to resolve a psychological conflict. He made the case that unconscious mental contents regained consciousness in disguised form in dreams and could be brought to consciousness through interpretation. More recently the neuroscientific consensus was thought to have disproved Freud's theory. EEG studies found that REM sleep in which dreaming was thought to happen was associated with ponto-geniculo-occipital waves. These were thought to activate the brain during dreaming generating hallucinatory phenomena which were epiphenomenal and of no significance [38, 39].

Mark Solms studied neurological and neurosurgical patients with brain lesions and impaired or absent dreaming using Luria's method of syndrome analysis to investigate the fundamental components of the functional system supporting dreaming [40]. He demonstrated the essential psychological processes of dreaming are mediated by higher structures rather than the brainstem nuclei which regulate REM sleep. Patients with brainstem lesions did not demonstrate cessation of dreaming whereas dreaming ceased altogether in patients with lesions affecting the inferior parietal and bilateral mediobasal frontal lobes. He concluded three factors mediated by these higher regions were essential to the conscious experience of dreams: (1) *symbolic operations*, (2) *spatial thought* and (3) *inhibitory mental control*. Damage to other parts of the brain led to other changes in the frequency and content of dreams such as increasing nightmares or loss of visual imagery. These findings cast doubt on the theory that core brainstem structures regulate the dream process.

Solms distinguished the physiological state of REM sleep from dreaming arguing that while REM sleep has a high statistical correlation with dreaming they were not the same thing. He demonstrated that anything which disturbed sleep gave rise to dreaming, REM activation being but one such phenomenon. Further to this he observed that the areas vital for dreaming include the limbic system linking dreaming closely to the processing of emotion. Solms concluded:

> in dreams, the primary "scene of action" of mental life shifts retrogressively, under the regulatory control of mediobasal frontal and anterior limbic systems, away from the dorsolateral frontal region which is the executive focus of normal waking cognition toward the parieto-occipital (perceptual-mnestic) systems. Nocturnal mentation is thus deprived of the characteristic goal-directedness of waking mental life, and the activating impulse is worked over symbolically in visuo-spatial consciousness [40].

The results of this study provide some striking corroboration of the classical theory of dreams introduced by Freud almost one hundred years before.

Conclusions

This small selection from the neuroscience literature demonstrates the correspondence with and differences between the findings of neuroscience research and psychoanalytic theory. It is apparent that the dual perspectives on the study of the brain, the objective brain in neuroscience and its subjective manifestation in the clinical study of the mind through psychoanalysis, facilitate the emergence of new ideas in both disciplines. This is of fundamental importance for academic and clinical psychiatry where the distinction between biological and psychological psychiatry now seems outdated. Further to this it is clear that psychoanalysis has an important contribution to make to neuroscience in building hypotheses to be tested. Conversely neuroscience can inform psychoanalysis, allowing a reappraisal of our metapsychology, informing clinical practice and perhaps most importantly bringing psychoanalysis back into the scientific mainstream.

References

1. Kandel ER. A new intellectual framework for psychiatry. *Am J Psychiatry* 1998; 155(4): 457–69.

2. Freud S. Project for a scientific psychology. In J Strachey, ed., *The Standard Edition of the Complete Psychological Works of Sigmund Freud, Volume I (1886–1899): Pre-Psycho-Analytic Publications and Unpublished Drafts*. London: Hogarth Press. 1966; pp. 175. (Original work written 1895)

3. Freud S. Instincts and their vicissitudes. In J Strachey, ed., *The Standard Edition of the Complete Psychological Works of Sigmund Freud, Volume XIV (1914–1916): On the History of the Psycho-Analytic Movement, Papers on Metapsychology and Other Works*. London: Hogarth Press. 1957; pp. 117–40. (Original work published 1915)

4. James W. What is emotion? *Mind* 1884; 9: 185–205.

5. Tomkins SS. *Affect Imagery Consciousness*. New York: Springer, 1962.

6. Fridlund AJ, Ekman P, Oster H. Facial expressions of emotion. In AW Siegman, S Feldstein, eds., *Nonverbal Behavior and Communication*. New Jersey: Lawrence Erlbaum Associates, Inc. 1987; pp. 143–223.

7. LeDoux JE. *The Emotional Brain*. New York: Simon and Schuster, 1996.

8. Panksepp J. *Affective Neuroscience: The Foundations of Human and Animal Emotions*. New York: Oxford University Press, 1998.

9. Watt DF, Panksepp J. Depression: an evolutionarily conserved mechanism to terminate separation distress? A review of aminergic, peptidergic and neural network perspectives. *Neuropsychoanalysis* 2009; 11(1): 7–51.

10. Yovell Y. Is there a drive to love? *Neuropsychoanalysis* 2008; 10(2): 117–44.

11. Yovell Y, Bar G, Mashiah M et al. Ultra-low dose buprenorphine a time limited treatment for severe suicidal ideation: a randomised controlled trial. *Am J Psychiatry* 2016; 173(5): 491–8.

12. Solms M. The conscious Id. *Neuropsychoanalysis* 2013; 15(1): 5–19.

13. Damasio A. *The Feeling of What Happens*. London: Heinemann, 1999.

14. Freud S. The ego and the id. In J Strachey, ed., *The Standard Edition of the Complete Psychological Works of Sigmund Freud, Volume XIX (1923–1925): The Ego and the Id and Other Works*. London: Hogarth Press. 1961; pp. 12–59. (Original work published 1923)

15. Smith R, Solms M. Examination of the hypothesis that *repression is premature automatization*: a psychoanalytic case

report and discussion. *Neuropsychoanalysis* 2018; 20(1): 47–61.

16. Fotopoulou A, Tsakiris M. Mentalizing homeostasis: the social origins of interoceptive inference. *Neuropsychoanalysis* 2017; 19(1): 3–28.

17. Garfinkel SN, Tiley C, O'Keeffe S et al. Discrepancies between dimensions of interoception in autism: implications for emotion and anxiety. *Biol Psychol* 2016; 114: 117–26.

18. Bowlby J. *Child Care and the Growth of Love*. London: Penguin Books, 1953.

19. Panksepp J. A neurochemical theory of autism. *Trends Neurosci* 1979; 2: 174–7.

20. Leboyer M, Bouvard MP, Launay J-M, et al. Brief report: a double-blind study of naltrexone in infantile autism. *J Autism Dev Disord* 1992; 22: 309–19.

21. Bacha CS. The first revolution: taking Jaak Panksepp seriously. Group Analysis and the neuroscience of emotion. *Group Anal* 2019; 52(4): 441–57.

22. Bosse T, Jonker CM, Treur J. Formalisation of Damasio's theory of emotion, feeling and core consciousness. *Conscious Cogn* 2008; 17(1): 94–113.

23. Uddin LQ, Iacoboni M, Lange C, Keenan JP. The self and social cognition. The role of cortical midline structures and mirror neurons. *Trends Cogn Sci* 2007; 11(4): 153–7.

24. Rizzolatti G, Fadiga L, Gallese V, Fogassi L. Premotor cortex and the recognition of motor actions. *Brain Res Cogn Brain Res* 1996; 3(2): 131–41.

25. Schore AN. *Affect Regulation and the Origin of the Self: The Neurobiology of Emotional Development*. London: Routledge, 1994.

26. Schore AN. Early organization of the nonlinear right brain and development of a predisposition to psychiatric disorders. *Dev Psychopathol* 1997; 9: 595–631.

27. Feldman R, Ilanit Gordon I, Zagoory-Sharon O. Maternal and paternal plasma, salivary, and urinary oxytocin and parent–infant synchrony: considering stress and affiliation components of human bonding. *Dev Sci* 2011; 14(4): 752–61.

28. Trevarthen C, Hubley P. Secondary intersubjectivity: confidence, confiding and acts of meaning in the first year. In A Lock, ed., *Action Gesture and Symbol: The Emergence of Language*. London: Academic Press. 1978; pp. 183–229.

29. Hobson RP. *The Cradle of Thought*. London: Pan Books, 2002.

30. Mizen CS. Neuroscience mind and meaning: an attempt at synthesis in a relational affective hypothesis. *Psychoanal Psychother* 2015; 29(4): 363–81.

31. Friston KJ. The free-energy principle: a unified brain theory. *Nat Rev Neurosci* 2010; 11: 127–38.

32. Holmes J. *The Brain Has a Mind of Its Own: Attachment, Neurobiology and the New Science of Psychotherapy*. Woodbridge: Confer Books, 2020.

33. Friston KJ. Hallucinations and perceptual inference. *Behav Brain Sci* 2005; 28(6): 764–6.

34. Freud S. Formulations on the two principles of mental functioning. In J Strachey, ed., *The Standard Edition of the Complete Psychological Works of Sigmund Freud, Volume XII (1911–1913): Case History of Schreber, Papers on Technique and Other Works*. London: Hogarth Press. 1958; pp. 213–26. (Original work published 1911)

35. Carhart-Harris RL, Friston KJ. The default mode, ego-functions and free energy: a neurobiological account of Freud's idea. *Brain* 2010; 133: 1265–83.

36. Carhart-Harris RL, Mayberg HS, Malizia AL, Nutt D. Mourning and melancholia revisited: correspondences between principles of Freudian metapsychology and empirical findings in neuropsychiatry. *Ann Gen Psychiatry* 2008; 7(9). https://doi.org/10.1186/1744-859X-7-9.

37. Freud S. The interpretation of dreams. In J Strachey, ed., *The Standard Edition of the Complete Psychological Works of Sigmund Freud, Volume IV (1900): The*

Interpretation of Dreams. London: Hogarth Press. 1953; p. 613. (Original work published 1900)

38. Hobson JA. The new neuropsychology of sleep: implications for psychoanalysis. *Neuropsychoanalysis* 1999; 1(2): 157–83.

39. Solms M. The new neuropsychology of sleep: commentary. *Neuropsychoanalysis* 1999; 1(2): 183–196.

40. Solms M. New findings on the neurological organization of dreaming: implications for psychoanalysis. *Psychoanal Q* 1995; 64: 43–67.

Psychedelic-Assisted Psychotherapy

Tim Read

The future may teach us to exercise a direct influence on the mind by means of particular chemical substances . . . . and there may be still other undreamt of possibilities for therapy as a result.

Sigmund Freud [1]

Why is This of Interest to Psychiatry and Psychotherapy?

In recent years there has been a resumption of research into the potential therapeutic benefits of psychedelic[1] drugs such as MDMA[2], psilocybin and LSD[3]. Clinical research suggests significant efficacy for psychiatric disorders that have traditionally been hard to treat. The evidence base has accumulated to the point that psychedelic-assisted psychotherapy appears to be moving from a fringe subject to a significant new treatment method that all psychotherapists should at least be aware of and that some may develop into a special interest.

Psychedelic substances and the psychological experiences associated with them do tend to challenge paradigms and elicit powerful reactions ranging from prohibition to evangelical enthusiasm. Neither of these positions predispose to the sober and thoughtful consideration of their clinical potential for psychiatric disorders, based on a developing evidence base. This would appear to be an important area of interest to psychiatry and psychotherapy inviting us to appraise potential benefits and risks, expand our models of therapeutic change, learn new skills and potentially take a leading role in the development of research and new treatments.

I will discuss the general principles of drug-assisted psychotherapy, the ways in which it differs from conventional psychotherapy, areas of therapeutic promise and implications for our understanding of the psyche.

Drug-assisted psychotherapy, as will be described here, involves the patient undergoing a short, time-limited course of psychotherapy, during which some of the sessions are enhanced by the acute action of a drug that has specific properties conducive to improving the efficacy of the psychotherapy. There is a class of powerful psychoactive substances, termed psychedelic drugs, that amplifies psychological material in a manner that can be used therapeutically. This is different to the use of psychoactive and mind-altering drugs as pharmacotherapy, such as ketamine for treatment-resistant depression.

Coined by the British psychiatrist Humphrey Osmond. Literally means mind manifesting – derived from Greek *psyche* and *delos*.
3,4-Methylenedioxymethamphetamine – Street name Ecstasy.   [3] Lysergic acid diethylamide.

The current psychedelic renaissance is necessarily driven by neuroscience and clinical research and is as yet less concerned in the complexity, topography and detail of the psyche that is uncovered. The clinical work of the first generation of psychedelic research in the 1950s and 1960s allowed a range of usage with different settings, variable dosages and greater numbers of sessions. Although much of the research from this era does not meet modern standards, it did allow a creative development of ideas leading to expanded models of the psyche to account for some of the phenomena that emerge in the psychedelic experience that could not be accounted for by existing models. I will discuss this briefly later.

The Crucial Elements of Psychedelic-Assisted Psychotherapy

Clinical outcome with therapeutic use of psychedelic substances depends on setting and integration as well as choice of substance and dosage. I will begin with a brief discussion of these critical factors.

The Set – is the mental state a person brings to the experience – thoughts, mood and expectations. The set needs to have the same qualities of curiosity, openness, therapist engagement and willingness to tolerate discomfort as in conventional therapy. There needs to be an additional psychoeducation process about the drug effects and how to tolerate and make therapeutic use of the intensity of the experience.

The Setting – is the physical and social environment, which is very different to the setting for conventional psychotherapy. The sober use of psychedelics as a method of treatment is a journey through the landscape of the interior. In properly supported psychedelic sessions, any contact with the everyday world or interpersonal communication is kept to a useful minimum. A relaxing non-clinical environment encourages a primary focus on the inner experience enhanced by optional use of eyeshades and music and accompanied by at least one sitter. The sitter is in a position of care and responsibility, and should have familiarity with the psychedelic territory and some of the mental states that may arise. The key role of the sitter is to support a naturally unfolding process that is assumed to have an intrinsic healing trajectory. The sitter takes a passive role and will not interfere with a person's process except on matters of care and safety, but is available to offer support if required. The support may be verbal, emotional or physical.

Integration – the drug session itself often has little verbal interaction. There follow structured meetings to process the content of the session, with additional support if required. This integrative process addresses emotional, intellectual and physical response to sessions, monitors risk and encourages self-caring activities and rest. The depth of the integration is enhanced by the therapist's preparatory work with the patient, the shared experience of the drug session and the therapist's experience and range of clinical skills.

Choice of drug – classical psychedelics such as LSD and psilocybin provide a range of emotional experiences ranging from sessions with a deeply positive spiritual (numinous) tone to more challenging encounters with previously hard to access psychological material. Empathogens/entactogens such as MDMA reliably provide positive affect and increased empathy that is a fundamental component of the current clinical research into treatment of post-traumatic stress disorder (PTSD) and was sometimes used in couple therapy before such treatment was made illegal in 1985.

Dosage – high-dose LSD was historically used to induce transpersonal/spiritual experiences thought to be the mutative factors in the treatment of alcoholism, addiction and terminal illness. Low to moderate dose LSD was used in *psycholytic* psychotherapy as a catalyst to access and amplify psychological material and places more emphasis on verbal interaction with the psychotherapist. There is developing research interest in *microdosing*, doses that are too low to have discernable clinical effects but may act as cognitive or emotional enhancers. In MDMA-assisted psychotherapy for PTSD there is accumulating evidence that a moderate dose of 75 mg has superior efficacy to a lower (30 mg) or higher dose (125 mg) [2].

MDMA-Assisted Psychotherapy for Treatment-Resistant Post-traumatic Stress Disorder

Researchers in the United States have led the field in developing MDMA as an adjunct to the psychological treatment of severe, treatment-resistant PTSD. The results have shown improvement that was sustained at follow-up. In August 2017 the USA Food and Drug Administration (FDA) granted Breakthrough Therapy Designation to MDMA for the treatment of PTSD. At time of writing phase 3 trials are underway with a view to making this treatment available for clinical use. So in the USA, MDMA-assisted psychotherapy appears likely to become a mainstream treatment.

The research is funded and coordinated by the Multidisciplinary Association for Psychedelic Studies (MAPS) and led by Dr Michael Mithoefer who is co-therapist with his wife Annie; a detailed treatment protocol can be found on the MAPS website [3]. The model of treatment in MDMA-assisted psychotherapy combines biological and psychotherapeutic approaches, which are applied synergistically to facilitate trauma processing, thereby decreasing or eliminating chronic hyperarousal and stress reactions to triggers. A key point in psychedelic-assisted psychotherapy is that the substance is seen as a catalyst for the process of therapeutic change – not as a pharmacological treatment in itself. The therapeutic effect is thought to flow from the interaction between those pharmacological effects, the therapeutic setting and the mindsets of the participant and the therapists. MDMA produces an experience that appears to temporarily reduce fear while increasing positive emotions and interpersonal trust, without clouding consciousness or reducing access to emotions.

MDMA may catalyse therapeutic processing by allowing participants to revisit traumatic experiences without being overwhelmed by anxiety or dissociating. This in turn enables a processing of the index trauma, as well as underlying vulnerability related to previous traumas. This trauma processing occurs both in the drug sessions and the non-drug sessions and the therapeutic process may be amplified by the enhanced therapeutic alliance with the therapists, which not only facilitates the processing of trauma but may also allow for an experience of secure attachment [3]

The British psychiatrist Ben Sessa describes MDMA as possessing all the required qualities to enhance psychotherapy. The drug is short-acting, has no dependence potential and is not toxic at therapeutic doses. It enhances the therapeutic alliance by amplifying a feeling of trust and closeness with the therapist, which in turn enables the addressing of trauma that may otherwise be too difficult. MDMA reduces depression and induces relaxation while simultaneously raising arousal levels for the therapy session with heightened sense of clarity, compassion and connectedness. It is consistent in its effects, almost always inducing positive affect and does not usually cause perceptual disturbances [4]. The effects last for between 6 and 8 hours.

The mechanism of action is incompletely understood, but MDMA is known to significantly decrease activity in the left amygdala [5]. This is compatible with some of the effects of MDMA such as reduction in fear or defensiveness and enhanced interaction with the therapist. Psychological models concerning the process of change and the interaction between substance, patient and therapist are developing. A psychoanalytic model of trauma and PTSD includes an overwhelming of the defences and loss of the ability to symbolise, so that the experience can only be repeated through flashbacks and nightmares rather than being processed. This can cause major challenges in establishing a therapeutic alliance when there is no longer any good object to call upon to help with the psychological tasks of facing a terrible reality and mourning one's former, untraumatised self. It appears that the euphoriant effect of the psychedelic substance enhances the potential to create a positive transference, which can allow some of the psychological work towards recovery that had previously not been possible.

The Treatment Programme for MDMA-Assisted Psychotherapy

The treatment programme in the research programme is carefully structured. Each participant has three preparatory sessions before the first drug session. There are usually three drug sessions in total over a three-month period and each drug session is followed by three integrative sessions. The therapeutic team comprises a male/female pair who are both present in all the drug and non-drug sessions, including the preparatory sessions.

The purpose of the preparatory sessions can be summarised as follows:

- Full history is taken together with exploration of client expectations and concerns
- Detailed explanation of the setting, the practical aspects of the treatment, the effects of MDMA, the structure of the sessions and the aftercare
- Explanation of the therapeutic approach, to try to stay with and tolerate emerging experiences, trust in the approach, focus on the body and inner processes
- Discussion of music, use of eyeshades, optional use of supportive touch from therapists if appropriate
- Agreement to stay in the treatment area, discussion of physical safety issues, anxiety management and support
- Establishment of therapeutic alliance, openness about any transference issues

The drug sessions have some important differences to conventional psychotherapy. There are two therapists throughout who are there in a supportive capacity. The effect of the male/female pair combined with the mood-enhancing effects of the drug has powerful transference implications. The patient is encouraged to lie on the couch, use eyeshades and maintain an inner focus. Music is carefully chosen to enhance the setting. There is regular monitoring of vital signs and this is an opportunity for the therapists to check in with the participant. Inevitably in this group of patients with PTSD the trauma will emerge and be available for discussion – at least to some extent. Anxiety management techniques allied with verbal emotional and physical support may be helpful.

The integration process is integral to the therapeutic process. Thus the participant is encouraged to use their own curiosity and tools in addition to the structures provided by the programme. Integration after the drug session begins with an informal recap of the session with the therapists. The participant spends the evening and night in a safe setting with recourse to additional support if required – this is a time for quiet and reflection. There follow three scheduled 90-minute integration sessions after each drug treatment using an active dialogue approach to uncover emotional, intellectual and physical response with consideration of emerging thoughts, feelings and concerns, risk assessment while encouraging self-caring activities and rest. Partners and important others are encouraged to participate – at least to some extent.

Mithoefer describes how the effects of MDMA can lead to profound insights about cognitive distortions with little or no intervention from the therapists; the largely non-directive approach often results in spontaneous cognitive restructuring resulting from qualities engendered by MDMA with increased mental clarity, confidence, and the courage to look honestly at oneself [6]. This cognitive restructuring is amplified and perpetuated in the integration sessions.

LSD-Assisted Psychotherapy in Terminal Illness

In 2014, Dr Peter Gasser's team in Switzerland published the first clinical research involving therapeutic use of LSD for over 40 years [7]. It is worth noting here that Switzerland has a major role in the history of psychedelic medicines. The Swiss chemist Albert Hofmann discovered LSD in 1943 and subsequently documented his first intentional LSD session [8]. Switzerland legalised psychedelic psychotherapy during the period 1988 until 1993 and this led to the training of psychedelic psychotherapists, including Dr Gasser, who have had a continuing influence in this field.

Using a controlled, randomised and blinded study design in 12 patients with distressing anxiety after the diagnosis of terminal cancer, Gasser's team found significant reductions in anxiety and the absence of significant side effects. End-of-life anxiety is notoriously difficult to treat but, as Gasser put it, 'with LSD assisted psychotherapy, the anxiety went down and stayed down'. The numbers of the patients involved in this study are too small to produce firm evidence, but it does provide proof of concept. Gasser's team provides an excellent model for the psychotherapeutic work required with LSD. Although LSD has different properties, a greater range of psychological effects and longer duration of action compared with MDMA, a similar programme was used. The characteristics are as follows:

- Ongoing psychotherapy over two to three months
- Two preparatory psychotherapy/explanatory sessions
- Two full day LSD sessions two to three weeks apart
- Moderate dose of LSD, i.e., 200 mcg – to avoid dissolution of ego structures
- Each LSD session accompanied by male/female therapist pair
- Participants were instructed to focus their awareness inwards, usually assisted by music
- Lengthy discussions between the participants and the co-therapists were discouraged during the acute effects of the LSD
- The therapeutic session ended after 8 hours followed by a brief review of the day's experiences
- Each LSD session was followed by three non-drug psychotherapy sessions over a few weeks
- Most of the participants stated a preference for more than two LSD sessions and a longer treatment period

Psilocybin-Assisted Psychotherapy for Depression

There is accumulating evidence for the possible efficacy of psilocybin in the treatment of depression. Psilocybin has considerable advantages compared with LSD due to shorter duration of action and arguably less historical stigma. It is a serotonin (5-HT) 2A receptor agonist and human imaging studies of psilocybin have shown changes in brain activity suggestive of antidepressant potential. In addition to any innate antidepressant effect it is assumed the occurrence of a profound, potentially transformative psychological experience is critical to the treatment's efficacy [9]. An open-label feasibility study of 12 people with treatment-resistant depression showed a significant reduction in depression at one week and three months after high-dose treatment. The drug was well tolerated and the study provided preliminary support for the safety and efficacy of psilocybin for treatment-resistant depression [10]. This first study provided basic psychological support rather than integrative psychotherapy. If further research confirms efficacy, subsequent studies will need to address the manner in which psychological approaches can be optimised in tandem with any biological antidepressant effect. The complexity of psychological experiences and the requirement for expert integration in psilocybin-assisted psychotherapy is likely to be of great interest to medical psychotherapy.

First-Generation LSD Research

The first generation of research into psychedelics came to an end when therapeutic use and clinical research using LSD was made illegal during the social and political turmoil of the 1960s.[4] There was a hiatus until the first decade of the twenty-first century when the clinical research was slowly resumed against the background of difficult legal and administrative barriers.

The psychedelic research conducted between 1950 and the mid 1960s published over 1000 scientific papers involving 40 000 patients. Many pioneers gave their careers to this field, hoping that psychedelic drugs could be to psychiatry what the microscope is to biology or the telescope is to astronomy; an essential tool to explore the parts of the internal world that are usually inaccessible. Although this research is almost entirely forgotten by modern psychiatry, there are some findings that may benefit from re-examination. Thus for abstinent alcoholics who were engaged in the recovery process, the LSD psychotherapy seemed particularly effective if the patient had a numinous or spiritual experience as a result of the psychedelic sessions, although the gains seemed to be lost with the passage of time [11] Thus, it is assumed that the numinous experience causes any therapeutic effect that results rather than the drug itself. Psychedelics may also be particularly useful for those people with anxiety about death associated with terminal illness. LSD research in the terminally ill found a reduced need for analgesics with improved mood and reduced fear of death in 60–70 per cent of cases. Again, the treatment response seemed to be correlated with the extent to which the patients experienced a mystical or transcendent state [12, 13].

LSD is remarkably safe when used with appropriate set, setting and attention to integration. A 1960 study of 5000 people who had taken LSD more than 25 000 times between them in clinical and research conditions found that only five of these people had suffered a psychotic reaction lasting more than 24 hours [14]. There is no evidence that psychedelic drugs are addictive or cause any recognised physical withdrawal syndrome. In animal models reliable self-administration does not occur [15]. Even when participants find the psychedelic experience to be intensely profound and valuable, very few had aspirations to repeat the experience again [16].

---

[4] Possession of LSD became illegal in the USA in 1968.

Psycholytic Psychotherapy

The Czech psychiatrist Stanislav Grof is widely regarded as the father of LSD psychotherapy. Grof developed an expanded model of psychological experience that emerges in LSD psychotherapy. As the only comprehensive model available as we move into the new era of clinical work with psychedelics, the next generation of psychedelic clinicians needs to have some familiarity with its basic principles.

Grof personally supervised an estimated 2500 LSD sessions in his clinical research between 1956 and 1972 and had access to material from a further 1300 sessions conducted by colleagues. Grof's seminal book *Realms of the Human Unconscious: Observations from LSD Research* was published in 1975. While current therapeutic work with psychedelics is limited by research parameters to two or three sessions, Grof's research shows us what may emerge with longer-term treatment with psychedelic-assisted psychotherapy. Essentially Grof found that serial sessions of LSD-assisted psychotherapy not only led to a deeper unfolding of psychic processes with trauma resolution and improvement in symptoms but also opened up areas of psyche that were not understood using any existing psychological models. Grof's original training was in Freudian psychoanalysis but he found that some of the phenomena encountered in his patients simply could not be explained in Freudian terms [17, p. 46].

Grof's first study involved the use of single sessions of LSD with 72 patients in a psychiatric ward in Prague. Grof found that rather than causing a toxic psychosis with the emergence of chaotic material from the psyche, LSD appeared to be a powerful catalyst that activated and amplified unconscious material that had previously been hidden or expressed as symptoms. As the British Jungian Margot Cutner put it – 'the material emerging under LSD, far from being chaotic, reveals, on the contrary, a definite relationship to the psychological needs of the patient at the moment of his taking the drug' [18].

Grof found that only 3 out of the 72 patients showed a dramatic and lasting improvement after a single session, some people showed temporary improvement or deterioration in mental function. But a crucial finding was that a few individuals had a series of five to eight consecutive sessions over a period of months, and for these cases there appeared to be a continuation of the process from session to session with an unfolding of deeper levels of the unconscious with some reliving and resolution of traumatic memories.

Grof's second study examined the unfolding effects of a series of LSD sessions in 52 patients with a variety of chronic neurotic and psychosomatic conditions. The study is described below as it may provide a model for future treatment of selected patients in specialist units for psychedelic-assisted psychotherapy. Grof's study excluded people with bipolar disorder or schizophrenia. The dose of LSD was in the moderate range, starting at 100 mcg and increasing by 25 mcg increments until the optimum dose was found that allowed emergence of psychological material without overwhelming ego function so that contact with the therapist could be maintained.

The patients had conventional psychotherapy before their LSD sessions and their therapist was with them throughout the LSD session and discussed the contents with them afterwards. The patient would leave the session to rejoin the ward to be supported by fellow patients who were in the LSD programme and nurses who had had their own training sessions with LSD. No one was left alone after an LSD session until at least 24 hours had passed. The patients had psychotherapy between the LSD sessions to discuss, analyse and integrate the content and discuss transference issues that emerged.

Grof noted that the single most important determinant of the LSD sessions themselves was the level of trust between patient and therapist. This therapeutic alliance made it possible to tolerate and make use of the challenging experiences that inevitably emerged during the course of treatment. Grof maintains that difficult psychedelic experiences are often caused by the emergence of traumatic memories and associated emotions from the unconscious. Because this unconscious material negatively impacts the person's life, difficult psychedelic sessions can become opportunities for healing when such material is properly worked with. Difficult and overwhelming experiential material described as a *bad trip* in an uncontrolled setting is exactly what is wanted in a controlled setting. For Grof, challenging experiences with LSD are merely an indication that psychological material yet to be processed has become accessible. These challenging experiences do not usually need intervention in the sessions themselves, but are seen as natural healing processes that need to be allowed to run their course – the role of the therapist is to prepare the mindset, provide support and facilitate integration.

Expanding Our Map of Psyche

Grof found that psychedelic experiences could be classified into the following four categories:

- Aesthetic
- Psychodynamic
- Perinatal
- Transpersonal

Aesthetic experiences represent the most superficial level. These are the visual imagery, often complex and fascinating, the synaesthesia and the various perceptual changes. While creatively stimulating they do not have psychodynamic significance and do not result in mutative change. The *psychodynamic* level refers to the range of biographical experience that is understandable in psychoanalytic terms. The *perinatal* and *transpersonal* levels represent important areas of psyche that emerge in psychedelic sessions that would not be familiar to most clinicians and thus need some introduction.

The fundamental characteristics of perinatal experience are described as the challenges of biological birth, physical pain and agony, ageing, disease and decrepitude, dying and death. Grof found that the visceral re-experiencing of this layer of psyche in psychedelic sessions was accompanied by an existential crisis. But if the experience was properly supported and allow to fully express itself, this not only led to significant symptom resolution but also a profound realignment of a person's relationship with their environment including convincing insights into the relevance of the spiritual dimension in the universal scheme of things [17, p. 95].

Grof's proposal that the trauma of birth had a residue in our personality development is not entirely original – Otto Rank was disfavoured by Freud after making such a proposal. Psychoanalytic thinking has traditionally assumed that the baby is born with pristine psyche, like virgin snow, but becomes immediately exquisitely tuned in to the nuance of the relationship with the primary object as the fundamental building block of personality. The recent work of Piontelli demonstrates the relevance of intrauterine life in subsequent personality development but has less to say about the impact of the birth experience itself [19].

From the perspective of the baby Grof proposed four stages of labour that he renamed *basic perinatal matrices (BPM)* to capture the complex emotional field associated with each stage. These stages progress from the serenity of the womb to the cataclysmic shock and existential threat associated with the onset of labour, the struggle through the birth canal and the exhausted relief of delivery. These four distinct meaning states are summarised below.

The **first perinatal matrix (BPM 1)** is the resting state that lasts until the onset of the contractions of labour. This is a peaceful state of fusion with needs being entirely met by mother. This resting state may become toxic, perhaps due to medication, metabolic issues or hypoxia.

The **second perinatal matrix (BPM 2)** is the physical onset of labour where the uterus contracts against a closed cervix. There is no available exit so this state involves an experience of constriction, entrapment and fear; the baby faces death.

The **third perinatal matrix (BPM 3)** represents the physical process of movement out of the constricted uterus through the opening cervix followed by the 'life or death struggle' through the birth canal.

The **fourth perinatal matrix (BPM 4)** is the birth, the emergence into the new world, the first intake of breath and the recovery phase for mother and baby.

In the psychological states that correspond to the perinatal experience, the first perinatal matrix involving good-womb experiences would equate to blissful oceanic feelings. A toxic womb state may be associated with paranoia. The second perinatal matrix carries feelings of profound hopelessness, existential despair and the encounter with death. This is often a profoundly challenging mental state that has high potential for psychological growth if fully supported and processed. The third perinatal matrix is the archetypal hero's journey, the call to arms, the tumultuous and perilous struggle. The fourth perinatal matrix holds themes of triumph, fortuitous escape from danger, revolution, decompression and expansion of space, radiant light and colour, but perhaps also the sense of loss of closeness to mother.

Psychedelic psychotherapy used higher doses of LSD, typically between 250 and 500 mcg, with the aim of facilitating religious or spiritual experiences that were thought to be mutative for some conditions, such as alcoholism or end of life anxiety. High-dose sessions frequently bypass the areas of psychodynamic conflict that are characteristic of psycholytic treatment but are more likely to induce transpersonal experiences. Grof found that in psycholytic sessions transpersonal experience was rare in the early sessions but occurred frequently in later sessions once psychodynamic and perinatal material had been worked through and integrated.

The transpersonal involves an expansion of conscious experience beyond normal ego boundaries and beyond the limitations of time and space. There is a wide variety of such experiences and a description of them goes beyond the remit of this chapter. But any clinician interested in this area really does need to have some knowledge of the transpersonal layer of psyche. People in psychedelic sessions often report strongly emotionally charged experiences centred on a specific theme (such as shame, abandonment or fear of annihilation) that permeates all these layers of psyche moving from biographical scenarios to the perinatal area and finally to a transpersonal or mythic flavour. Processing these experiences as fully as possible may be the key to long-term symptom resolution.

References

1. Freud S. An outline of psycho-analysis. In J Strachey, ed., *The Standard Edition of the Complete Psychological Works of Sigmund Freud, Volume XXIII (1937–1939). Moses and Monotheism, An Outline of Psycho-Analysis and Other Works*. London: Hogarth Press. 1964; pp. 139–208. (Original work published 1938)

2. Mithoefer MC, Mithoefer AT, Feduccia AA et al. 3,4-methylenedioxymethamphetamine (MDMA) psychotherapy for post-traumatic stress disorder in military veterans, firefighters, and police officers: a randomised, double-blind, dose-response, phase 2 clinical trial. *Lancet Psychiatry* 2018; 5(6): 486–97.

3. Mithoefer M, Mithoefer A, Jerome L et al. A manual for MDMA-assisted psychotherapy in the treatment of PTSD (version 8). http://www.maps.org/researc h/mdma/mdma-research-timeline/4887-a-manual-for-mdma-assisted-psychotherapy -in-the-treatment-of-ptsd [Accessed 23/ 11/2020]

4. Sessa B. *The Psychedelic Renaissance*, 2nd ed. London: Muswell Hill Press. 2017; p. 41.

5. Carhart-Harris RL, Murphy K, Leech R et al. The effects of acutely administered 3,4-methylenedioxymethamphetamine on spontaneous brain function in healthy volunteers measured with arterial spin labeling and blood oxygen level-dependent resting state functional connectivity. *Biol Psychiatry* 2015; 78(8): 554–62.

6. Mithoefer M. MDMA-assisted psychotherapy: how different is it from other psychotherapy? MAPS Bulletin Special Edition, Spring 2013. www .maps.org/news-letters/v23n1/v23n1_p10-14.pdf> [Accessed 23/11/2020]

7. Gasser P, Holstein D, Michel Y et al. Safety and efficacy of lysergic acid diethylamide-assisted psychotherapy for anxiety associated with life-threatening diseases. *J Nerv Ment Dis* 2014; 202(7): 513–20.

8. Hoffman A. *LSD My Problem Child*, 2nd ed. Sarasota FL: MAPS, 2005.

9. Roseman L, Nutt D, Carhart-Harris RL. Quality of acute psychedelic experience predicts therapeutic efficacy of psilocybin for treatment-resistant depression. *Front Pharmacol* 2018; 8: 974.

10. Carhart-Harris RL, Bolstridge M, Rucker J et al. Psilocybin with psychological support for treatment-resistant depression: an open-label feasibility study. *Lancet Psychiatry* 2016; 3(7): 619–27.

11. Kurland A, Savage C, Pahnke WN, Grof S, Olsson JE. LSD in the treatment of alcoholics. *Pharmacopsychiatry* 1971; 4(2): 83–94.

12. Kast E. LSD and the dying patient. *Chic Med Sch Q* 1966; 26(2): 80–7.

13. Pahnke WN, Kurland AA, Goodman LE, Richards WA. LSD-assisted psychotherapy with terminal cancer patients. *Curr Psychiatr Ther* 1969; 9: 144–52.

14. Cohen S. Lysergic acid diethylamide: side effects and complications. *J Nerv Ment Dis* 1960; 130: 30–40.

15. Griffiths RR, Bigelow GE, Henningfield JE Similarities and animal and human drug-taking behaviour. In NK Mello, ed., *Advances in Substance Abuse*. Vol. 1. Greenwich: JAI Press. 1980; pp. 1–90.

16. Griffiths RR, Richards WA, McCann U, Jesse R. Psilocybin can occasion mystical-type experiences having substantial and sustained personal meaning and spiritual significance. *Psychopharmacology* 2006; 187: 268–83.

17. Grof S. *Realms of the Human Unconscious Observations from LSD Research*. New York: Viking, 1975.

18. Cutner M. *Analytic work with LSD*. *Psychiatr Q* 1969; 33: 715–57.

19. Piontelli A. *From Fetus to Child: Observational and Psychoanalytical Study*. Hove: Routledge, 1992.

Chapter 29

Psychotherapeutic Development through the Life of the Psychiatrist

William Burbridge-James

The Human Seasons
Four Seasons fill the measure of the year;
There are four seasons in the mind of man:
He has his lusty Spring, when fancy clear
Takes in all beauty with an easy span:
He has his Summer, when luxuriously
Spring's honied cud of youthful thought he loves
To ruminate, and by such dreaming high
Is nearest unto heaven: quiet coves
His soul has in its Autumn, when his wings
He furleth close; contented so to look
On mists in idleness–to let fair things
Pass by unheeded as a threshold brook.
He has his Winter too of pale misfeature,
Or else he would forego his mortal nature
                                        John Keats, 1818

Introduction

Life is a cycle as Keats' poem beautifully illustrates.[1] We progress through the seasons of life as we do with our professional lives, intertwining with our more private lives and our personal development. Shakespeare wrote about the seven ages of man [1] in *As You Like It* in the famous speech of Jacques when he compares the world to a stage and roles that we occupy as we pass through life. The psychoanalyst Eric Erikson developed his theory of the stages of psychosocial development [2] where we experience conflicts at each stage of development that need to be negotiated to feel a sense of mastery and develop a strong sense of self. Many of us would have come across Shakespeare and Erickson linked together in Brown and Pedder's *Introduction to Psychotherapy* [3] where we also read about Freud and his psychosexual developmental stages, where Freud described how we can become fixated at a stage in our development that we can regress to in times of stress.

As we progress through our lives and careers, as doctors and psychiatrists, we have to negotiate transitions which invariably involve a letting go of old certainties and identities as we move on to the next stage; from medical student to doctor, from trainee to consultant

---

Keats trained as a doctor, having experienced early losses in his life, before poetry became his calling. He died young at the age of 25 from TB but he could anticipate the inexorable progress of time.

and through to retirement. This entails feeling insecure and being able to tolerate uncertainty while we find our feet in the next phase of our career, and the right kind of nurturing facilitative support to enable a process of establishing ourselves in our developing professional roles. This needs time and space for reflection, to enable working through of loss, and renewal, if we are not to become stuck in a repetition of an earlier developmental struggle, burnt out or ossified in our professional lives.

The chapter starts with the nature of Freud's beginning of his psychoanalytic discovery with his articulation of the unconscious nature of mental life. It then touches on relevant developments by psychoanalysts that came after him, and discusses how these can help us think about our own professional developmental life cycle, and how this relates to our potential to develop as psychotherapeutic psychiatrists.

Johnston defines psychotherapeutic psychiatry in his paper 'Learning from the cradle to the grave' [4], as being 'a frame of mind' where psychotherapy is seen 'less an activity of others but more a therapeutic way of thinking about patients and a vital part of *our psychiatric*[2] professional identity', where we are able to see the 'person beyond the diagnosis and problem'. Johnston describes how this therapeutic frame of mind, which he terms 'therapeutic attitude', is both a reflective and reflexive intersubjective examination of the mind. The mind of the patient, which is 'on examination', affects the mind of the psychiatrist, which will also be in part a reflection of the psychiatrist's 'own life experience and personality'.

> It is a remarkable thing that the Ucs (unconscious) of one human being can react upon that of another, without passing through the Cs (conscious). Sigmund Freud, 1915 [5]

A reflective capacity and therapeutic attitude may be difficult to achieve and maintain because it means being and remaining open, and alive to our emotional responses; being disturbed by forgotten aspects of ourselves that emotional contact with our patients resonates with. This can feel antithetical to the carapace of a dispassionate professional, 'scientific and technical approach to psychiatry [6].

The chapter takes readers on their passage alongside the psychiatrist in his/her developmental stages through the lifespan of a professional career to illustrate the developmental challenges that are faced by all of us who seek to be compassionate self-aware clinicians. This is a task not to be underestimated given that however much we might like to see ourselves as working independently we are inevitably interdependent on the settings within which we work, and the socio-political cultural environment within which we and our patients live.

Beginnings

We are all drawn to medicine for our own reasons and some of these are more unconscious than conscious. It may be that these hidden reasons, alongside our rational explanations, underlie our motivation that brought us to study medicine and then on to specialise in psychiatry. If the practice of medicine is about the alleviation of suffering combined with a wish to heal and make better; we can link this on a personal level with our own experience and those that are or have been close to us, who have been subject to illness, loss, separation, death and trauma of one kind or another, that are woven into the tapestry of our lives. It is these experiences that have emotionally and psychologically deeply affected us that may

---

[2] Author's addition in italics.

have initiated us on our medical journeys. They function like a kernel, a motive agent, hidden or less hidden, that lives on as a chrysalis in the psyche, motivating our curiosity, and appetite for knowledge and understanding, described by Melanie Klein (1928) [7] as the epistemophilic instinct in her observation of young children.[3] It is this instinct, in the German '*Trieb*', that underlies the maturational development of a nascent psychotherapeutic psychiatrist. This is alongside identifications with significant others, parents or other aspirational role models who have been or are doctors.

Concepts: Transference, Projection and Identification

Freud's research into hysteria, a condition encompassing the psyche and the soma, at the end of the nineteenth century building on the work of Charcot and Janet, and the mental mechanisms which repressed unacceptable mental contents from conscious articulation, led to his discovery of dynamic mental processes. He continued to elaborate these in his evolving models of the mind. From his initial affect-trauma model through to the topographical and structural models, continuing to develop his theories throughout his life.

However, Freud, as perhaps many of us do, initially struggled with his discovery of the transference seeing this as a resistance to free association and an obstacle to therapy. This is movingly described in the case of Anna O with his colleague Joseph Breuer.[4] He later recognised transference as a ubiquitous phenomenon; and a tool to be used in the service of the psychotherapy, 'the transference, which, whether affectionate or hostile, seemed in every case to constitute the greatest threat to the treatment, becomes its best tool' [8]. The transference is a position we immediately unconsciously occupy as a medical student, doctor and psychiatrist. We become a subject in our patients' unconscious representations, taking on a significance that is beyond how we consciously perceive ourselves. As such our representation is coloured and shaped by our patients' projections and we become '*facsimiles*' [9], characters, of our patients' internal worlds represented in the here and now of the encounter.

These projections that we are subject to, ubiquitous in other parts of our lives, not only shape us but actually take up residence within us. Our receptivity to the impact of these projections depends on our own experiences, sensitivities and vulnerabilities. A projection is in search of a receptor, much as we might think of a drug that will have a greater affinity for certain receptors than others, which Wilfred Bion in his study of groups described as 'valency'[5] [10]. On locating the receptor, the receptor responds to accommodate the projection. It is this accommodation that then evokes a response in us; our identification with the projection. Our receptivity is at its most open as infants, or comparably when we come into medicine as students or when we start as new trainees in psychiatry, before we have built up our defensive structures which may be both personal and systemic.[6]

Klein linked the epistemophilic instinct with aggression and early 'Oedipus tendencies', and curiosity of the contents of mother's body, and feelings of fear and guilt. [7, p. 188]

Anna had developed a positive erotic transference to Breuer, and a phantom pregnancy, which led to Breuer abandoning his treatment of Anna and going on a second honeymoon with his wife.

Initially a word borrowed from physics valency is used by Bion as expressing 'a capacity for instantaneous voluntary combination with another for sharing or acting on a basic assumption'.

See Isabel Menzies Leith for a good description of systemic defences, The Functioning of Social Systems as a Defence Against Anxiety. *Hum Relat* 1959; 13: 95–121.

When we enter medicine and psychiatry we are sensitive and thin-skinned,[7] newly exposed to the full range, highs and lows, of human experience from birth, the impact of illness and disability, to facing terminal illness and death. The latter may be sudden and unexpected, and we have to deal with the effect of sharing the news with families and loved ones.

'Bodily Beginnings' at the End of Life

Uniquely in medical training before this we are exposed to the cadaver in the study of anatomy through dissection in groups as a shared experience. We are brought face to face with death and the frailty of human existence at this sensitive stage in our professional development that has a rite of passage symbolic quality [11]. However, the context is often one where the past life of the person who inhabited the cadaver is split off and medicalised under the scientific umbrella of anatomy. Nevertheless in this exposure to mortality medical students will often be forced to reconnect with the embodied personhood of their cadaver through an aspect of their physical form, perhaps a small detail that allows for an imaginative leap into the person's life and death.

> *The first body had a notable tattoo on his arm. Seeing him first reminded me that every cadaver is individual, although some might look quite similar. They'd all lived their own complex lives.*
> Toyin Jesuloba [12]

Thus it is through this experience of dissection that as medical students we are confronted with the deep connection with our being and mortality, the psyche and the soma; and for generations of doctors this is their first exposure to a dead person that is out of the ordinary that needs to be digested and made sense of. The danger is that instead of being digested this experience can remain split off, deflected with black humour or distanced by inventive unflattering 'cadaver naming' [13], and stoicism can become 'the litmus test for professionalism' [14]. Medical schools are increasingly recognising the importance of humanising the experience of dissection [15], where the cadaver is seen as the first patient, or 'Silent Mentor' [16], and their identity revealed with contact with the donors' families either before the start of dissection, or at the end with a memorial service where their contribution is recognised with families and loved ones invited. These contacts with lives of the donors and ceremonies help students to cultivate a sense of empathy and express their feelings.

These early experiences in a medical career received and taken in by the receptive medical student are ones that serve as a prototype for subsequent experiences in clinical encounters. We are affected and have to digest and make sense of encounters with our patients and it is this internal experience that percolates, in psychoanalytic language our countertransference, for which we need to have time and space to be able to acknowledge and recognise. Countertransference can be thought about as the totality of our experience that our work evokes in ourselves, it can be subtle, like a spontaneous thought or association or a bodily feeling, such as a 'gut reaction', which can then be used to help us in our contact with our patients and to deepen our understanding.

Starting with our early experiences in the dissecting room, we can begin to understand the shock and revulsion evoked present in many encounters when looking after patients; the

---

[7] A capacity that we need to maintain while developing a professional second skin. See Ester Bick, The experience of the skin in early object relations. *Int J Psychoanal* 1968; 49(2): 484–6.

smell of gangrene and bodily excreta; or the sight of a severe self-inflicted wound; are understandably things that we may seek to avoid because of their emotional and sensory impact. These gross manifestations of contact with others can be represented at more subtle levels.

For example a young male medical student who has struggled with his experience of brittle asthma during his childhood, and whose mother also had a chronic medical condition, found himself caring for an elderly man with breathing difficulties on one of the older people's medical wards. He was often asked to go and take bloods from the gentleman and the older man clearly appreciated the time despite the intrusion, and would chat about his life to the young student. The student then learned during the ward round that his patient had been diagnosed with terminal lung cancer. He struggled to go and see him although he wanted to, and it was not until his attendance in his Balint group could he talk about how his grandfather had died of dementia and he had felt guilty for not going to see him when he was in his nursing home. He also spoke of his own experience of asthma in childhood and could then start to recognise that his avoidance of his elderly patient on his placement had very personal resonances for him. He was able to return to see his patient on the ward, who was pleased to see him and they were able to continue a conversation about a mutual love of art.

In common with his initial concerns about transference Freud had first thought that this experience of countertransference was something to be 'conquered', a problem for the analyst – just as in the example of the medical student, 'the patient represents for the analyst an object of the past onto whom past feelings and wishes are projected' [17], and that can lead to problems. This would now be viewed as a communication from the patient that occurs in an intersubjective space. As such it needs to be digested by the receptive doctor/student, made available for thought, and then used as a helpful fragment of information that can enrich our understanding of what might be taking place in the here and now of the relationship.

These developmental steps in psychoanalytic theory evolved with the work of Melanie Klein and her development of the concept of projective identification. For Klein this was a phantasy where parts of the self are projected into the mother, or other, and evoke the feelings of the phantasies that are being projected. Klein viewed this as a defence, that is these were aspects of the self, self-objects and associated affects, which for whatever reason could not be contained by the projector. These could be either good or bad, depending on the underlying phantasy for the projection, and what might be internally threatening and therefore need to be projected.

For example, a patient who felt very ambivalent about her relationship with her father who was both abandoning and longed for and had suddenly died prematurely in her adolescence. In her session shortly after a break in the psychotherapy her therapist found she was feeling very uncomfortable and felt there was something missing in her contact with the patient, although the patient was outwardly pleased to be back in her psychotherapy. It was only later in the session when the patient was able to express her ambivalence to her therapist whom she suspected of selfish motives could she be open about her phantasy that she had killed her father with her long-standing hatred.

In its original sense projective identification tends to be viewed as pathological and not normative, that is part of life. It was Bion who extended Klein's concept of projective identification and highlighted the communicative aspects of projective identification viewing it as a primitive non-verbal communication that babies used as a way of communicating with their mother. Bion liked to think in terms of mathematical formula and wrote about how primitive beta elements projected by the baby were by the mother's process of reverie, which he termed alpha function, turned into 'alpha elements' that were available for thought. The baby can then re-introject his projections modified by understanding and also introject the experience of the mother as a container capable of dealing with his anxiety.

Early Medical Years

Therefore, we might consider how can this process be provided for doctors in training? We might think of creating a space where this process of maternal alpha function, to use Bion's terminology, can enable these experiences to be digested and made sense of. In order to do this safe spaces need to be created to be able to talk about these feelings. Exposure to psychological disturbance early in the psychiatric career, such as depression, self-harm, suicide, substance misuse, emotional turmoil and psychosis, evokes powerful emotional responses, anxieties and identifications at both conscious and unconscious levels. Fear of contagion by madness may underly the stigmatisation of psychiatric patients and those that work with them [18].

The wish to heal which motivates many of us to train in medicine also applies to psychological wounds. We are drawn to psychiatry for complex personal and psychological developmental reasons, and a wish to understand, care and make better.

Identification Separation and Mourning

When a village grows into a town or a child into a man, the village and the child become lost in the town and the man.
Sigmund Freud, 1915 [19]

In psychiatry therefore the difficulties faced by our patients may have an unconscious familiarity that resonates with us on a personal level. Being able to identify with our patients is helpful in establishing empathy; we can place ourselves in the shoes of another – 'Einfühlung' coined by Edward Titchner [20] and translated into the English word empathy comes from the Greek Em – into and Pathos – feeling.

This can be used to the therapeutic benefit of patients but there is a risk. If we are too closely identified then it can become difficult to distinguish ourselves from our patients who are then no longer viewed as separate from ourselves. It can then become hard to make difficult decisions that are in their best interests, or we can go to extreme lengths to help them which can be exhausting and emotionally draining to the detriment of the doctor's well-being. Differentiation between self and other is needed as a prerequisite to maintain our capacity for thinking.

Developing as a psychotherapeutic psychiatrist requires us to acknowledge our identifications which bring us into contact with our patients and then being able to differentiate ourselves from them, and acknowledge our own vulnerabilities, needs, wishes, desires and feelings. This can be through self-reflection, use of supervision, Balint groups, or in our own psychotherapy and psychoanalysis.

This is a complex task. Klein articulated in her conceptual development of the depressive position a constellation of anxiety and defences that the infant experiences from about six months of age, when he perceives the loved object as a whole separate object. The infant's anxiety focusses on concern for the welfare of the object which leads to a remorseful guilt for hateful feelings to the object, and painful feelings of sadness. The recognition of the object as separate leads to pining for what has been lost and the wish to repair and the process of reparation provides a means to overcome the despair for the damage done.[8]

> The ego feels impelled–by its identification with the good object–to make restitution for all the sadistic attacks that it has launched on that object.   Klein, 1935 [22]

> The depressive position is 'also the experience at any stage of life, of guilt and grief over hateful attacks and over the damaged external and internal objects' [23].

Henri Rey the psychiatrist and psychoanalyst expanded on Freud's discovery in 'Mourning and Melancholia' that the link between the two conditions was the identification of the self with the lost object. So in melancholia the lost object is retained within the self and attacked in the depressive recrimination that the patient makes towards him/herself. He then links it to Klein's notion of reparation. Rey suggests that one of the reasons for keeping the object alive like this is not only guilt suggested by Freud, but also to allow for reparation of the object [24].

We can then perhaps start to understand how feelings of helplessness, or unbearable psychic pain and anguish can motivate clinicians to evermore heroic attempts to care for their patients, rather than face these experiences within themselves and endure the discomfort that they arouse.

It is this discomfort which may often not only be coming from the patient but from the team within which the trainee works. The nascent psychiatrist on-call will be the de-facto representative of the consultant, and thus the medical lead. She or he will then be under significant pressures coming from the nursing team who have the most direct contact with inpatients. Often the nursing team's push is for the doctor to take action. Sanction a self-discharge, provide prn medication and act on the behalf of the nursing team's feelings to the patient, that is their anxiety, hostility, feelings of helplessness and vulnerability, rather than on behalf of the patient. These dilemmas have been recurring themes in Balint groups for trainee psychiatrists.

Inhabiting professional authority and the development of this is an integral part of the development of the psychotherapeutic psychiatrist. Being able to resist the pressure to act, and engage with the patient to find out what is behind the team's requests is not only about good medical practice, but also keeping an open mind and remaining curious, which is a developmental process that has to be negotiated.

Growth versus Stagnation

It is our formative experiences beginning at medical school that remain fundamental to continued growth as we progress during our careers. That is, how can we remain open to experience, rather than feeling overwhelmed, or becoming complacent, closed off, more rigid and ossified?

At the heart of this as with our trainee-selves is the maintenance of a reflective space which can contain and allow us to metabolise our anxiety (Figure 29.1). This may be represented as a triangular space, where we need the presence of an other to contain our anxiety and thus to maintain our capacity for curiosity and deepen our understanding.

Freud viewed doctors' wishes to make reparation as a reaction formation to their sadism; and in an autobiographical reflection he thought that his 'sadistic disposition was not very strong, and so I did not need to develop its derivatives' [21].

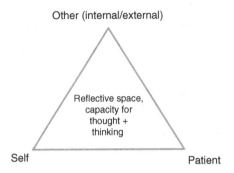

Figure 29.1 Triangular space.

Developmentally this may be seen as tolerating the persecutory anxieties from our internal damaged self-objects, who we are failing to repair, by recognising our identifications with our patients, and taking ownership for them.

It is being able to take up the third position – the triangulation of the dyadic relationship with the patient. This can be both internal and external. Externally can be though continued supervision – in peer groups, or individual supervision, or through continued attendance in Balint groups.

On an internal level this is through the build-up of experience of supervision and reflection. The internalisation of our supervisors who have been helpful to us who then become the internal supervisor [25], alongside our theoretical model that serves to frame our thought, and that we use to relate to in our minds. This internal observing other-self is able to reflect on internal experiences while still being present in the here and now of an interaction.

This observing part of ourselves might then recognise the feelings that suddenly arise in a clinical scenario or the thoughts that go through our mind; these may seem more or less connected with our patient, but giving an internal voice to these is the start of deciphering the projective processes that we are part of.

A patient, for example, may be describing a painful traumatic event in a detached but detailed descriptive way when we suddenly feel intruded upon by the unpleasant traumatic imagery – we can then start to get a feel for the painful intrusion experienced by our patient that has been split off and projected – and at the same time in the retelling there is an unconscious identification with the aggressor – perhaps not only to maintain a distance from the experience but also to gain some control of the traumatic experience.

Or another example may be that we feel detached and unemotional when another patient talks about themselves and jokes about their suicidal intent – we might then reflect how our own experience might relate to the patient's need to be detached from a vulnerable suicidal self – and for us to collude with a jokey cruel self that wants to kill off any concern for the vulnerable self.

Establishing these levels of maturity where it is possible to achieve this third position is part of the development of the psychiatrist and the importance of having a frame to establish this through exposure to undertaking psychotherapeutic experience as an integral part of their training.

The Psychotherapy Long Case

At the heart of this experience is the psychotherapy long case which is part of the core psychiatric curriculum for psychiatric trainees in the UK. This alongside attendance at a Balint group and undertaking a short psychotherapy case form the foundation of developing psychotherapeutic capabilities in UK psychiatric training. The long case has tended to be psychoanalytic/psychodynamic psychotherapy (69%) and the short case cognitive behavioural psychotherapy (35%) [26].

The significance of the experience of the psychotherapy long case is that for trainees it means inhabiting a transitional space[9] for the analytic hour a week when they are with their patient in a psychotherapy. The trainee psychiatrist has to temporarily set aside their developing identity as a psychiatrist with its illusory security and learn to inhabit a new uncertain identity for that moment as a psychotherapist. It is then through the qualitative experience of being with a patient over a consistent period of time in this protected space that has value for the patient first and foremost,[10] but also for the trainee's development of the capabilities that go with their developing psychotherapeutic identity. It is this experience of being with patients in a psychotherapy where we deepen our learning of the experience of being able to listen, to both conscious and unconscious aspects of communication. Undertaking the psychotherapy long case has been shown to be a creative developmental experience helping trainee psychiatrists not only developing their capacity to listen, but also to empathise with their patients, and manage professional boundaries and challenging interactions [28].

Burnout and Ossification

Inevitably though when we think about the setting in which we work it is one where we can also see that third position is not just related to the patient but also the workplace and our relationship to the organisations within which we work.

Creating and sustaining a supportive reflective space is vital to mitigate the effects of burnout 'an experience of physical, emotional, and mental exhaustion, caused by long-term involvement in situations that are emotionally demanding' [29]. Burnout can be characterised by feelings of cynicism and detachment from the work, and a sense of ineffectiveness and lack of autonomy and accomplishment. We struggle to realise our work-related ideals and we are exposed to the repeated traumas of our patients, and their ongoing disturbance and dependency needs.

This is hard to bear and we can retreat into defensive responses doing things by rote that ally with the unspoken systemic culture to keep the emotional demands of our work at bay, and to decrease the cognitive dissonance [30] that we experience. The culture of community psychiatry has become one where fragmentation has unwittingly become part of the model [31] and the therapeutic value of continuity of relationships between clinicians and their patients degraded.

---

[9] D. W. Winnicott in his paper Transitional Objects and Transitional Phenomena (1951, 1971) used the term transitional to describe the 'intermediate' or 'third area', where fantasy and reality overlap, that creativity, including the basis for adult cultural life, and play originate. He compared this with the therapeutic situation, where the worlds of the patient and analyst overlap [27].

[10] For many of the patients referred to NHS Psychotherapy services this is their first experience of being attentively listened to and feeling that another person is interested in them, their life stories, and how these have shaped them.

The strains of working within the system that fails to meet the needs of their patients and professional aspirations propels clinicians to think about ways that they can reduce clinical commitments and take retirement, the latter being an exit strategy rather than the culmination of a satisfying career.

Other factors can mitigate against burnout. One of the most significant of these is being involved in training of the next generation psychiatrists. As with the experience of being a parent being a trainer gives an opportunity for the older generation to continue a process of rediscovering themselves through the development of their trainees, and thus participate in a regenerative cycle that can help reinvigorate them. Trainees challenge us and keep our capacity for thinking alive in relation to our theoretical and clinical framework and thus continue to expand a triangulated space for thought that can otherwise feel to be constricting.

Endings

However, knowing when to retire from the frontline of clinical practice is a very personal choice [32] related to hopes and plans for retirement, but also dependent on the settings in which we work. The stress of working in psychiatry was previously recognised by the potential to take early retirement in the UK at 55 [33] through mental health officer status with pension benefits. This incentive alongside tribulations of working within the NHS and the pressures of revalidation introduced for doctors in the UK in 2012 can force choices on mature clinicians which would otherwise not have been made [34]. For the up and coming generation it is expected that like other medical specialties psychiatrists will remain in post until 65.

Experienced older clinicians who may have retired from the frontline have a significant contribution to make with their accumulated clinical wisdom and ability to continue to provide perspectives to others who are engaged at that level [35]. This is a valuable perspective for it is knowing when not to actively intervene that is often the hardest decision that doctors have to make, where a longitudinal view can be of great help. At a systemic level this means respecting the contributions that senior clinicians can make in providing meaningful supervisory containment for the younger generations of clinicians who are following in their footsteps.

In psychiatric practice this means knowing patients and their families, partners or carers over a long period of time; their vulnerabilities and highs and lows, and travelling on a shared journey with them. It is this depth of contact that can inform sensitive decision-making on whether to act or not. When a consultant retires this knowledge is lost that is difficult to replace. Leaving the workplace can feel like a bereavement, letting go of the familiar and saying goodbye to the 'team' of colleagues who have been like a second family, as well as to patients who may have become part of the fabric of one's life and psyche especially if in a post for many years. Norman Clemens a US psychiatrist and psychoanalyst writes movingly about ending his practice in his late 70s.

> *longstanding patients on long-term medication and low frequency psychotherapeutic maintenance will never be free of need for psychiatric help to sustain a decent quality of life and healthy functioning. It is usually hard to part with these old-timers, with whom there is a real bond based on many years of confronting mental life together. I found that there were very few, if any, with whom parting was a relief rather than a moment of sorrow.* Clemens, 2011 [36]

Returning to Johnston's reflexive intersubjective understanding of psychotherapeutic psychiatry at an individual level for the psychiatrist retirement is a process involving a letting go of professional status and psychiatric identity, as well as patients. Being able to go through the sorrow of losing these and face the destabilising transition rather than defend against it through manic defences of denial and a need to keep busy can allow for a productive creative phase of life shaped by accrued experience and contact with human mental life.

Summary

A psychiatrist is drawn to psychiatry, as with other doctors to their chosen specialties, by a multitude of factors but it is the unconscious drive to care for, repair and make amends to our internal objects that underlies this motivation alongside our aspirational identifications. The psyche and the soma have a complex interrelationship and cannot be separated. To develop as a psychotherapeutic psychiatrist requires psychiatrists to become aware of their necessary identifications with their patients, without which they would not be empathetic, so that they can maintain a capacity for thought while remaining open to new experience. This is a career-long endeavour that inevitably goes through cycles like the seasons – there may be periods of drought and mourning but the rain will come and times for renewal at all stages of a career and it's being able to take in nourishment when it arrives that is vital for growth even at the end of a career.

References

1. Shakespeare W. *As You Like It*, Act II Scene VII Line 138, Publishes 1623, first folio.

2. Erikson EH, Erikson JM. *The Life Cycle Completed: Extended Version*. New York: W. W. Norton & Company, 1998.

3. Brown D, Pedder J. *Introduction to Psychotherapy: An Outline of Psychodynamic Principles and Practice*. London: Tavistock Publications, 1979.

4. Johnston J. Learning from the cradle to the grave: the psychotherapeutic development of doctors from beginning to end of a career in medicine and psychiatry. Occasional Paper 102, Royal College of Psychiatrists, 2017.

5. Freud S The unconscious. In J Strachey, ed., *The Standard Edition of the Complete Psychological Works of Sigmund Freud, Volume XIV (1914–1916): On the History of the Psycho-Analytic Movement, Papers on Metapsychology and Other Works*. London: Hogarth Press. 1957; p. 194. (Original work published 1915)

6. Hinshelwood R. The difficult patient: the role of 'scientific psychiatry' in understanding patients with chronic schizophrenia or severe personality disorder. *Br J Psychiatry* 1999; 174(3): 187–90. doi:10.1192/bjp.174.3.187.

7. Klein M. The early stages of the Oedipus conflict. Reprinted in *Love, Guilt and Reparation and Other Works 1921–1945: The Writings of Melanie Klein*. Vol. 1. London: The Hogarth Press and the Institute of Psycho-Analysis. 1975; pp. 188, 190–1, 193. (Original work published 1928)

8. Freud S. *Introductory Lectures on Psychoanalysis* (Penguin Freud Library Vol. 1). London: Penguin Books Ltd. 1991; p. 496. (Original work published 1917)

9. Freud S. Fragment of an analysis of a case of hysteria. In J Strachey, ed., *The Standard Edition of the Complete Psychological Works of Sigmund Freud, Volume VII (1901–1905): A Case of Hysteria, Three Essays on Sexuality and Other Works*. London: Hogarth Press. 1953; p. 115. (Original work published 1905)

10. Bion WR. *Experiences in Groups*. London: Tavistock Publications, 1961; pp. 117–19.

11. Fox RC. *In the Field: A Sociologist's Journey*. New Brunswick: Transaction Publishers, 2011; p. 100.

12. Jesuloba T. First experiences with cadaveric dissection. The Medic Portal blog.

13. Williams AD, Greenwald EE, Soricelli RL, DePace DM. Medical students' reactions to anatomic dissection and the phenomenon of cadaver naming. *Anat Sci Educ* 2014; 7(3): 169–80. doi: 10.1002/ase.1391.

14. Allen JT. Learning Empathy from the Dead. *The Atlantic*, July 28, 2015.

15. Kumar Ghosh S, Kumar A. Building professionalism in human dissection room as a component of hidden curriculum delivery: a systematic review of good practices. *Anat Sci Educ* 2019; 12: 210–21. doi:10.1002/ase.1836.

16. Santibañez S, Boudreaux D, Tseng G et al. The Tzu Chi Silent Mentor Program: application of Buddhist ethics to teach student physicians empathy, compassion, and self-sacrifice. *J Relig Health* 2016; 55: 1483–94. https://doi.org/10.1007/s10943-0 15-0110-x

17. Reich A, quoted in Casement P. *Further Learning from the Patient*. London: Routledge. 1997; p. 177.

18. Cutler JL, Harding KJ, Mozian SA et al. Discrediting the notion "working with 'crazies' will make you 'crazy'": addressing stigma and enhancing empathy in medical student education. *Adv Health Sci Educ* 2009; 14: 487–502. https://doi.org/10.1007 /s10459-008-9132-4

19. Freud S. Thoughts for the times on war and death. In J Strachey, ed., *Standard Edition of the Complete Psychological Works of Sigmund Freud, Volume XIV (1914–1916): On the History of the Psycho-Analytic Movement, Papers on Metapsychology and Other Works*. London: Hogarth Press. 1957; pp. 273–300. (Original work published 1915)

20. Titchener EB. Introspection and empathy. *Dial Phil Ment Neuro Sci* 2014; 7: 25–30.

21. Freud S. The question of lay analysis. Postscript. In J Strachey, ed., *Standard Edition of the Complete Psychological Works of Sigmund Freud, Volume XX (1925–1926): An Autobiographical Study, Inhibitions, Symptoms and Anxiety, Lay Analysis and Other Works*. London: Hogarth Press. 1959; p. 253. (Original work published 1915)

22. Klein M. *Love, Guilt and Reparation and Other Works 1921–1945*. London: Vintage. 1998; p. 265.

23. Bott Spillius E, Milton J, Garvey P, Couve C, Steiner D. *The New Dictionary of Kleinian Thought*. Hove: Routledge, 2011.

24. Rey HJ. That which patients bring to analysis. *Int J Psychoanal* 1988; 69(Pt 4): 457–70.

25. Casement P. *On Learning from the Patient*. London: Routledge, 1985.

26. Johnston J. *The UK Psychotherapy Training Survey*. Royal College of Psychiatrists, 2013.

27. de Mijolla A (ed.). *International Dictionary of Psychoanalysis*. Detroit: Macmillan Reference USA, 2005.

28. McGrady C, Le Grice C, Slater H, Burbridge-James W. Survey of Trainees' Views on the Impact of Psychotherapy Long Case on their Professional Development and Broader Clinical Practice. Poster presented at: RCPsych International Congress; 2019; London.

29. Mateen FJ, Dorji C. Health-care worker burnout and the mental health imperative. *Lancet* 2009; 374(9690): 595–7.

30. Festinger L. *A Theory of Cognitive Dissonance*. Standford, CA: Standford University Press, 1957.

31. Tyrer P. A solution to the ossification of community psychiatry. *Psychiatrist* 2013; 37: 336–9. doi: 10.1192/pb.bp.113.042937.

32. Taylor K, Lambert T, Goldacre M. Future career plans of a cohort of senior doctors working in the National Health Service. *J R Soc Med* 2008; 101(4): 182–90. https:// doi.org/10.1258/jrsm.2007.070276

33. Mears A, Kendall T, Katona C, Pashley C, Pajak S. Retirement intentions of older consultant psychiatrists. *Psychiatr Bull* 2004; 28(4): 130–2. doi:10.1192/ pb.28.4.130.

34. Dale J, Potter R, Owen K et al. The general practitioner workforce crisis in England: a qualitative study of how appraisal and revalidation are contributing to intentions to leave practice. *BMC Fam Pract* 2016; 17: 84. https://doi.org/10.1186/s12875-016-0489-9

35. Draper B, Winfield S, Luscombe G. The Senior Psychiatrist Survey II: Experience and psychiatric practice. *Aust N Z J Psychiatry* 1999; 33: 709–16.

36. Clemens NA, A psychiatrist retires: an oxymoron? *J Psychiatr Pract* 2011; 17(5): 351–4.

Index

Printed in the United States
by Baker & Taylor Publisher Services